The Conquest of Cancer

Guy Faguet

The Conquest of Cancer

A distant goal

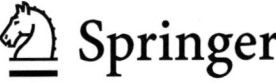

Springer

Guy Faguet
Daytona Beach Shores
FL, USA

ISBN 978-94-017-9164-9   ISBN 978-94-017-9165-6 (eBook)
DOI 10.1007/978-94-017-9165-6
Springer Dordrecht Heidelberg New York London

Library of Congress Control Number: 2014949244

© Springer Science+Business Media Dordrecht 2015
This work is subject to copyright. All rights are reserved by the Publisher, whether the whole or part of the material is concerned, specifically the rights of translation, reprinting, reuse of illustrations, recitation, broadcasting, reproduction on microfilms or in any other physical way, and transmission or information storage and retrieval, electronic adaptation, computer software, or by similar or dissimilar methodology now known or hereafter developed. Exempted from this legal reservation are brief excerpts in connection with reviews or scholarly analysis or material supplied specifically for the purpose of being entered and executed on a computer system, for exclusive use by the purchaser of the work. Duplication of this publication or parts thereof is permitted only under the provisions of the Copyright Law of the Publisher's location, in its current version, and permission for use must always be obtained from Springer. Permissions for use may be obtained through RightsLink at the Copyright Clearance Center. Violations are liable to prosecution under the respective Copyright Law.
The use of general descriptive names, registered names, trademarks, service marks, etc. in this publication does not imply, even in the absence of a specific statement, that such names are exempt from the relevant protective laws and regulations and therefore free for general use.
While the advice and information in this book are believed to be true and accurate at the date of publication, neither the authors nor the editors nor the publisher can accept any legal responsibility for any errors or omissions that may be made. The publisher makes no warranty, express or implied, with respect to the material contained herein.

Printed on acid-free paper

Springer is part of Springer Science+Business Media (www.springer.com)

To Anaïs and Margot

Preface

In *The War on Cancer: An Anatomy of Failure, A Blueprint for the Future* [1], I documented the stagnation of advanced cancer treatment after several decades of clinical trials shaped by changing theories on the origin and progression of cancer but always using drugs that, in addition to being cancer nonspecific, exhibit a plateau for efficacy but not for side effects. This indicting conclusion was based on detailed analyses of treatment outcome benchmarks that included cure rates, 5-year survival rates, and quality of life as recorded through 2004. An analysis of the root causes of the stagnation, which is implied in *An Anatomy of Failure*, the book's first subtitle, was followed by a *Blueprint for the Future* proposal that called for a fundamental paradigm shift in cancer management based on a trifold approach: "prevention, early diagnosis, and, when these fail, on controlling the aberrant molecular genetic pathways underlying the development, growth, and dissemination of cancer" [2].

The current book revisits the status and outcome of cancer management 10 years later. The chapter on theories on the origin and treatment of cancer through the ages has been greatly expanded. Likewise, coverage of molecular biology, genetics, and epigenetics of cancer was brought up to date, and sections on the role of carcinogens in cancer development and incidence and of alternate methods to combat cancer were included. I now show that, despite momentous progress in our understanding of the origin, progression, and dissemination of cancer, translational applications of this knowledge to the clinical setting have been slow, with little impact on any of the outcome benchmarks of cancer treatment. The impact of the increasing commercialization of medicine on the quality and cost of cancer care is highlighted by the growing trend of placing profit ahead of patients' needs, where providers and suppliers drive demand often unrelated to patient needs and where the extremely high cost of new agents is rarely matched by commensurate outcomes fostering a supply-driven industry, the largest in the country and a major contributor to budget deficits [3].

Cancer incidence rates rose by 16 % overall between 1975 and 2009, while death rates declined by 15 % and 5-year survival improved by 19 % between 1975 and 2008. However, because the modest gains in the latter two outcomes are attributable mostly to smoking cessation, early-stage diagnosis, and improvements in medical support measures rather than efficacious treatment, I propose a radical paradigm shift in cancer control. It calls for a break with the past at all levels of the cancer "enterprise." The new paradigm would entail a three-pronged approach: national cancer prevention campaigns initially aimed at cancer-promoting lifestyles responsible for two-third of new cancers and one-third of cancer deaths in the USA pursued concomitantly with coordinated national efforts, akin to the Manhattan project and the Apollo program, involving thousands of scientists in cancer-related fields focused on designing efficient tools for detecting surgically curable early-stage disease and on developing cancer-specific therapies capable of controlling advanced cancer. In the meantime, patients with advanced cancer would be offered the best available management while abiding by the four cardinal principles of ethical medical care: ensuring beneficence, reducing maleficence, and respecting patients' autonomy to remain in control of their own destiny while observing the principle of justice that seeks an equitable distribution of limited health-care resources.

Daytona Beach Shores, FL, USA   Guy Faguet

Acknowledgments

I thank Dr. Brian Druker (Director, OHSU Knight Cancer Institute, JELD-WEN Chair of Leukemia Research, and Professor of Medicine) and Dr. Kanti Rai (Joel Finkelstein Cancer Foundation Professor of Medicine and Professor of Molecular Medicine, Hofstra North Shore-LIJ School of Medicine) for helpful comments. All remaining errors are mine.

Contents

Part I An Historical Overview of the War on Cancer

1 The Four-Decade Journey to the National Cancer Act of 1971 3

Part II Cancer Through the Ages

2 An Historical Overview: From Prehistory to WWII 13
    2.1 From Prehistory to Ancient Egypt 13
    2.2 From Ancient Egypt to Greece and Rome 14
    2.3 From Rome to the Middle Age 20
    2.4 From Medieval Europe to World War II 23

3 Our Current Knowledge 35
    3.1 The Genetic Bases of Cancer 35
        3.1.1 First the Basics 35
        3.1.2 More Details 38
    3.2 How Does Cancer Arise? 54
        3.2.1 First the Basics 54
        3.2.2 More Details 56
    3.3 How Does Cancer Spread? 62
        3.3.1 First the Basics 62
        3.3.2 More Details: The Invasion-Metastasis Cascade 64

4 Environmental Carcinogens 69
    4.1 First the Basics 69
    4.2 More Details 71
        4.2.1 Smoking 72
        4.2.2 Obesity 73
        4.2.3 Alcoholism 76

Part III Cancer Statistics

5 Assessing the Enormity of the Problem 83
    5.1   Origin, Purpose, and Data Collection 84
    5.2   Incidence and Mortality Statistics:
           Reporting and Interpretation 85
    5.3   Cancer Incidence and Mortality Rates, US 2013 Estimates 85
    5.4   Probability of Developing and Dying
           of Advanced Cancer, 2007–2009 87
    5.5   Cancer Prevalence, US 2009 88
    5.6   Trends in Cancer Incidence and Mortality, US 1975–2009 89
    5.7   Historical Trends in Cancer Survival 91

6 An Uncontrolled Problem 95

Part IV How Is Advanced Cancer Treated?

7 The Cancer Cell-Kill Paradigm and Beyond 101
    7.1   An Historical Overview 101
    7.2   Nitrogen Mustard: Cytotoxic Chemotherapy Is Born 107
    7.3   Drug Discovery: Five Decades of Trial & Error 111
    7.4   Attempts to Surmount Cancer Drug Inefficacy:
           Five Decades Lost 113
    7.5   The New Targeted Therapeutics 123

8 Complementary and Alternative Medicine 129

9 The Cell-Kill Paradigm: Bleak Outcomes 135

Part V Stakeholders' Role in the Status Quo

10 The Role of the National Cancer Institute 145
    10.1   Current Organization, Role, and Influence 145
    10.2   NCI's Cancer Centers Program Network 146
    10.3   NCI's Clinical Trials Program Network 147
    10.4   Clinical Trials: Types, Phases, Design,
            and Interpretation 149

11 Factors that Impact Oncology Research and Practice 155
    11.1   Oncologists Qualifications 155
            11.1.1   Training and Board Certification 155
            11.1.2   Continuing Medical Education 156
    11.2   Factors that Influence Oncology Practice 158
            11.2.1   Standard of Care 159
            11.2.2   Overutilization of Services and the Chemotherapy
                        Concession 161
            11.2.3   Medical Malpractice 164

	11.2.4	Clinical Researchers and Publications	166
	11.2.5	Pharmaceutical Companies	168
	11.2.6	The Media	171

12 The Complex Physician-Patient Interaction: Expectations *vs.* Reality ... 173
    12.1 From the Patient's Perspective ... 173
        12.1.1 First the Basics ... 173
        12.1.2 More Details ... 174
    12.2 From the Caregiver's Perspective ... 181
        12.2.1 Facing Difficult Decisions ... 181
        12.2.2 Managing Cancer Patients at the End of Life ... 186

Part VI A Paradigm Shift in Cancer Management

13 Prevention and Early Detection ... 193

14 The Holistic Management of Advanced Cancer: A Three-Stage Blueprint ... 199
    14.1 Redesigning the Search for New Cancer Agents ... 201
    14.2 Restructuring the Treatment of Advanced-Stage Cancer ... 202
    14.3 Reviving the Art of End of Life Care ... 205

Conclusions ... 207

References ... 211

Index ... 241

About the Author

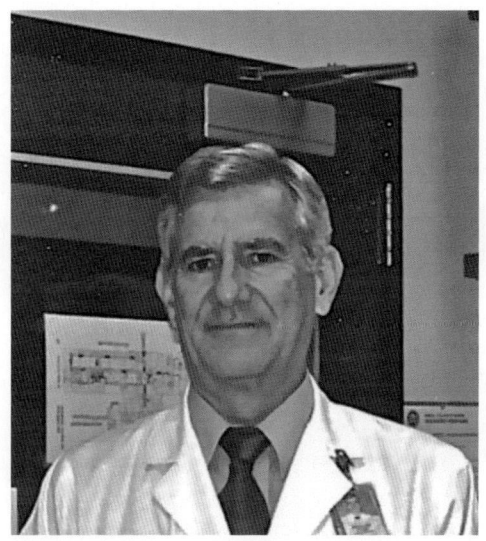

Dr. Faguet retired from the Medical College of Georgia (of the Georgia Regents University) after a 30-year academic career that included clinical and bench research funded by the National Institutes of Health and the Department of Veterans Affairs, respectively. He was a member of numerous scientific societies; a consultant for the National Institutes of Health, the Department of Veterans Affairs, the National Science Foundation, and the American Cancer Society; and a reviewer for several prestigious scientific journals. He authored numerous peer-reviewed publications and seven book chapters and edited two books: *Hematologic Malignancies* (The Humana Press, 2000) and *Chronic Lymphocytic Leukemia* (The Humana Press, 2003). Since retiring, Dr. Faguet has authored three books on public and health policy: *The War on Cancer* (Springer, 2005), *Pain Control and Drug Policy* (Praeger, 2010), and *The Affordable Care Act* (Algora, 2013). For more information, please visit www.faguet.net.

Part I
An Historical Overview of the War on Cancer

Chapter 1
The Four-Decade Journey to the National Cancer Act of 1971

> To authorize a reward for the discovery of a successful cure for cancer, and to create a commission to inquire into and ascertain the success of such a cure.
>
> – Senator Matthew M. Neely's cancer bill (1927).

Congressional attempts to address cancer at the national level began in the 1920s, but were ill-conceived and naive mainly because of prevailing misconceptions about the nature and causes of cancer and lawmakers' lack of sophistication. For example, on February 4, 1927, Senator Matthew M. Neely (D-WV) introduced the first cancer bill (S. 5589), offering a $5 million reward for anyone finding the cure for cancer [4] Although Congress did not act upon the bill, mention of a reward triggered a deluge of outlandish letters to Congress by the usual assortment of quacks, charlatans, snake-oil healers, and other unsavory characters claiming a right to part of the reward pie. Recognizing that offering a reward was an "imperfect if not utterly futile" means for tackling cancer, and after seeking medical guidance, Senator Neely introduced S. 3554 a year later (March 7, 1928), authorizing the Academy of Sciences to seek ways for the federal government to lead research into cancer. The new bill fared no better despite the eloquent plea he addressed to his colleagues on May 18, 1928,

> During the last Congress we appropriated $10,000,000 to eradicate the corn borer. For the present fiscal year we appropriated for the investigation of tuberculosis in animals more than $5,000,000; for meat inspection, more than $2,000,000; for the improvement of cereals, more than $700,000; for the investigation of insects affecting deciduous fruits, vineyards, and nuts more than $130,000; I favored and supported all of these appropriations…But in view of our unequaled liberality in protecting our domestic animals against every sort of disease and pest, and in view of the vast expenditures we have made in protecting every species of food-yielding plant and tree, and in further view of the fact that the Government has never yet appropriated a dollar for the particular purpose of combating cancer, I beg, in the name of all the vast hosts of cancer victims living and dead, for an appropriation that will make it possible for the work of rescuing suffering and perishing humanity from this frightful scourge immediately to begin [5].

When Senator Neely was defeated for re-election, his friend William J. Harris (D-GA) took up the fight by introducing bills S. 466 and S. 4531 on April 23 and May 29, 1929, respectively, and in 1930, spear-headed a committee of five Senators to draft a cancer bill, all unsuccessfully.

However, in the mid-1930s, cancer acquired a certain notoriety thanks to major newspaper stories raising the public's dread of a mysterious disease that kills slowly and painfully, letter-writing campaigns organized by prominent activist physicians to persuade Congress to support research on cancer and other diseases, a national campaign by the American Society for the Control of Cancer (precursor to today's American Cancer Society-ACS), and the popularity of Social Security enacted in 1935, a federal program to help those that can't help themselves. Hence, several members of Congress took notice and introduced bills to established a national cancer center, including Senator Homer T. Bone (D-WA), who introduced S. 2067 on April 2, 1937, the first of two thoughtful and well-conceived cancer bills; the other (HR 6767) was introduced on April 29, 1937 by Representative Maury Maverick (D-TX). Representatives John F. Hunter (D-OH) and Warren Magnuson (D-WA) introduced similar bills in the same time frame. Senator Bone, who managed to secure co-sponsorship by all of his colleagues, a congressional first, was motivated by his belief that cancer victimized the poor and needy who lacked access to healthcare and hence required federal assistance [6]. In drafting his bill, Representative Maverick received advice from Public Heath Service (PHS) legal experts, guidance from Drs. Dudley Jackson Sr., of San Antonio, Texas, and George W. McCoy, Director of the National Institutes of Health (NIH), and strong support from U.S. Surgeon General Thomas J. Parran, Jr., an influential public figure and an expert on venereal diseases. Maverick swayed many congressional colleagues to support the cancer project declaring,

> One out of eight persons over 40 will die, die of cancer. As most of us are over 40, I have figured there will be around 60 of us who thus meet deaths [7].

Dr. Jackson conducted research on dogs in hopes of unraveling the nature of human cancer, and once transplanted live cancer cells into himself to disprove the theory that cancer is contagious [8]. Struggling financially, he had applied for research funds to the same PHS that belittled his research but eventually rewarded his tireless persistence with a meager $1,000 award in 1935 [9]. Unwilling to accept defeat, he enlisted the support of his friend Congressman Maverick to sponsor a federal institute for cancer research and subsequently testified enthusiastically at House hearings. He is credited as the major mover of the legislation. Surgeon General Parran embraced and strongly supported the national cancer center project for he favored an activist government role in public health, which is best exemplified by a speech in which he stated,

> We have reached a stage when we must accept as a major premise citizens should have an equal opportunity for health as an inherent right with the right of liberty and the pursuit of happiness… whatever path we take, inevitably will conform to the governmental framework [10].

Opposition to the bills came from many quarters including promoters of folk medicine and healers afraid of losing followers, private physicians fearing a takeover by the government, and even some noted cancer researchers apprehensive about what was called a "General Motors approach to science". In the end, competing bills were reconciled in the Senate and the House, and President Franklin D. Roosevelt signed into law the National Cancer Act (Public Law 244) on August 5, 1937 [11] "to provide, aid, and coordinate research relating to cancer; to establish the National Cancer Institute [NCI]; and for other purposes" [12]. An annual budget of $700,000 was appropriated. The first Director of the new institute, who was to report directly to the US Surgeon General, was Swiss-born Carl Voegtlin, Ph.D., head of Pharmacology at the PHS. Upon assuming his new post, Voegtlin merged his group with researchers at the Office of Cancer Investigations of Harvard University to establish the first core of NCI researchers, and issued the first 13 research fellowship grants. Construction of the first independent home for the NCI began in June 1939 and was dedicated with great fanfare by President Roosevelt on October 31, 1940, to house the Institute's first 100 staff members. That same year, Voegtlin launched the *Journal of the National Cancer Institute*, serving as its first editor. However, despite numerous legislative, organizational, and research initiatives, the overall impact of the NCI on the understanding and treating of cancer over the ensuing 30 years was minimal.

Fast-forward 30 years. At the urging of Senator Ralph W. Yarborough, (D-TX), "the People's Senator" [13], chairman of the Senate Labor and Public Welfare Committee, on April 27, 1970, the Senate approved the creation of the National Panel of Consultants on the Conquest of Cancer. On November 25, 1970, 7 months after receiving its mandate, the Panel submitted to the Senate its report entitled "National Program for the Conquest of Cancer", and on December 4, 1970, Senator Yarborough introduced S. 4564, "A bill which would establish a National Cancer Authority for the purpose of devising and implementing a national program for the conquest of the world's most dreaded disease – cancer" [14]. The power behind the cancer project was Mary W. Lasker (1900–1994). Born in Watertown, Wisconsin, Mary studied at the University of Wisconsin and at Ratcliff College, where she graduated with a major in art history. After postgraduate studies at Oxford, she moved to New York City, where she worked for art dealer Paul Reinhart, whom she married in 1926 and divorced in 1934. In 1940, she married Albert D. Lasker, who, as owner of the Lord & Thomas advertising agency, had pioneered branding through the use of logos and slogans that became linked to individual brands. After selling the agency, the Laskers turned their full attention to national health issues through political activism and philanthropy. They established the Lasker Foundation in 1942 to promote healthcare research through yearly awards to honor prominent basic science and clinical researchers, and were staunch supporters of the American Cancer Society. Encouraged by her well-connected husband, Mary became a,

> Catalyst for the rapid growth of the biomedical research enterprise in the United States after World War II. Called '*a matchmaker between science and society*' by Jonas Salk, Lasker was a well-connected fundraiser and astute lobbyist who through charm, energy, and skillful use of the media persuaded donors, congressmen, and presidents to provide greatly increased funds for medical research as the main means of safeguarding the health and welfare of Americans [15].

After her husband's death from colon cancer in 1952, Mary became convinced that only the resources of the Federal government could confront the cancer challenge. Using her extensive network of political, business, medical, and social contacts, and the considerable financial resources of her husband's estate, ironically boosted by the "*reach for a Lucky instead of a sweet*" advertising campaign to convince women to smoke, Mary launched an assault on cancer campaign. She and her followers believed that if American ingenuity was capable of putting a man on the moon within a decade, the conquest of cancer seemed a goal attainable by the nation's Bicentennial. However, her access to the White House, facilitated by partially funding Jacqueline Kennedy's White House redecoration project and subsequently by the expansive spending of the Lyndon Johnson administration came to an end when Richard M. Nixon became President. Given Nixon's preoccupation with inflation and pressures on the US Congress to limit spending, she adopted a two-prong strategy: she surrounded herself with high-profile medical researchers such as Sidney Farber, Scientific Director of the Children's Cancer Research Foundation in Boston and former President of the American Cancer Society, and with business leaders such as Benno Schmidt Sr., a lawyer and venture capitalist, who would later co-Chair with Farber the Senate's National Panel of Consultants. She also befriended influential politicians, especially Senator Yarborough, chairman of the powerful Senate Labor and Public Welfare Committee who, on June 2, 1970, appointed her to the Committee of Consultants to "conduct a study of research activities in cancer to determine what legislation and new Federal programs are necessary for the conquest and elimination of cancer" [16]. Her political savvy served her well becoming,

> Director, Chairman, or trustee of the American Cancer Society, the United Cerebral Palsy Research and Education Foundation, the National Committee for Mental Hygiene, and a range of other medical and cultural organizations. She received over three-dozen honorary degrees and awards, chief among them the Presidential Medal of Freedom, the nation's highest civilian honor, in 1969, and a special Congressional Gold Medal in 1989 [17].

Farber, who became famous but controversial when he reported the first remissions in acute childhood leukemia [18], believed, as did Solomon Garb, author of the book *Cure for Cancer* [19], that the cure could be achieved with little further research, if concerted efforts and sufficient funds were allocated to its eradication. He forcefully argued before the Senate Labor and Public Welfare Committee,

> The whole history of the NIH in the clinical application and investigation has been one of slow progress, in part because of the belief on the part of many scientists in the country too that only by basic research yielding a full understanding of the nature of cancer can proper clinical treatment of cancer be achieved. We cannot wait for full understanding; The 325,000 patients with cancer who are going to die this year cannot wait; nor is it necessary, in order to make great progress in the cure of cancer, for us to have the full solution of all the problems of basic research....the history of Medicine is replete with examples of cures obtained years, decades, and even centuries before the mechanism of action was understood for these cures [20].

Likewise, Randolph L. Clark, a cancer researcher and editor of the *Year Book of Cancer*, declared, "With a billion dollars a year for 10 years we could lick cancer". Such views, as unorthodox then as they are now, were not shared by many of Farber's own colleagues at Harvard, including Francis Moore, surgeon-in-chief at the Peter Bent Brigham Hospital in Boston. Moore correctly argued that most breakthroughs in medical science have originated from creative, independent researchers, not from organized, centrally-directed research as was being proposed. Likewise, many researchers at the NIH were privately dismayed at Farber's views, and at the goals being set they knew to be unattainable within the timeframe contemplated. Additionally, the medical establishment was vehemently opposed to the plan, arguing that a cancer program outside the NIH would be isolated from other biomedical research potentially useful in the fight against cancer. As objections from skeptics and critics mounted, Lasker countered by organizing a grass-roots cancer advocacy group called the Citizens' Committee for the Conquest of Cancer. In December 1969, her committee initiated a public relations campaign aimed at influencing the US President and the US Senate, where the National Cancer Act was being debated. A full-page advertisement published on December 9, 1969 by the New York Times (Fig. 1.1) urged the President,

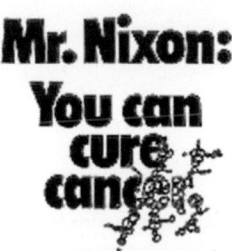

"If prayers are heard in Heaven, this prayer is heard the most, 'Dear God, please, not cancer'. Still more than 318,000 Americans died of cancer last year. This year, Mr. President, you have it in your power to begin to end this curse"[21].

Fig. 1.1 Lasker cancer advocacy group's New York Times advertising

Other ads by the Lasker group read "This year, Mr. President, we are so close to the cure of cancer. We lack only the will and the kind of money…that went into putting a man on the moon. Why don't we try to conquer cancer by America's 200th birthday?". Moreover, she enlisted the help of her good friend, syndicated columnist Ann Landers, who urged her nationwide readers to write their representatives in support of the bill. An estimated 300,000 letters landed at Congress' doorsteps as it debated the merits of the National Cancer Act. Members of the Senate Labor and Public

Welfare Committee opposing the bill received individual letters threatening that their reelection would be opposed if they did not reconsider their opposition to the cancer act.

Seizing an opportunity for political gain, President Nixon embraced the cancer cause, and in his January 22, 1971 State of the Union address declared,

> The time has come in America when the same kind of concentrated effort that split the atom and took man to the moon should be turned toward conquering this dread disease. Let us make a total national commitment to achieve this goal. America has long been the wealthiest nation in the world. Now it is time we became the healthiest nation in the world [22].

In October 1971, he converted the Army's Fort Detrick, Maryland from a biological warfare facility to a national cancer research center, now called the Frederick Cancer Research and Development Center. In the meantime, Senator Edward Kennedy had become Committee Chairman and co-sponsor of the final bill when Senator Yarborough lost his bid for reelection in 1970. Fearing that Kennedy might oppose him in the presidential race of 1972, President Nixon, who had lost the presidential race to John F. Kennedy in 1960, opposed the Kennedy name on that important legislation. Eventually, Senator Kennedy withdrew his name as sponsor of the bill and President Nixon signed into law the National Cancer Act on December 23, 1971, calling it "A Christmas gift to the nation", adding, "I hope in the years ahead we will look back on this action today as the most significant taken during my Administration" [23]. The law established the NCI within the NIH, but with a budget to be submitted directly to the President for approval, thus bypassing the NIH and the Department of Health, Education, and Welfare. Its director became a presidential appointee. The Act also created a President's Cancer Panel, composed of two scientists and one management specialist charged with submitting to the President yearly progress reports on the status of research at NCI. The act also replaced the National Advisory Cancer Council with an 18-member National Cancer Advisory Board of scientists and laypersons empowered to guide and advise the NCI on all initiatives. Since then, numerous legislative amendments have maintained, complemented, and expanded the NCI's authority and dominance, scope in basic and clinical cancer research according to perceived needs and evolving priorities leading to the current 14 intra- and extramural National Cancer Programs. Some of the most inclusive extramural initiatives include the Comprehensive Cancer Centers program (1973), comprising 67 centers to "integrate a diversity of research approaches to focus on the problem of cancer," CancerLine (1974), a computerized service jointly established with the National Library of Medicine to provide scientists with the latest published research and clinical cancer data, and the Community Clinical Oncology Program (1983), which is designed to bring clinical research to cancer patients in their own communities. Perhaps the intramural initiative that, in time, will have the greatest impact on human health is the Cancer Genome Anatomy Project (1997) [24]. As its scope and reach expanded, the NCI budget grew from $492.2 million in 1973 to $6.2 billion in fiscal year 2011 [25], or approximately 8 % average annual increase after inflation. Yet, the fiscally watchful Republican-led House of Representatives recently approved spending packages that substantially reduce spending for fiscal years 2011 and 2012 though, at this writing, both budgets remain under continuing resolution. Given its enormous and ever-expanding budget and reach, the NCI has the financial resources to, and does in fact, fund most of the nation's non-private cancer research at any given time. This financial muscle, backed by an excellent and far-reaching organizational infrastructure, gives the NCI the power to "plan, prioritize, direct, coordinate, evaluate, administer, and serve as the focal point" for most of the nation's basic and applied cancer research. It is ironic that the country that stands the tallest among nations for the free flow of ideas leads its War on Cancer through a central bureaucracy whose mandate is to control the type and direction of nearly all cancer research. According to its own mission statement [26], NCI currently:

- Supports and coordinates research projects conducted by universities, hospitals, research foundations, and businesses throughout this country and abroad through research grants and cooperative agreements.
- Conducts research in its own laboratories and clinics.
- Supports education and training in fundamental sciences and clinical disciplines for participation in basic and clinical research programs and treatment programs relating to cancer through career awards, training grants, and fellowships.
- Supports research projects in cancer control.
- Supports a national network of cancer centers.
- Collaborates with voluntary organizations and other national and foreign institutions engaged in cancer research and training activities.
- Encourages and coordinates cancer research by industrial concerns where such concerns evidence a particular capability for programmatic research.
- Collects and disseminates information on cancer.
- Supports construction of laboratories, clinics, and related facilities necessary for cancer research through the award of construction grants.

Thus, given NCI's extraordinary reach and influence on the direction of basic and applied cancer research, it must be credited for major advances in molecular biology and genetics of cancer, but also held accountable for several decades of stagnation in cancer treatment outcomes. But first, let us look at how our ancestors perceived cancer.

Part II
Cancer Through the Ages

Chapter 2
An Historical Overview: From Prehistory to WWII

The only true wisdom is in knowing you know nothing.

– Socrates

2.1 From Prehistory to Ancient Egypt

Cancer has afflicted humanity from pre-historic times, though its prevalence has markedly increased in recent decades in unison with rapidly aging populations and, in the last half-century, increasingly risky health behavior in the general population and the increased presence of carcinogens in consumer products and in the environment. The oldest credible evidence of cancer in mammals consists of tumor masses found in fossilized dinosaurs and human bones from pre-historic times. Perhaps the most compelling evidence of cancer in dinosaurs emanates from a recent large-scale study that screened by fluoroscopy more than 10,000 specimens of dinosaur vertebrae for evidence of tumors and assessed abnormal vertebrae by computerized tomography (CT) [27]. Of the various species of dinosaurs surveyed, only *cretaceous hadrosaurs* (duck-billed dinosaurs) that lived approximately 70 Ma ago exhibited tumors, and although most were benign (hemangiomas,[1] desmoplastic fibromas,[2] and osteoblastomas[3]), malignant metastatic cancers also were detected in 0.2 % of specimens tested.

The earliest written record of what is generally agreed to have been human cancer appeared in ancient Egyptian manuscripts discovered in the nineteenth century, especially the Edwin Smith and George Ebers papyri that describe surgical, pharmacological, and magical treatments. They were written between 1500 and 1600 BCE, possibly based on material from thousands of years earlier. The Smith papyrus, possibly written by the physician-architect Imhotep, who designed and built the step pyramid at Sakkara in the thirtieth century BCE under Pharaoh Djoser, is believed to contain the first reference to breast cancer (case 45) when referring to tumors of the anterior chest. It postulates that when such tumors are cool to touch, bulging, and

---

[1] Benign vascular tumors.
[2] Benign fibrous tumors of bone.
[3] Rare benign bone tumors.

have spread over the breast, no treatment can succeed [28]. It also provides the earliest mention of suturing wounds and using a "*fire drill*" to cauterize open wounds. In ancient times, gods were thought to preside over human destiny, including health and disease, medicine and religion were intertwined and practiced by priests and sages, and famous physicians were thought to be gods' intermediaries. For instance, in case 1 of the Edwin Smith papyrus, physicians are called "lay-priests of Sekhmet." Sekhmet, the feared lion-headed "lady of terror" and one of the oldest Egyptian deities, was known as the "lady of life" patron of physicians and healers [29].

The earliest cancerous growths in humans were found in Egyptian and Peruvian mummies dating back to approximately 1500 BC. The oldest scientifically documented case of disseminated cancer was that of a 40–50 year-old Scythian king who lived in the steppes of Southern Siberia approximately 2,700 years ago. Modern microscopic and proteomic techniques confirmed the cancerous nature of the lesions throughout his entire skeleton and their prostatic origin [30]. Half a millennium later and half a world away, a Ptolemaic Egyptian was dying of cancer [31]. Digital radiography and multi-detector CT scans of his mummy, kept at the Museu Nacional de Arqueología in Lisbon, determined that his cancer was disseminated. The morphology and distribution of his lesions (spine, pelvis, and proximal extremities), and the mummy's gender and age favor prostate as the most likely origin.

2.2 From Ancient Egypt to Greece and Rome

Following the decline of Egypt, Greek and Roman medicine became preeminent, especially with Hippocrates of Kos (460–c.360 BC), an island off the coast of Turkey, and Claudius Galenus (AD 129–c.216), better known as Galen of Pergamum (modern-day Bergama, Turkey). Their writings, describing their life-long experience and observations, became the foundation and repository of medical knowledge for the ensuing 1,500 years.

Although little is known with certainty about who he was, what he thought and wrote, and how he practiced medicine, the image we now have of Hippocrates emerged in the sixteenth century after "…[being] constantly invented and reinvented; constructed, deconstructed, and reconstructed; molded and remolded, according to the cultural, philosophical, social, and political context, or the private and moral background" [32]. According to that image, Hippocrates emerged from a group of illustrious teachers at the famed medical school in the island of Kos in the Aegean Sea, during the Age of Pericles. As a seat of learning and the provincial seat of the museum of Alexandria, Kos was an educational center and a playground for the princes of the Ptolemaic dynasty. Its market place was one of the largest in the ancient world and its well-fortified port gave it prominence in Aegean trade. Much of what we know about Hippocrates we owe to Soranus of Ephesus (a second century AD Greek physician), his first biographer, and to Aristotle (384 BC–322 BC), who mentions him in his writings as *The Great Hippocrates*. The medical legacy associated with Hippocrates' name and the imagery it conjures up have become legendary. Hippocrates is called the *Father of Medicine* more for rejecting prevailing views on the supernatural causes of disease and their cure through rituals and offerings, for promoting a rational approach to medicine, and for his famous Oath, than for the so-called Hippocratic Corpus, a collection of 60 "books"[4] of medical writings on a variety of medical topics, including "On air, water, and places", "On ancient medicine", "On epidemics", "On surgery", "On the sacred disease", "On ulcers", "On fractures", "On Hemorrhoids", "Aphorisms" [33], "The oath", and many others of which he might have written only 12–14, according to scholars' best estimates (Fig. 2.1).

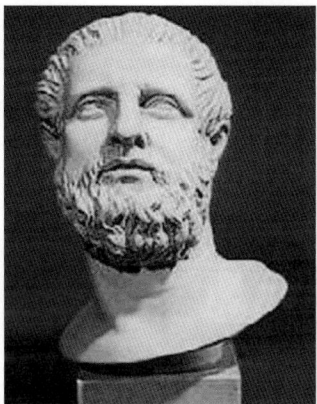

Fig. 2.1 Hippocrates of Kos

The Hippocratic Oath, sworn upon a number of healing gods, required new physicians to be trained and to uphold a number of professional ethical standards. Today, few medical schools adhere to this ancient rite of passage. The Oath:

> I swear by Apollo the physician, Asclepius, Hygieia, Panacea, and all the gods and goddesses as my witnesses, that, according to my ability and judgment, I will keep this Oath and this contract:
> 1. To hold him who taught me this art equally dear to me as my parents, to make my teacher a partner in life, and to fulfill his needs when required; to look upon his offspring as equals to my own siblings, and to teach them this art, if they shall wish to learn it, without fee or contract; and that by the set rules, lectures, and every other mode of instruction, I will impart a knowledge of the art to my own sons, and those of my teachers, and to students bound by this contract and having sworn this Oath to the law of medicine, but to no others.
> 2. I will use those dietary regimens which will benefit my patients according to my greatest ability and judgment, and I will do no harm or injustice to them.
> 3. I will not give a lethal drug to anyone if I am asked, nor will I advise such a plan; and similarly I will not give a woman a pessary to cause an abortion.
> 4. In purity and according to divine law will I carry out my life and my art.
> 5. I will not use the knife, even upon those suffering from stones, but I will leave this to those who are trained in this craft.
> 6. Into whatever homes I go, I will enter them for the benefit of the sick, avoiding any voluntary act of impropriety or corruption, including the seduction of women or men, whether they are free men or slaves.

---

[4] Essay-length. For instance, the "book" of *Aphorisms* is only 14,426 words-long in its English translation.

7. Whatever I see or hear in the lives of my patients, whether in connection with my professional practice or not, which ought not to be spoken of outside, I will keep secret, as considering all such things to be private.
8. So long as I maintain this Oath faithfully and without corruption, may it be granted to me to partake of life fully and the practice of my art, gaining the respect of all men for all time. However, should I transgress this Oath and violate it, may the opposite be my fate [34].

The Hippocratic Oath is remarkable for it promotes both a system of accreditation requiring a period of apprenticeship and an ethical professional code of conduct that differentiate knowledgeable and trustworthy physicians from improvised healers, whether this was intended or not.

Hippocrates' approach to diagnosing diseases was based on careful observations of patients and on monitoring their symptoms. For instance, in "On forecasting diseases", he advises,

> First of all the doctor should look at the patient's face. If he looks his usual self this is a good sign. If not, however, the following are bad signs – sharp nose, hollow eyes, cold ears, dry skin on the forehead, strange face color such as green, black, red or lead colored. If the face is like this at the beginning of the illness, the doctor must ask the patient if he has lost sleep, or had diarrhea, or not eaten [35].

In his book "On epidemics", he advises to record patients' symptoms and appearance on a day-to day-basis in order to forecast disease progression or recovery. He believed that health resulted from the balance and disease from the imbalance in the main four body fluids or humors: *black bile*, *yellow bile*, *phlegm*, and *blood*, each originating in a different organ and each corresponding to a personal temperament, a physical earthly element, and a specific season (Table 2.1). However, while Hippocrates subscribed to the theory that was later adopted by Greek, Roman, and Muslim physicians, its true origins are controversial.

Table 2.1 Hippocrates' humoral system of health and disease

Humor	Organ	Temperament	Element	Season
Blood	Heart	Sanguine	Air	Spring
Black bile	Spleen	Melancholic	Earth	Summer
Yellow bile	Liver	Choleric	Fire	Fall
Phlegm	Brain	Phlegmatic	Water	Winter

The relative dominance of one of the humors determined personality traits and their imbalance resulted in a propensity toward certain diseases. Thus, the aim of treatment was to restore balance through diet, exercise, and the judicious use of herbs, oils, earthly compounds, and occasionally heavy metals or surgery. For instance, a phlegmatic or lethargic individual (one with too much phlegm) could be restored to balance by administering citrus fruit thought to counter phlegm. The Hippocratic Corpus deals at length with diseases that produced masses (*onkos*), and coined the word *karkinos* to describe ulcerating and non-healing lumps that in retrospect included lesions ranging from benign processes to malignant tumors. He advocated diet, rest, and exercise for mild illnesses, followed by purgatives, heavy metals and surgery for more serious diseases, especially *karkinomas*. His stepwise treatment approach is summarized in one of his *Aphorisms*, "That which medicine does not heal, the knife frequently heals; and what the knife does not heal, actual cautery often heals; but when all these fail, the disease is incurable" [36]. To his credit, he recognized the relentless progression of deep-seated karkinomas and the often-negative effect of treatment when he wrote: "Occult cancers should not be molested. Attempting to treat them, they quickly become fatal. When unmolested, they remain in a dormant state for a length of time" (Aphorism 38 [37]). Hippocrates died at Larissa, in Thessaly, at the probable age of 100.

Aulus Cornelius Celsus (25 BC–50 AD), a Roman physician and one of Hippocrates' most prominent successors, also held the view that "the excised carcinomas have returned and caused death" [38]. He described the evolution of tumors from *cacoethes* followed by *carcinos* (which he later called *carcinomas*) without ulceration, then fungated ulcers and is credited as the first to have performed reconstruction surgery following excision of cancer [39]. Celsus believed that cacoethes were treatable by surgical resection, whereas more advanced lesions were unresponsive and should be left alone. He wrote,

> It is only the cacoethes which can be removed; the other stages are irritated by treatment; and the more so the more vigorous it is. Some have used caustic medicaments, some the cautery, some excision with a scalpel; but no medicament has ever given relief; the parts cauterized are excited immediately to an increase until they cause death [40].

Yet, he acknowledged that only time could differentiate the stage of a particular tumor,

> No one, however, except by time and experiment, can have the skill to distinguish a cacoethes which admits of being treated from a carcinoma which does not [41].

He vividly described the invasive nature of advanced cancer,

> This also is a spreading disease. And all these signs often extend, and there results from them an ulcer which the Greeks call phagedaena, because it spreads rapidly and penetrates down to the bones and so devours the flesh [42].

Archigenes of Apamea, Syria (75–129 AD), who practiced in Rome in the time of Trajan, also stressed the importance of early stage diagnosis when various remedies can be successful but advised surgery for advanced cancer as absolutely necessary but only in strong patients able to cope with the harshness of the operation, warning, "if it has taken anything into its claws it cannot be easily ripped away." However, Hippocrates' most prominent successor and the one who propelled his legacy for nearly 15 centuries was Galen.

Galen was born of Greek parents in Pergamum, the ancient capital of the Kingdom of Pergamum during the Hellenistic period, under the Attalid dynasty (281–133 BC). In Galen's time, Pergamum was a thriving cultural center famous for its library second only to Alexandria's and its statue of Asclepius (Aesculapius in Latin), the Greek god of medicine and healing. His prosperous patrician architect father, Aelius Nicon, oversaw Galen's broad and eclectic education, which included mathematics, grammar, logic, and inquiry into the four major schools of philosophy of the time: the Platonists, the Peripatetics, the Stoics, and the Epicureans. He started medical studies in Smyrna and Corinth at age 16 and later lived in Alexandria for 5 years (152–157 AD), where he studied anatomy and was exposed to the practice of autopsy as a means to understanding health and disease. Years later he wrote, "look at the human skeleton with your own eyes. This is very easy in Alexandria, so that the physicians of that area instruct their pupils with the aid of autopsy" [43]. In 157 AD, his appointment as physician of the gymnasium attached to the Asclepius sanctuary of Pergamum brought him back to his hometown, where he became surgeon to local gladiators. When civil unrest broke out, Galen moved to Rome, where his talents and ambition soon brought him fame but also numerous enemies that forced him to flee the city in 166, the year the plague (presumably smallpox) struck.

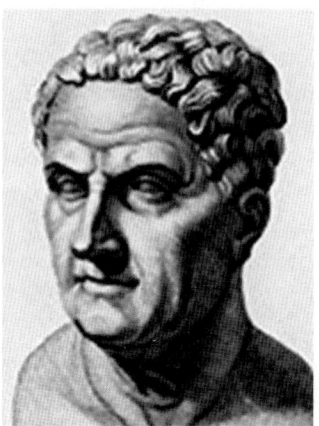

Fig. 2.2 Galen of Pergamum

Two years later, Roman Emperors Marcus Aurelius and Lucius Verus recalled him to serve as army surgeon during an outbreak among troops stationed at Aquileia (168–169), and when the plague extended to Rome, he was named personal physician to Emperor Marcus Aurelius and his son Commodus, adding luster and fame to his fast rising career. While medical practitioners of the time disagreed on whether experience or established theories should guide treatment, Galen applied Aristotelian empiricism by ensuring that established theories gave meaning to personal observations and relied on logic to sort out uncertainties and discover medical truths. He viewed himself as the best interpreter of Hippocratic thought. His pioneering anatomical studies, based on dissecting pigs and primates, were only surpassed by Andreas Vesalius' pivotal 1543-work *De humani corporis fabrica* that described and illustrated human dissections. He was the first to recognize the difference between arterial (bright) and venous (dark) blood, which he postulated to be distinct systems originating from the heart and liver, respectively. He used vivisections to study body functions. For instance, when he cut the laryngeal nerve of a pig, the animal stopped squealing; this nerve is now known as *Galen's Nerve*. Likewise, he showed that urine came from kidneys by tying the ureters, and that severing spinal cord nerves caused paralysis. He performed audacious and delicate operations, such as removal of the lens to treat cataracts, an operation that would become commonplace only 2,000 years later. Galen's prolific writings include 300 titles, of which approximately half have survived wholly or in part. Many were destroyed in the fire of the Temple of Peace (AD 191). In *On My Own Books*, Galen himself indicated which of the many works circulating under his name was genuine, though "several indisputably genuine texts fail to appear in them, either because they were written later, or because for whatever reason Galen chose to disown them" [44].

The influence of Galen's work in the west went into decline after the collapse of the Roman Empire, for no Latin translations were available and few scholars could read Greek, but Greek medical tradition remained alive and well in the Eastern Roman (Byzantine) Empire. This is because interest in Greek science and medicine by Arab Muslims during the Abbasid period led to translations of Galen's work into Arabic, many of them by Syrian Christian scholars. The need to be fluent in Greek or Arabic limited the number of later scholars capable of translating Galen's work into modern languages. Perhaps the most complete and authoritative compendium of Galen's work is the one compiled by Karl Gottlob Kühn of Leipzig between 1821 and 1833. It assembled 122 of Galen's works into 22 volumes (20,000 pages in length), translated from the original Greek into Latin and published in both languages. In addition to contributing to understanding anatomy, physiology, pathology, neurology, pharmacology, and other disciplines, Galen bridged the Greek and Roman medical worlds by enshrining Hippocratic principles and his own as the foundation of all medical knowledge that lasted through the Middle Ages. Indeed, many of the later medical scholars, teachers, and practitioners referred to Galen as the source of all medical knowledge, including Oribasius of Pergamum, Aëtius of Amidenus, Alexander of Tralles, and Paulus Ægineta. Professor Vivian Nutton, a renowned Galen expert, called him, "The most prolific writer to survive from the ancient world, whose combination of great learning and practical skill imposed his ideas on learned doctors for centuries" [45]. With respect to cancer, Galen addressed tumors of various types and origins, distinguishing *onkoi* (lumps or masses in general), *karkinos* (including malignant ulcers), and *karkinomas* (including non-ulcerating cancers) [46]. His greatest contribution to advancing our understanding of cancer was the classification that graded lumps and growths into three categories ranging from the most benign to the most malignant. The *De tumoribus secondum naturam* (tumors according to nature) included benign lumps and physiologic processes, such as the growth of breasts during puberty, or even a pregnant uterus. *De tumoribus supra naturam* (tumors beyond nature) comprised processes such as abscesses and swelling from inflammation he compared to a "soaking-wet sponge" for "if the inflamed part is cut, a large quantity of blood can be seen flowing out". Not surprisingly, bloodletting was the preferred treatment of these conditions. *De tumoribus praeter naturam* (tumors beyond nature) included lesions considered cancer today. Galen's classification of lumps and growths is the first and only written document of antiquity devoted exclusively to tumors both cancerous and non-cancerous. Not surprisingly, despite his decisive role in shaping Greek medical tradition and his influence on medical practice lasting nearly 1,500 years, Galen's original contributions to understanding and treating cancer were essentially nil. He died in Rome at the probable age of 87 [47].

2.3 From Rome to the Middle Age

With the collapse of Greco-Roman civilization after the fall of Rome in 476 AD, medical knowledge in the Western Roman Empire stagnated and many ancient medical writings were lost. Nevertheless, prominent physician-scholars emerged during the Eastern Roman or Byzantine Empire by the end of the fourth century, including Oribasius of Pergamum (325–403), Aëtius of Amidenus (502–575), and Paulus Ægineta (625?–690?), all of whom wrote about cancer. Oribasius stressed the painful nature of cancer and described cancers of the face, breast, and genitalia. Aëtius is attributed the observation that swollen blood vessels around breast cancer often look like crab legs; hence the term cancroid (resembling a crab). He believed that surgery for uterine cancer was too risky but advocated that approach for more accessible cancers, such as breast. In his writings, he upheld observations on breast cancer made by Leonides of Alexandria (second century AD),

> Breast cancer appears mainly in women and rarely in men. The tumor is painful because of the intense traction of the nipple…[avoid operating when] the tumor has taken over the entire breast and adhered to the thorax…[but] if the scirrhous tumor begins at the edge of the breast and spreads in more than half of it, we must try to amputate the breast without cauterization [48].

A century later, Paulus Ægineta published seven books he described as a treatise that,

> Contain[s] the description, causes, and cure of all diseases, whether situated in parts of uniform texture, in particular organs, or consisting of solutions of continuity, and that not merely in a summary way, but at as great length as possible [49].

In book IV, section 26, he states that cancer "occurs in every part of the body…but it is more particularly frequent in the breasts of women…". In book VI, section 45, he quotes Galen's surgical treatment for breast cancer, which he advocates as the treatment of choice for all operable cancers,

> If ever you attempt to cure cancer by an operation, begin your evacuations by purging the melancholic humor, and having cut away the whole affected part, so that a root of it be left, permit the blood to be discharged, and to not speedily restrain it, but squeeze the surrounding veins so as to force out the thick part of the blood, and then cure the wound like other ulcers [50].

He called attention to the presence of lymph nodes in the armpits of women with breast cancer and advocated poppy extracts to combat pain. Although these authors and their contemporaries contributed little to our knowledge of medicine and cancer, through their writings, they ensured the preservation of Greek-Roman medical tradition accumulated by their predecessors. Paulus Ægineta clearly acknowledges its dominance over medical practice of his time in the introduction of the preface to his seven books,

> It is not because the more ancient writers had omitted anything relative to the Art that I have composed this work, but in order to give a compendious course of instructions; for, on the contrary, everything is handed by them properly, and without any omissions…[51].

2.3 From Rome to the Middle Age

Greek scientific tradition spread widely, first through Christian Syriac writers, scholars, and scientists reaching Arab lands mainly via translations of Greek texts into Arabic by "Nestorians" [52]. Followers of Nestorius, Patriarchy of Constantinople, Nestorians' teachings were eventually condemned as heretical at the Council of Chalcedon (451 AD). Nestorianism spread throughout Asia Minor through churches, monasteries, and schools where Nestorian monks came into close contact with Arabs. Pivotal to the adoption of Greek thought by the Arabs was the pro-Greek penchant of Ja'far Ibn Barmak, minister of the Caliph of Bagdad, along with like-minded members of the Caliph's entourage. "Thus the Nestorian heritage of Greek scholarship passed from Edessa and Nisibis, through Jundi-Shapur, to Baghdad" [53] Islamic physician-scholars and medical writers became preeminent in the early middle Ages, including the illustrious and influential Abu Bakr Muhammad Ibn Sazariya Razi, also known as Rhazes (865?–925?), Abū 'Alī al-Ḥusayn ibn 'Abd Allāh ibn Sīnā, known as Avicenna (980–1037), Abū-Marwān 'Abd al-Malik ibn Zuhr or Avenzoar (1094–1162), and Ala-al-din abu Al-Hassan Ali ibn Abi-Hazm al-Qarshi al-Dimashqi known as Ibn Al-Nafis (1213–1288). The latter described the pulmonary circulation in great detail and accuracy, as told in *Commentary on the Anatomy of Canon of Avicenna*, a manuscript discovered in the Prussian State Library of Berlin. Ibn Al-Nafis stated,

> The blood from the right chamber of the heart must arrive at the left chamber but there is no direct pathway between them. The thick septum of the heart is not perforated and does not have visible pores as some people thought or invisible pores as Galen thought. The blood from the right chamber must flow through the vena arteriosa (pulmonary artery) to the lungs, spread through its substances, be mingled there with air, pass through the arteria venosa (pulmonary vein) to reach the left chamber of the heart and there form the vital spirit... [54].

He also understood the anatomy of the lungs explaining,

> The lungs are composed of parts, one of which is the bronchi; the second, the branches of the arteria venosa; and the third, the branches of the vena arteriosa, all of them connected by loose porous flesh [55].

And he was the first to describe the coronary circulation and its function, "The nourishment of the heart is through the vessels that permeate the body of the heart" [56].

Of greatest interest to us is Avenzoar, who first described the symptoms of esophageal and stomach cancer in his book *Kitab al-Taysir*, and proposed feeding enemas to keep alive patients with stomach cancer [57], a treatment approach unsuccessfully attempted by his predecessors. He insisted that the surgeon-to-be receive hands-on training before being allowed to operate on his own. By the end of the fourteenth century, Avenzoar had become well-known in university circles at Padua, Bologna, and Montpellier where he was considered one of the greatest physicians of all time. Successive publications of his *Kitab al-Taysir* and of translations ensured his influence through the seventeenth century when Paracelsus' new treatment paradigm emphasizing chemical ingredients rather than herbs, disseminated in the vernacular rather than in Greek or Latin, set in motion the decline of Greco-Roman medical tradition. In the meantime, the Mongolian capture and sacking of Bagdad, the capital of the Abbasid Caliphate, in 1258, and the defeat of the Emirate of

Granada in 1492 by Isabel "The Catholic", Queen of Castile and León and her husband Ferdinand II of Aragón, completing the centuries-long recapture of the Iberian Peninsula from the Arabs, marked the decline of the Islamic world that accelerated the demise of traditional Hippocratic and Galenic medicine.

Meanwhile, new religious fervor, especially in Christian France, and the early success of the crusades contributed to the proliferation of Christian monasteries and health centers across Europe becoming the repositories of Greek medicine where monks copied ancient manuscripts and attended the sick, as Nestorian monks had done centuries earlier, giving rise to a network of *hospitiums*[5] throughout Western Europe that,

> Flourished during the times of the Christian crusades and pilgrimages that were found mostly in monasteries where monks extended care to the sick and dying, but also to the hungry and weary on their way to the Holy Land, Rome, or other holy places, as well as to the woman in labor, the needy poor, the orphan, and the leper on their journey through life [58].

Perhaps the most famous Hospitium was the ninth century *Studium* of Salerno, a coastal town in southern Italy, key to trade with Sicily and other Mediterranean towns. Although this humble dispensary was initially sustained by the needs of thousands of pilgrims en route to the Holy Land, the Studium soon became the first formal association of physicians that eventually grew into the *Schola Medica Salernitana*. Fostered by its Greek past, the dispensary and the town rose in fame with the arrival at a nearby abbey in 1060 of Constantine Africanus, a Benedictine monk and native of Carthage whose medical guide for travelers titled *Viaticum* and his translations and annotations of Greek and Arabic texts led Salerno to be known as *Hippocratica Civitas* (Hippocrates Town). By the end of the eleventh century, the fame of the Studium had spread across Europe thanks to the erudition of its teachers and scholars, women as well as men, and of their writings still anchored in the Hippocratic-Galenic tradition. Prominent and best known medical writings arising from the Studium in that period include the *Breviary on the Signs, Causes, and Cures of Diseases* by Joannes de Sancto Paulo, the *Liber de Simplici Medicina* by Johannes and Matthaeus Plantearius, and *De Passionibus Mulierum Curandorum,* a compilation of women's health issues attributed to Trotula, the most famous female physician of her time. Given its widespread fame and its eclectic teaching merging Greek, Latin, Jewish, and Arab medical traditions, the Studium became a Mecca for students, teachers, and scholars between the eleventh and thirteenth centuries. And although the *Studium* had little direct impact on the progress of medicine, it is noteworthy mainly as the precursor of the *Schola Medica Salernitana*, the first university of medicine in the world, and as a model for the greatly influential and enduring pre-Renaissance medical schools at Montpellier (1150), Bologna (1158), and Paris (1208) that through local and relocated scholars became European meccas for the study and practice of medicine.

---

[5] Precursors to today's hospices.

2.4 From Medieval Europe to World War II

The early-Renaissance period witnessed a revival of interest in Greek culture fostered by the arrival in Western Europe of many Greek scholars who fled Constantinople after the Turks conquered Byzantium in 1453, thus enabling western scholars to abandon Arabic translations of the Greek masters. This and other transcendental events of that time, such as the invention of the printing press, the discovery of America, and the Reformation, brought about a change in direction and outlook; a desire to escape the boundaries of the past and an eagerness to explore new horizons. This inquisitiveness was broad-based, encompassing all areas of human knowledge and endeavor from the study of anatomy to the scrutiny of the skies that culminated in the publication of two revolutionary and immensely influential treatises of that period: *"De Humani Corporis Fabrica Libri Septum"* (*Seven Books on the Fabric of the Human Body*) [59] by Andreas Vessalius (1514–1564), and *"De Revolutionibus orbium coelestium"* (*On the Revolutions of the Celestial Orbs*) by Nicolaus Copernicus (1473–1543) [60]. Likewise, progress was made in surgical techniques and treatment of wounds, thanks to Ambroise Paré (1510–1590), surgeon to the French Armies, private physician to three Kings of France and the father of modern surgery and forensic pathology, whose extensive experience on the battlefields of France's Armies and ingenious prostheses reduced surgical mortality and accelerated rehabilitation [61]. He is said to have turned butchery into humane surgery. However, this burst of Renaissance knowledge did not extend to cancer, leading Paré to call all cancers *Noli me tangere* (do not touch me) and to declare, "Any kind of cancer is almost incurable and…[if operated]…heals with great difficulty" [62].

Nonetheless, some of the physical attributes of cancer began to emerge. Gabriele Fallopius (1523–1562) is credited with having described the clinical differences between benign and malignant tumors, a distinction largely applicable today. He identified malignant tumors by their woody firmness, irregular shape, multilobulation, adhesion to neighboring tissues (skin, muscles, and bones), and by congested blood vessels often surrounding the lesion. In contrast, benign tumors were said to be softer masses of regular shape (often round) that are movable and do not adhere to adjacent structures. Like his predecessors, he advocated a cautious approach to cancer treatment, "Quiescente cancro, medicum quiescentrum" (If a cancer doesn't bother, leave it alone). More importantly, for the first time in 1,500 years, Galen's black bile theory of the origin of cancer was challenged and new hypotheses were formulated. For example, Wilhelm Bombast von Hohenheim (1493–1541), best known as Paracelsus, proposed substituting Galen's black bile with *"ens"* (entities): *ens astrorum* (cosmic entities); *ens veneni* (toxic entities); *ens naturale et spirituale* (physical or mental entities); and *ens deale* (providential entities). Similarly, Johannes Baptista van Helmont (1577–1644) envisioned a mysterious *"Archeus"* system [63]. While these hypotheses were throwbacks to pre-Hippocratic beliefs in supernatural forces governing human health and disease, it was at this time that René Descartes (1590–1650) published his *"Discours de la méthode pour bien conduire sa raison et chercher la verité dans les sciences"* (Discourse on rightly conducting one's reason for seeking the truth in the sciences) [64]. This seminal philosophical treatise on the method of systematic doubt, beginning with *cogito ergo sum* (I think, therefore I exist), was pivotal in guiding thinkers and researchers in their quest for the truth. Then, the discovery of chyle (lymph) by Gaspare Aselli (1581–1626) [65] and of its circulation and final drainage into the blood system through the thoracic duct later discovered by Jean Pecquet (1622–1674), and the circulation of blood in a system that included the heart, arteries, and veins, discovered by William Harvey (1578–1657), led scholars to conclude that Galen's black bile implicated in cancer could be found nowhere, whereas lymph was everywhere and was therefore suspect. For instance, French physician Jean Astruc (1684–1766) was key to the demise of the bile-cancer link. In 1759, he compared the flavor of cooked slices of beef and breast cancer, and finding no appreciable difference, concluded breast tissue contained no additional bile or acid. Based on this new lead, Henri François Le Dran (1685–1770), one of the best surgeons of his time, postulated that cancer developed locally but spread through lymphatics, becoming inoperable and fatal [66], an observation as true today as it was then. His contemporary, Jean-Louis Petit (1674–1750), advocated total mastectomy for breast cancer, including resection of axillary glands (lymph nodes), which he correctly judged necessary 'to preclude recurrences' [67, 68]. Three and a half centuries later, the practice survives as a prognostic indicator rather than as a preventive measure. Petit's surgical approach to breast cancer surgery is still current today after many modifications made possible by enormous progress achieved in surgical techniques, anesthesia, antibiotics, and general medical support.

How cancer began and what its causes were remained a puzzle, and several scientific institutions promoted the search for an answer. For example, in 1773, the Academy of Lyon, France offered a prize for the best scientific report on "Qu'est-ce que le cancer" (What is cancer?). It was won by Bernard Peyrilhe's (1735–1804) doctoral thesis; the first investigation to explore systematically the causes, nature, patterns of growth, and treatment of cancer [69] that catapulted Peyrilhe as one of the founders of experimental cancer research. He postulated the presence of an *"Ichorous matter"*, a cancer-promoting factor akin to a virus, emerging from degenerated or putrefied lymph. To test whether the *Ichorous matter* was contagious, he injected breast cancer extract under the skin of a dog, which he kept at home under observation. However, his servants drowned the constantly howling dog, thus cutting short the experiment. Peyrilhe also subscribed to the notion of the local origin of cancer and called disease emerging distally as *consequent cancers*. Like Petit's, his surgical approach to breast cancer included removal of the axillary lymph nodes but added the pectoralis major muscle; an operation further augmented by William Stewart Halsted (1852–1922), a New York surgeon, who in 1882 popularized the "radical mastectomy", which consisted of removing the breast, the axillary nodes, and the major and minor pectoralis muscles in a single *en bloc* procedure [70]. Yet more aggressive twentieth century surgeons added prophylactic oophorectomy, adrenalectomy, and hypophysectomy[6] to breast cancer surgery, procedures

---

[6] Removal of the ovaries, adrenal glands, and hypophysis (or pituitary) gland, respectively.

that have been abandoned as ineffective and mutilating. The term *metastases* to describe cancer arising distally to the primary lesion was coined in 1829 by Joseph Recamier, a French gynecologist better known for advocating the use of the vaginal speculum to examine female genitalia. Meanwhile, Giovanni Battista Morgagni (1682–1771) contributed greatly to understanding cancer pathology through his monumental *"De Sedibus et Causis Morborum per Anatomen Indigatis"* (On the Seats and Causes of Diseases as Investigated by Anatomy), which contains careful descriptions of autopsies carried out on 700 patients who died from breast, stomach, rectum, and pancreas cancer. On another front, recognizing that the special needs of cancer patients were not being met, Jean Godinot (1661–1739), canon of the Rheims cathedral, bequeathed a considerable sum of money to the city of Rheims to erect and maintain in perpetuity a cancer hospital for the poor. The *Hôpital des cancers* became functional in 1740 amidst strong protestations by local inhabitants. It initially welcomed 8 cancer patients; 5 women and 3 men [71]. However, the fear that cancer might be contagious was such that cancer patients were avoided, as were lepers, and the inhabitants of Rheims eventually succeeded in having the hospital relocated outside the city in 1779.

In the meantime, Bernardino Ramazzini (1633–1714), born in Capri, focused on workers' health problems from his medical school years, visiting workplaces in attempts to determine whether workers' activities and environment impacted their health. After years of painstaking field observations, he published *De morbis artificum diatriba* (Diseases of workers) [72], first in Modena (1700) and later in Padua (1713). His exhaustive workplace surveys produced the first persuasive empiric evidence of a link between work activity and environment and human diseases. The inclusion of detailed descriptions of 52 specific occupational illnesses and their link to a particular work activity or work environment, supported by literature surveys, and complemented by suggested remedies won him the title *Father of modern occupational medicine* [73] and, three centuries later, to the Colegium Ramazzini, an international organization dedicated to the advancement of occupational and environmental issues [74]. In 1713, he reported a virtual absence of cervical cancer but a higher incidence of breast cancer in nuns relative to married women and thought there might be a connection to their celibacy, a notion challenged in 1991 [75]. Surprisingly, he suggested a lack of sexual activity as the possible cause for both. Yet, he couldn't have known that refraining from sexual activity lowered nuns' exposure to the virus responsible for the vast majority of cervical cancers. Indeed, we now know from empiric evidence that over 90 % of cases of cervical cancers worldwide are caused by sexually transmitted human papillomaviruses (HPV), especially HPV-16 [76]. Hence, life-long celibate women, whether nuns or not, are not exposed to genital HPVs and should be spared of developing cervical cancer. Years later (1761), John Hill (1716?–1775?) warned of the dangers of the then popular tobacco snuff, stating "No man should venture upon Snuff who is not sure that he is not so far liable to a cancer: and no man can be sure of that" [77], and in 1775, Percivall Pott (1714–1788) called attention to scrotum cancer in chimney sweepers. In his *Chirurgical observations relative to the Cataract, the Polypus of the Nose, and the Cancer of the Scrotum, etc.*, he accurately noted,

> Ramazzini has written a book De morbis artificum; the Colic of Poictou[7] is a well-known distemper, and every body is acquainted with the disorders to which painters, plummers, glaziers, and the workers in white lead are liable; but there is disease as peculiar to a certain set of people, which has not, at least to my knowledge, been publickly noticed; I mean chimney-sweepers' cancer. It is a disease which always makes its first attack on, and its first appearance in, the inferior part of the scrotum; where it produces a superficial, painful, ragged, ill-looking sore, with hard and rising edges. The trade call[s] it soot-wart [78].

Pott was well aware of the progressive nature of the disease, of the benefits of early intervention, and of the questionable outcome of late surgical intervention, for he advised,

> If there is any chance of putting a stop to, or prevent this mischief, it must be the immediate removal of the part affected…for if it be suffered to remain until the virus has seized the testicle, it is generally too late for even castration. I have many times made the experiment; but though the sores…have healed kindly, and the patients have gone from the hospital seemingly well yet, in the space of a few months…they have returned either with the same disease in the other testicle, or glands of the groin, or with…a disease state of some of the viscera, and which have soon been followed by a painful death [79].

He also suspected the chemical origin of scrotum cancer, noting, "The disease, in these people, seems to derive its origin from a lodgment of soot in the rugae of the scrotum…" [80] Two centuries later, scrotal cancer in chemeney sweepers was linked to absorption of polycyclic aromatic hydrocarbons [81]. In his Chirurgical observations book, Pott states not having encountered any case under the age of puberty. Yet, his editor added a footnote regarding an 8-year old 'chimney sweeper apprentice' whose scrotum cancer was confirmed by Pott [82]. A century later (1875), an Act of the British Parliament, passed in 1840, was finally enforced. It provided for chimneysweepers to be licensed and forbade both chimney climbing before age 21 and apprenticeship before age 16 [83].

Notwithstanding a better understanding of certain aspects of cancer, other baffling observations of that time included recurrence at sites distal to the original cancer, multiple cancers in a single individual, and families with a high incidence of cancer. Such occurrences were explained by a certain cancer predisposition or *diathesis* as first invoked by Jacques Delpech (1772–1835) and Gaspard Laurent Bayle (1774–1816) [84], later re-energized throughout Europe by Pierre Paul Broca (1824–1880), Sir James Paget (1814–1899), and Carl von Rokitansky (1804–1878). Believers in the *diathesis* hypothesis viewed cancer as a clinical manifestation of an underlying constitutional defect. Yet, different medical writers often used the terms diathesis, predisposition, and even cachexia interchangeably. For instance, pathologist Jean Cruveilhier (1791–1874) considered cancer diathesis and cancer cachexia as different manifestations of the same process caused by cancerous impregnation of venous blood. Consequently, there was a generally nihilistic attitude regarding therapy, as cancer relapses were considered nearly inevitable unless resected very early. However, the observation that at least some cancers were surgically curable

---

[7] Chronic lead poisoning by lead-containing wine first diagnosed in the Poitou region of France.

convinced Peyrilhe and followers that cancer was a local disease, and that relapses after surgery were either local re-growth of remnant disease or unrecognized early dissemination through lymphatic or blood vessels. This view was widely embraced by prominent physicians and medical writers of the time, including anatomist Heinrich von Waldeyer-Hartz (1836–1931), famous for his work on the pharyngeal lymphoid tissue or *Waldeyer's ring* and for coining the words *chromosome* and *neuron*, surgeon Franz König (1832–1910), who is credited for first using X-rays to visualize a sarcoma in an amputated leg [85], and Broca, whose *Mémoire sur l'anatomie pathologique du cancer* (Essay on the pathologic anatomy of cancer) [86] provided an empiric foundation for cancer staging and hence prognostic assessment that endures today.

Zacharias Jansen (c. 1580–c. 1638) is credited as inventor of a prototype to the microscope but scholars believe his father Hans must have played a key role, for they worked together as spectacle makers in Middleburg, the Netherlands, and Zacharias was just an adolescent at the time of the invention, circa 1590 [87]. Three centuries later, Vincent Chevalier (1771–1841) and his son Charles (1804–1859) developed the first distortion-free (achromatic) objectives that served as a basis for the younger Chevalier to introduce, in 1842, the first commercially achromatic microscope with great success in France and abroad. In Chevalier's catalogue, the instrument, item No. 238, is described as,

> Vertical achromatic microscope, small model, simple and compound with three achromatic lenses, two Huygens oculars, two doublets, accessories, mahogany case, from 180 to 250 [francs] [88].

As microscopes improved in power and resolution, cells were recognized as the fundamental structural and functional unit of plants and animals, setting the stage for new hypotheses about cancer to emerge, with some dissenters. For example, Johannes Müller (1801–1858) devoted his efforts to the microscopic study of tumors, and in 1839, published *On the fine structure and forms of morbid tumors*. He postulated that cancer originated not from normal tissue, but from "*budding elements*", which his 500-fold magnifying microscope failed to identify. Alternatively, Adolf Hannover (1814–1894) fancied that cancer arose from a mysterious "*cellula cancrosa*" that was different from a normal cell in size and appearance. However, Rudolph Virchow (1821–1902) and his followers were unable to confirm the existence of such a cell [89], a view first articulated by Alfred Armand Louis Marie Velpeau (1795–1867). After examining 400 malignant and 100 benign tumors under the microscope, Velpeau concluded, as if he had correctly anticipated the genetic bases of cancer,

> The so-called cancer cell is merely a secondary product rather than the essential element in the disease. Beneath it, there must exist some more intimate element which science would need in order to define the nature of cancer [90].

Robert Remak (1815–1865), best known for his embryological studies that determined which organ derives from each embryonic germ layer, took another step forward by postulating that all cells derive from binary fusion of pre-existing cells, and that cancer was not a *new formation* but a *transformation* of normal tissues, which resembles or, if degeneration ensues, differs from the tissue of origin. He wrote,

> These findings are as relevant to pathology as they are to physiology…I make bold to assert that pathological tissues are not, any more than normal tissues, formed in an extracellular cytoblastem, but are the progeny or products of normal tissues in the organism [91].

On the other hand, he dedicated much of his clinical practice to galvano-therapy that was considered unscientific by the medical establishment and led the medical faculty and the Cultural Ministry to refuse his application for a position at the Charité clinic in Berlin [92]. Barred from practicing at the Charité, and his post at the University being, as a Jew, unpaid, he was forced to rely on income generated from patients he attended at his home, where he also conducted research. It is of interest that the famous Rudolf Virchow, a German physician, pathologist, and politician, who in his three-volume work, *Die Krankhaften Geschwulste* had postulated that cancer originated in changes in connective tissues, initially rejected Remak's work, but soon changed his mind and published it as his own [93]. He is attributed the phrase *omnis cellula e cellula* (every cell derives from another cell), previously coined by François Vincent Raspail (1794–1878), a French chemist, politician, and President of the Human Rights Society. Remak's cell division observations were expanded by Louis Bard (1829–1894), who proposed also correctly that normal cells are capable of developing into a mature differentiated state, whereas cancer cells suffer from developmental defects that result in tumor formation [94]. Remak's and Bard's notions on cell division are significant in providing clues on the genetic origin of cancer and serving as precursors to today's histologic classification of many cancers into *well differentiated, moderately differentiated*, and *poorly differentiated* subtypes, a stratification still useful today to plan treatment and to gage prognosis. Another notable scientist who bridged Velpeau's views on the probable cause of cancer to our present knowledge was Theodor Boveri (1862–1915). In an essay entitled *Zur Frage der Entstehung maligner Tumoren* (The Origin of malignant tumors) [95], Boveri first proposed a role for somatic mutations in cancer development based on his observations in sea urchins. He found that fertilizing a single egg with two sperm cells often led to anomalous progenitor cell growth and division, chromosomal imbalance, and the emergence of tissue masses. Thus, it had taken 50 years of progress for Boveri to validate Velpeau's intuition, and it would take another half a century for the emergence of molecular biology and molecular genetics to confirm Boveri's initially ignored views on the nature of cancer.

While small pieces of the cancer puzzle were slowly falling into place, the true nature of cancer and the code governing its development, growth, and dissemination remained a mystery and remedies continued whimsical and inefficacious. Indeed, Oliver Wendell Holmes (1809–1894), addressing the Massachusetts Medical Society in 1860, summed up the status of drugs at the time as follows,

> If the whole materia medica, as now used, could be sunk to the bottom of the sea, it would be all the better for mankind – and all the worse for the fishes [96].

As this statement resonated in America, progress in bacteriology and parasitology was having a profound impact on cancer theory and cancer therapeutics of the nineteenth century. Interest in a possible bacterial or parasitic link to cancer, first raised in the seventeenth and eighteenth centuries, led to equating cancer invasion to bacterial infections and to adopting the bacteria-eradication concept as a model for treating cancer, a notion that still prevails today. Between the 1880s and the 1920s, the hunt for cancer-causing microorganisms was obstinate and relentless, as summed up by Sigismund Peller (1890–1980),

> In the first period, every conceivable group of microorganisms was the search target: worms, bacilli, cocci, spirochetes; molds, fungi, coccidiae; sporozoa, ameba, trypanosomas, polimorphous microorganisms, and filtrable viruses. It was like fishing in a well-stocked pond. Most fishermen became victims of self-deception... [97].

The zenith of this particular saga was reached when Johannes Andreas Grib Fibiger (1867–1928) was awarded the 1926 Nobel Prize in Physiology or Medicine *for his discovery of the Spiroptera carcinoma*. In the presentation speech, the Dean of the Royal Caroline Institute stated,

> By feeding healthy mice with cockroaches containing the larvae of the spiroptera, Fibiger succeeded in producing cancerous growths in the stomachs of a large number of animals. It was therefore possible, for the first time, to change by experiment normal cells into cells having all the terrible properties of cancer [98].

The long-held hypothesis of a link between microorganisms and cancer is of historic significance, as it exemplifies how generations of scientists, researchers, and scholars, misguided by flawed hypotheses, often commit their talents and energy, as well as considerable human and financial resources to the unproductive pursuit of a false lead. While the determined pursuit of a worthy goal by many is often necessary, overly enthusiastic adherence to a single hypothesis by many is self-reinforcing and can obfuscate good judgment while dismissing the unwelcome views of isolated dissenters. As our knowledge about both the causes of cancer and cancer genetics improved, the hypothesis of the bacteriological basis of cancer eventually lost much of its luster, but not before it had established another, more pervasive and counterproductive parallel with infectious diseases: that cancer cells, like bacteria, are foreign invaders that must be eradicated at any cost. In turn, this has lead to the development of ever more powerful cytotoxic drugs and increasingly aggressive anti-cancer treatment approaches but few cures. As will be described in Chap. 7, cancer drug development remained hostage, at least initially, to the bacteria-cancer link hypothesis. Indeed, some early unacceptably toxic agents, developed as antimicrobials, were thought suitable for treating cancer and some demonstrated anti-cancer activity. This was the case of the antibiotic agent *daunarubicin*, isolated concomitantly by a French and an Italian laboratory in the 1950s from a new strain of *Streptomyces peucetius* that exhibited good activity against murine tumors. The name daunarubicin derives from *Dauni*, a pre-Roman tribe that lived in the region of Italy where the bacteria were obtained, and *Ruby*, the French word describing the red pigment produced by the bacterium. Daunarubicin is a prototype anthracycline antibiotic from which over 500 derived analogs have been evaluated in the NCI's anti-cancer screening program [99]. The hydroxy derivative of daunarubicin, Doxorubicin, is sold under the trade names of Adriamycin® and Doxil®. The former is an intravenous preparation effective in the treatment of several cancers, especially leukemia and lymphoma, alone or in combination chemotherapy. The latter is a liposome-encapsulated formulation available in the US in limited supplies. Another legacy of this period is a drug development strategy by trial and error, pioneered by Ehrlich in his 7-year quest for antimicrobials, a simplistic approach not suited for cancer drug development that unfortunately persists today, as discussed in Chap. 7. Finally, after 150 years of inconclusive evidence on the bacteria-cancer link, inflammation and mutagenic bacterial metabolites are now invoked as causing several cancers. Examples of the former are gastric carcinoma [100] and MALT[8] [101] that have been linked to the bacterium *Helicobacter pylori*, leading the International Agency for Research on Cancer to classify *H. pylori* as a Group 1 human carcinogen in 1994, and many physicians to attempt its eradication. However, recent data suggest that MALT might straddle between malignancy and inflammation [102]. Moreover,

> Evidence links the lack of *H pylori* with gastro-oesophageal reflux disease, Barrett's oesophagus, and the risk of adenocarcinoma of the oesophagus and gastric cardia. In particular, it seems that cag+strains exert a protective effect whereas cag–strains have essentially no effect... suggest[ing] that clinicians should not eliminate *H pylori* from everyone [103].

In fact,

> ...screening for and treatment of *H. pylori* infection as a strategy for secondary prevention of gastric cancer remains controversial. The controversy is amplified by data indicating benefits by preventing esophageal adenocarcinoma, asthma, diarrhoea, and even tuberculosis [104].

Colon cancer is cited as possibly being linked to mutagenic bacterial metabolites. A corollary of the bacteria-cancer link hypothesis is the suggestion that cancer could be treated with bacteria or their products, a concept that goes back more than a century when William B. Coley (1862–1936) inoculated a cancer patient with erysipelas [105]. Eventually, he treated more than 1,000 patients with various bacteria and bacterial products, claiming excellent results, raising doubts and criticism, and leading to the abandonment of the practice [106]. Today, BCG[9] administered intravesically, with or without percutaneous boosting, is the only FDA-approved bacterial agent for the non-surgical treatment of carcinoma *in situ* of the bladder. It has been reported to reduce tumor progression and recurrences, and to prolong survival [107].

The discovery of anesthesia in 1842 by Crawford W. Long (1815–1878) [108] and of asepsis in 1867 by Joseph Lister (1827–1912) [109] propelled surgery to the forefront of early stage cancer management with slowly increasing cure rates paralleling progress in fields underlying surgical success, including effective antibiotics, new powerful and safe anesthetic agents, refinements in surgical techniques, and general medical support. Likewise, the discovery of X-rays in 1895 by Wilhelm

---

[8] Mucosal-Associated Lymphoid Tissue that can lead to a low-grade non-Hodgkin's Lymphoma.
[9] Bacillus Calmette Guerin; and attenuated Bacillus Bovis.

Conrad Röentgen (1845–1923) [110], uranium by Henri Becquerel, and radium and polonium by Marie Sklodowska-Curie (1867–1934) and her husband Pierre Curie (1859–1906) [111] marked the dawn of modern diagnostic and therapeutic radiology and of nuclear medicine, raising expectations that the successful treatment of cancer was at hand.

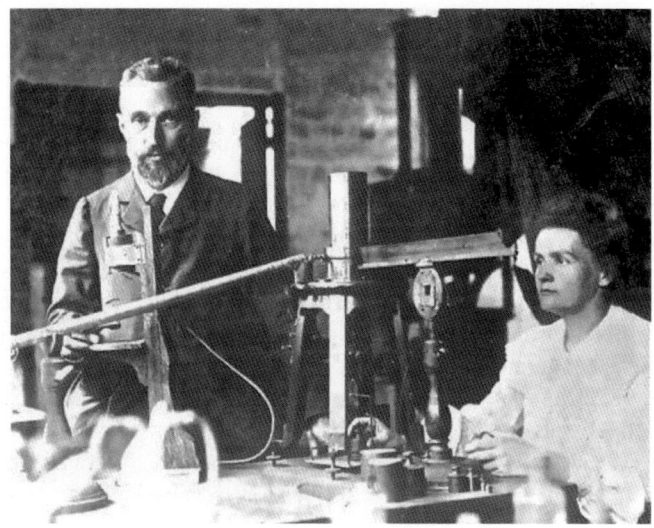

Fig. 2.3 Pierre and Marie Curie in their dilapidated laboratory, circa 1903

It began when Pierre's skin burns from handling radioactive samples, the evolution of which he carefully recorded and reported, led him to seek the collaboration of eminent physicians to further delineate the power of radioactivity in experimental animals. Their results showed that radium could cure growths, tumors, and some cancers; a therapeutic method that became known as *Curietherapy*. Several clinicians applied the method to diseased individuals with "encouraging results" [112]. No longer restricted to research, radioactivity would become central to an entire industry. In 1903, Marie and Pierre were awarded the Nobel Prize in Physics, "in recognition of the extraordinary services they have rendered by their joint researches on the radiation phenomena discovered by Professor Henri Becquerel", who shared the Prize [113]. At his award address, Pierre questioned whether new discoveries such as theirs in the wrong hands would be harmful to the world, but concluded, "I am one of those who believe with Nobel that mankind will derive more good than harm from the new discoveries." Eager to exploit radioactivity for the treatment of disease and facing inertia from the French state and her university, Marie decided to spearhead the efforts herself by sending gas emanations from radium to hospitals for therapeutic purposes and established a program at the Radium Institute, founded in 1911, to train technicians and physicians in their safe use. After an entirely altruistic dedication to science, Pierre died on April 19, 1906, run over by a horse-drawn wagon. Although sexism and xenophobia had prevented her from being admitted to the French Academy of Science in 1911, Marie received that year's Nobel Prize in Chemistry "in recognition of her services to the advancement of chemistry by the discovery of the elements radium and polonium, by the isolation of radium and the study of the nature and compounds of this remarkable element" [114]. She was the first woman to win a Nobel Prize, the only woman to win two Nobel Prizes, and one of two persons to win Nobel Prizes in more than one scientific discipline; the other being Linus Pauling (Chemistry and Peace). Indeed, Marie's major and unparalleled achievements include formulating the theory of radioactivity (a term she coined), techniques for isolating radioactive elements from pitchblende,[10] and the discovery of Radium and Polonium. The couple's daughter, Iréne Joliot-Curie, and her husband, Frédéric Joliot, were awarded the 1935 Nobel Prize in chemistry for the synthesis of new radioactive elements. On July 4, 1934, Marie died of aplastic anemia from exposure to the very radioactivity that brought her fame. Indeed, she had been exposed to the then unknown damaging effects of ionizing radiation in her ramshackle laboratory (compared to a stable or potato cellar by a visiting colleague) from test tubes containing radioactive pellets she carried in her pockets and kept in her desk drawer and from unshielded x-ray equipment she used while serving as a volunteer radiologist in field hospitals during WWI [115]. She had admitted, "one of our pleasures was to enter our workshop at night; then, all around us, we would see the luminous silhouettes of the beakers and capsules that contained our products."

During the early part of the twentieth century, the introduction of innovative research tools enabled medical investigators to systematically explore old and new hypotheses on the origin and nature of cancer, leading to incremental progress on many fronts. For example, John Hill's suspicion in 1761 that tobacco induced cancer in heavy snuffers and Percivall Pott's 1775 suggestion of a tar-cancer link in chimney sweepers were confirmed in 1915 by Katsusaburo Yamagiwa (1863–1930) and his assistant Koichi Ichikawa, who were able to induce squamous cell carcinoma in rabbits' ears chronically exposed to coal tar. Likewise, the virus-cancer link was confirmed in 1910 by Peyton Rous (1879–1970) who succeeded in inducing cancer in healthy chickens injected with a cell-free filtrate of a tumor from a cancer-stricken fowl. Because the filtrate had been put through filters of small size pores that removed bacteria, Rous correctly concluded the cancer-causing agent must be a virus. In his 1910 report, Rous stated,

> In this paper is reported the first avian tumor that has proved transplantable to other individuals. It is a spindle-celled sarcoma of a hen, which has thus far been propagated to the fourth generation… [116].

Rous' findings were initially rejected by much of the medical establishment for they challenged the prevailing view of the genetic heredity of cancer, and he was

---

[10] A uranium-rich mineral and ore.

ostracized for many years. Fifty years later, he was awarded the 1966 Nobel Prize for Physiology or Medicine for his momentous discovery, now known as the *Rous sarcoma virus*. Likewise, the carcinogenicity of radiation and of numerous non-radioactive agents found in the environment (e.g., radon), in industrial products (e.g., asbestos), and in consumer products (e.g., tobacco), was established, and the list keeps growing As these health risks and other aspects of cancer became known, growing public awareness and interest triggered a response by policy makers which eventually prompted the US Congress to enact the National Cancer Act of 1937, the first major attempt to address cancer at the national level. However, the first reports demonstrating the efficacy of an anticancer drug in humans, albeit modest, took place towards the end of World War II [117, 118]. Ironically, that drug was derived from mustard gas, a blistering agent first introduced as a chemical warfare agent by the Imperial German Army that was widely utilized by both Germany and the Allies as a standard weapon in WWI. It was know as *Yellow Cross* by the Germans (the name inscribed on shells containing the gas), *HS* (Hun Stuff) by the British, and *Yperite* (after Ypres, the Belgian town where the gas was first used in 1915) by the French. Although effective countermeasures limited the death rate from mustard gas to 7.5 % of 1.3 million total WWI deaths [119], it was the most-feared weapon of the war, for it caused slow and agonizing death, as witnessed by a British nurse. She reported,

> They cannot be bandaged or touched. We cover them with a tent of propped-up sheets. Gas burns must be agonizing because usually the other cases do not complain, even with the worst wounds, but gas cases are invariably beyond endurance and they cannot help crying out [120].

Remarkably, mustard gas would launch the era of cytotoxic chemotherapy that, along with x-ray and to a lesser extent radium, was to become the bases of today's treatment of advanced cancer, as described in Chap. 7.

Chapter 3
Our Current Knowledge

> *Beneath it* [the cancer cell] *there must exist some more intimate element which science would need in order to define the nature of cancer*
>
> – Alfred Velpeau (1795–1867)

Because cancer arises from the interaction of multiple factors not yet fully understood, this Chapter will describe the status of our still incomplete knowledge.

3.1 The Genetic Bases of Cancer

3.1.1 First the Basics

In the popular mind, cancer conjures up notions of pain, despair, and finality. However, cancer is not a single disease but an assortment of more than 300 very diverse malignancies that can arise from all tissues and organs (broadly divided into *leukemias* arising from blood cells and *solid tumors* emerging from solid organs), become clinically manifest at various stages of development, and exhibit a wide spectrum of biological and progression patterns, each impacting the bearer's survival. Additionally, more than one type of cancer can originate from an organ or tissue, as dramatically exemplified by the over 120 types of brain and central nervous system tumors both benign and malignant and the 70 types of lymphomas according to the 2008 World Health Organization's (WHO) classification [121]. From a clinical standpoint, cancers can exhibit slow growth patterns compatible with long and symptom-free survival, such as indolent lymphomas and chronic lymphocytic leukemia (CLL) [122], or quickly progress to death in only a few months, as exemplified by pancreatic cancer [123]. Likewise, some cancers spread distally from the site of origin, including colon, prostate, and lung cancers that often metastasize to liver, bone, and brain, respectively, whereas others tend to invade locally as is the case of head and neck cancers. Yet, despite their heterogeneous origin, distinct clinical features, and vastly different clinical course and outcome, the underlying genetic processes identified to date leading to their development, growth, and dissemination are broadly similar, mainly mutations occurring in proto-oncogenes,[1] tumor suppressor genes[2] or microRNA genes.[3]

The master blueprint that determines the structure and function of all organisms, including man, is called the *genome*. Each of the approximately 30 trillion cells that make a human being contains a copy of the entire genome and its approximately 20,000–25,000 *genes*, neatly packaged in 46 microscopic units called *chromosomes* found bundled in the cell *nucleus*. Genes are deoxyribonucleic acid (DNA) sequences that contain the code for cells to produce proteins, which are the signals that control the structure and function of each cell, of each organ, and ultimately of the entire organism. These cell-produced, cell-targeted protein signals are at the center of the interdependent relationship that characterizes both the harmonious function of normal cells and the aberrant behavior of cancer cells. Thus, the genome can be thought of as the book of life where chromosomes are chapters and genes are the carefully crafted sentences made of precise words spelled with *nucleotide bases* (letters), all sequentially arranged on the DNA molecule. During the process of cell division and of human reproduction the entire genome must be duplicated and passed from cell to cell and from parent to offspring, respectively. While this process is prodigiously accurate, *spelling* errors do occur. DNA repair genes correct minor, non-lethal alterations. Major errors activate *gatekeeper* genes that block cell replication and force the cell to commit suicide (*apoptosis*). The role of DNA repair and gatekeeper genes is to ensure genomic integrity as cells advance through their replication cycle (*cell cycle*). However, occasional non-lethal alterations escape detection, repair, or blockade and are transmitted from a replicating cell to its daughter cells, giving rise to a genetically abnormal cell line. Transmitted alterations of DNA sequences outside of genes, called *polymorphism*, are neither beneficial nor harmful to the cell or the host. Conversely, transmitted alterations within gene sequences, called *mutations*, are responsible for approximately 4,000 human diseases, including cancer. When mutations affect a sex cell or gamete (egg or sperm), they can be transmitted to future generations, resulting in familial predisposition to diseases such as hemophilia, and to some cancers such as retinoblastoma. At present, the genetic fingerprints of most cancers are not known mainly because insensitive detection techniques of the pre-genomic era uncovered mostly structural chromosomal abnormalities visible by light microscopy that are seldom disease-specific. While diagnostically and prognostically valuable in the clinical setting, such gross abnormalities seldom provide insight into the genetic defects responsible for the development, growth, and dissemination of cancer.

Recognizing that the genome occupied a central role in health and disease, in 1987, the "Health and Environmental Research Advisory Committee (HERAC), recommends a 15-year, multidisciplinary, scientific, and technological undertaking to map and sequence the human genome. Department of Energy designates

---

[1] Growth-promoting genes.
[2] Growth-inhibiting genes.
[3] Genes that regulate gene expression.

multidisciplinary human genome centers" [124]. A year later the NIH received congressional authority and funding to coordinate and support genomics activities in cooperation with other federal agencies, academia, and international groups. An independent NIH institute, named The National Human Genome Research Institute (NHGRI), was created to that effect. Francis Collins M.D., who had participated in the discovery of several elusive genes including those linked to cystic fibrosis, neurofibromatosis, and Huntington's disease, was chosen as its head. The overall project goal was to identify the position and sequence of the three-billion nucleotide bases that make up the human genome. However, because the book of life is written as a continuous string of sequential letters without separation or punctuation between words, sentences or paragraphs, deciphering the position and sequence of the nucleotide bases would still be unreadable and uninterpretable. Thus, another major goal was to identify all human genes (the *words* and *sentences* made up of strings of *letters*) and determine their location. The project formally began on October 1, 1990, cosponsored by the DOE and the NIH, as a $3 billion, 15-year effort. The first 5-year plan, intended to guide research between 1990 and 1995, was revised in 1993 due to unexpected progress. The second, third and final 5-year plans outlined goals through 1998 and 2003, respectively. Some 18 countries participated in the worldwide effort, with significant contributions from research centers in the United Kingdom, Germany, France, and Japan. However, in direct competition with this multinational group of government and academic research centers arose Celera Genomics, a biotechnology company established in May 1998 by J. Craig Venter, Ph.D., founder of the Institute for Genomic Research at the NIH, with venture capital funding from Perkin-Elmer Corp. Using a faster DNA sequencing strategy known as the *whole-genome shotgun* sequencing method, and highly automated sequencing machines that require human attention only 15 min per day despite running continuously, Celera (*swift* in Latin) was able to publish, in February 2001, a working draft of the human genome sequence [125]. The same month, the International Human Genome Sequencing Consortium published its own draft, 10 years in the making and at ten times Celera's cost [126]. These publications marked the end of a race punctuated by "acrimonious feud between the public and private teams" and their American leaders [127]. Although heralded as the crown jewel of twentieth century biology when it was first proposed, the Human Genome Project (HGP) was greeted by many scientists and researchers as, "Absurd, dangerous, and impossible…who noted that the technology did not exist to sequence a bacterium, much less a human…" [128]. The human genome sequence was completed in April 2003. However, many years will pass before this information is translated into tangible benefits in the clinical arena, for it will require uncovering the genetic bases of disease and designing targeted agents to prevent, reverse, or control the defective genes, or to modulate or block their encoded protein products, an endeavor far more complex than anticipated. In the meantime, government- and industry-sponsored initiatives have made substantial progress, particularly speeding DNA sequencing, and gene identification and mapping. For example, while it took Dr. Lap-Chee Tsui's team 9 years to discover the cystic fibrosis gene in 1989 [129], the Parkinson's disease gene was mapped in only 9 days by Dr. Robert Nussbaum's team 9 years later [130]. Likewise, the cancer gene-discovery process also proceeded at a rapid pace as demonstrated by the fact that over just a few years,

> ...more than 1,000 somatic mutations found in 274 megabases (Mb) of DNA corresponding to the coding exons of 518 protein kinase genes in 210 diverse human cancers...[of which] there was evidence for 'driver' mutations contributing to the development of the cancers studied in approximately 120 genes [131].

As our knowledge in cancer genetics continues to accrue and deepen, the post-genomic period will be remembered as the era when the genetic defects that render normal cells malignant were uncovered and when that knowledge was exploited for designing means to prevent, control, and reverse the genetic defects responsible for the development, growth, and dissemination of cancer.

Further details on the basic aspects on the genetics and epigenetics of cancer follow. However, Readers not especially interested in such details can bypass this segment and advance to the section *How does cancer arise?*, starting on page 54.

3.1.2 More Details

3.1.2.1 DNA

On March 7th, 1953, Francis Harry Crick, a 35-year old graduate student at the Cavendish laboratory of the University of Cambridge, England, walked into the Eagle pub and declared, "we have found the secret of life". He was referring to his and James Dewey Watson's discovery of the structure of DNA that explained transmission of genetic information from cell to cell and from parent to offspring, and helped understand how genetic mutations are produced. Theirs was a brilliant interpretation of another investigator's published and, reportedly, still unpublished research data. Crick's career had evolved from physics to chemistry and biology. On the other hand, the 23-year old Watson had received a B.S degree from the University of Chicago and a Ph.D. degree in zoology from Indiana University. However, as a research fellow at the Cavendish laboratory, he abandoned his chosen field for *the pursuit of glory*, as he recounts in his memoirs entitled *The double Helix: A personal account of the discovery of the structure of DNA*, first published in 1968 [132]. In that self-serving account of the momentous discovery, he described his obsession with the DNA molecule and his anticipation that unraveling its structure would bring the Nobel Prize. After attending a 1951 lecture where the gifted Rosalind Franklin presented X-ray crystallography data and her helical concept of the DNA molecule, Watson and Crick built a three-chain DNA molecule model with the backbone on the inside that drew sharp criticism. The head of the Cavendish laboratory, Sir Lawrence Bragg, ordered the unlikely pair to leave DNA to King's College where Franklin and her rival Maurice Hugh Wilkins were assigned the task. However, when Linus Pauling, the world's leading structural chemist who would be awarded Nobel Prizes for Chemistry in 1954 and for Peace in 1962, and the odds-on favorite to solve the structure of DNA published a wrong structure for DNA, it became evident to them that someone else might soonlay claim to "the most important of all scientific prizes" [133]. According to a special report published on August 17, 1998 [134], "When Watson came calling in January 1953, Wilkins [who Watson described as 'a beginner' in X-ray diffraction work, wanted some professional help and hoped that 'Rosy', a trained crystallographer, could speed up his research], revealed he had been quietly copying Franklin's data. He showed one of her x-ray photos" (Fig. 3.1).

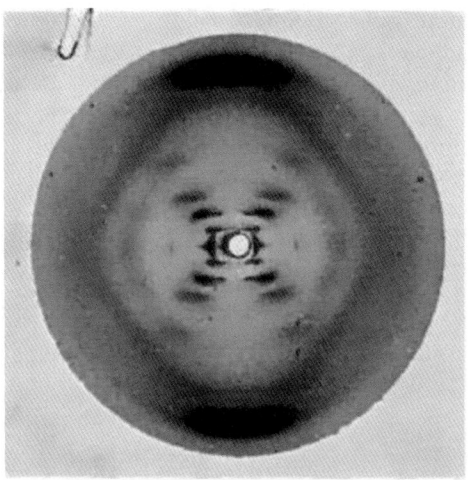

Fig. 3.1 Rosalind Franklin's crystallography photo #51

Watson was so impressed that he later wrote, "The instant I saw the picture my mouth fell open and my pulse began to race.... the black cross of reflections which dominated the picture could arise only from a helical structure... mere inspection of the X-ray picture gave several of the vital helical parameters" [135]. Watson's own admission, the fact that neither he nor Crick conducted bench research on DNA, relying instead on other investigators' data to draw diagrams and construct tri-dimensional models, and the short time between this episode and the publication of their report leads to the inescapable conclusion: Franklin's work was pivotal in their inferring the correct molecular structure of DNA. Their highly acclaimed and universally accepted model included two helical chains made of sugar-phosphate backbones, as Franklin's work revealed, held together by complementary pairs of four nitrogen bases interlocked between them. Thus, Watson's and Crick's failure to acknowledge Franklin's crucial role in their formulation of the structure of DNA reported in the April 2, 1953 *Nature* article [136] where he and Crick disclosed their final model is a most regrettable episode in the annals of great discoveries. To add insult to injury, Watson ridiculed Franklin in his book, stating, "So it was quite easy to imagine her the product of an unsatisfied mother who unduly stressed the desirability of professional careers that could save bright girls from marriages to dull men". Franklin's biographer adds "'Rosy' was depicted as an aggressive, perhaps belligerent, female subordinate with no respect for her superiors" who "refused to think of herself as an assistant to Wilkins" [137]. Crick, Watson, and Wilkins received the 1962 Nobel Prize for Physiology or Medicine "for their discoveries concerning the molecular structure of nucleic acids and its significance for information transfer in living material" [138]. Watson went on to receive the most honors and recognition, including honorary degrees from 22 universities. Franklin died of ovarian cancer in 1958, age 37.

From an anatomical standpoint, the genome is contained in tightly coiled strands of DNA organized in chromosomes, which are housed in the cell nucleus. To illustrate the minuscule size of the DNA, suffice it to say that, if unwound, the DNA of a single cell (one million cells fit on the head of a pin) would stretch 5 ft but would be only 50 trillionth of an inch wide. Stretching all the DNA of a human being would reach the sun and back. A human DNA molecule (Fig. 3.2) consists of two strands that wrap around each other like a twisted ladder or a spiral staircase, the

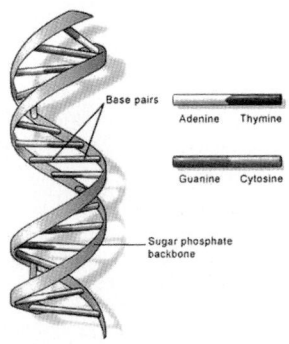

Fig. 3.2 The structure of DNA (Reproduced from the US National Library of Medicine [139])

so-called *double helix*, whose sugar and phosphate sides connect to each other by rungs of nitrogen-containing chemicals called bases. Each strand is a linearly repeated sequence called nucleotides, made of one sugar, one phosphate, and one nitrogenous base. There are four different bases: adenine (A), thymine (T), cytosine (C), and guanine (G). The order of the bases along the sugar-phosphate backbone, called the DNA sequence, is like a barcode that encrypts the genetic instructions necessary for the structural and functional integrity of an organism with its array of unique traits. Weak bonds between bases forming base pairs, of which there are approximately three billion in the human genome, hold the two DNA strands together. Each time a cell divides, its genome is duplicated by DNA replication, a complex process initiated by DNA polymerase, an enzyme that breaks the weak bonds between base pairs, unwinding the *helix* to allow separation of the two DNA

3.1 The Genetic Bases of Cancer

strands. Once separated, each strand directs the synthesis of a complementary DNA strand, including matching bases following strict base pairing: adenine with thymine (A-T pair) and cytosine with guanine (C-G pair). Each daughter cell receives one parental and one new DNA strand, thus minimizing chances of errors (mutations) in gene transfer.

At the functional cellular level, genetic information encoded in nuclear DNA ultimately leads to production of regulatory proteins in the cell cytoplasm. This process requires an intermediary molecule, called ribonucleic acid (RNA). RNA polymerase first *unzips* a section of nuclear DNA and transcribes (copies), base-by-base, a given sequence of exposed bases, and moves into the cell cytoplasm as messenger RNA (mRNA) where it translates the genetic code (or message) into synthesis of the particular protein encoded in the exposed DNA.

3.1.2.2 Genes

Johann Mendel (Fig. 3.3), born in Hynčice, Moravia (in the Austro-Hungarian Empire) in 1822, entered religious life at the seminary of the Abbey of St. Augustine in Brünn, Moravia's capital (Brno in today's Czech Republic) in 1843, taking the name Gregor. He worked on the side as a substitute teacher in a secondary school in Znaim, near Brünn, and tried to upgrade to regular teacher but failed the certification examination. Paradoxically, his lowest mark was in biology. Sponsored by his Abbot, František Cyril Napp (1824–1867), himself an accomplished scholar, Mendel enrolled at the University of Vienna in 1851 where he studied physics, chemistry, mathematics, zoology, and botany. He returned to the abbey in 1853 and

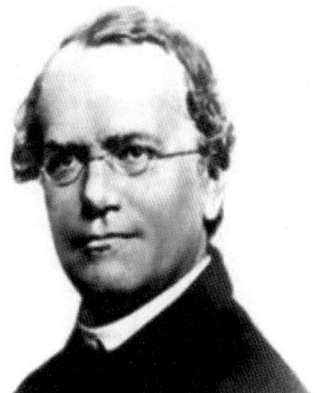

Fig. 3.3 Johann (Gregor) Mendel

became its Abbot in 1867, a demanding responsibility that effectively ended his research career. Although he worked alone, Mendel did not operate in a vacuum, for he drew inspiration from his former teachers Friedrich Franz and Karl Nestler, and his scientific interests and pursuits were supported by a good library at the monastery, by other monks, most notably Aurelius Thaler, a botanical expert who in 1830 had established an experimental garden at the monastery, and by colleagues at the Brünn's Natural Science Society. Mendel's now famous paper entitled *Versuche über pflanzenhybriden* (Experiments with plant hybridization), describing his work on heredity, was presented orally before the Society in February 1865, and published in the Society's transactions in 1866 [140]. From his modest monastery garden, Mendel had unraveled the secrets of heredity that would earn him the title of *father of modern genetics*. Yet, his contemporaries failed to understand the importance of Mendel's work on genetics and his observations fell into oblivion to the point that, for several decades, they were unknown to the public and to scientists, including Charles Darwin [141].

Mendel's success in choosing seemingly rudimentary techniques applied to the study of ordinary garden peas (*Pisum sativum*) leading to deciphering the secrets of genetics that rest on carefully designed experiments, painstakingly collecting large amounts of data, analyzing results in light of a starting hypothesis, and testing results at each step with a new set of experiments. Choosing garden peas was a carefully considered decision that demonstrated his genius. Indeed, he selected inexpensive and easily available peas of distinct shapes and colors with a short generation time that produce many offspring, enabling him accurately and systematically to sort sequential generations of cross-pollination results. Moreover, in addition to an anatomy designed for self-pollination that prevents cross-pollination, garden peas can be cross-pollinated at will by the experimenter by placing pollen from one plant on the female flowers of another [142]. Mendel selected seven traits or characteristics for study involving various colors and shapes, but first grew the plants for 2 years to ensure a pure line. That is, all offspring produced by 2 years of self-pollination would be identical with regards to each trait under study. His first major observation contradicted the then popular notion known as *blending inheritance* that assumed that all traits were inherited by the first generation offspring (F_1) as a blend or average of the parents' (P). Thus, crossing a tall plant with a short one, for example, was expected to produce a medium-sized offspring plant. When Mendel pollinated tall or short plants within themselves, offspring plants remained tall or short, as expected. Curiously, when he cross-pollinated plants with green pea pods with plants that had yellow pods, he noticed that all offspring hybrid plants (F_1) exhibited green pea pods, as if the yellow pea pod trait had vanished. Yet, when he pollinated two (F_1) hybrid plants between themselves, some of their offspring (F_2) exhibited yellow pods and others had green pods. This phenomenon reappeared regardless of the trait studied and did so at a constant ratio of approximately 3:1 (Table 3.1). Mendel correctly concluded that hereditary traits are discrete packets or particles that pass unchanged from one generation to the next, although each trait might not be expressed in each generation. He called these packets *elemente* (elements), and called *dominant* those elements that appeared in the first offspring (F_1)

3.1 The Genetic Bases of Cancer

and *recessive* those that were hidden in the first generation but re-surfaced in the second (F_2). He further concluded, also correctly, that paired traits pass from one generation to the next as separate and independent elements, each inherited from one parent. While genetics, particularly human genetics, is more complex, with each trait, physical and otherwise, generally being influenced by more than

Table 3.1 Mendel's cross-pollination results (Adapted from [143])

Parental trait	F_1	F_2	F_2 trait ratio
Round × wrinkled seeds	All round	5474 round – 1850 wrinkled	2.96:1
Yellow × green seeds	All yellow	6022 yellow – 2001 green	3.01:1
Purple × white petals	All purple	705 purple – 224 white	3.15:1
Inflated × pinched pods	All inflated	882 inflated – 299 pinched	2.95:1
Green × yellow pods	All green	428 green – 152 yellow	2.82:1
Axial × terminal flowers	All axial	651 axial – 207 terminal	3.14:1
Long × short stems	All long	787 long – 277 short	2.84:1

one gene, Mendel's concept of elements, which we now call *alleles*, and his notion that elements are *paired* and inherited as *separate* and *independent* entities from one another in a *dominant* or *recessive* fashion remain largely accurate. Yet, despite being pivotal to understanding genetics, Mendel's momentous work fell into oblivion until 1900 when his article *Experiments with plant hybridization* was simultaneously re-discovered by Hugo De Vries of the University of Amsterdam, Carl Correns of the Kaiser Wilhelm Institute for Biology in Berlin, Erik von Tschermak of the University of Vienna, and British botanist William Bateson. The latter became a fervent advocate of Mendel's, published a book in defense of his work [144] extending his conclusions to animals and demonstrating that, contrary to Mendel's findings, certain traits are inherited together by genes located in close proximity on the same chromosome, a phenomenon now known as *linkage*. Mendel died at the monastery in 1884, where his tombstone reads, "Scientist and biologist in charge of the Augustinian monastery in Old Brno. He discovered the laws of heredity in plants and animals. His knowledge provided a permanent scientific basis for recent progress in genetics."

Genes are the fundamental physical and functional units of heredity that are passed from parent to offspring. They are made of specific sequences of DNA bases located on a particular chromosome that encode (contain information for) the production of specific proteins that serve as cellular signals. The size of genes varies widely, from approximately 10,000–150,000 base pairs. However, only a fraction (10 %) of the three billion base pairs that constitute the genome represents protein-encoding sequences (*exons*) of genes, the rest being intercalated sequences (*introns*) with no known coding function. Additionally, only a small fraction of the approximately 25,000 human genes are *expressed* in any particular cell. For example, hemoglobin genes are expressed in red blood cell precursors, not in muscle or brain cells. Yet, the very presence of all genes in every cell makes each of them a potential source for cloning virtually any cell lineage, under the right conditions. Gene expression begins with the synthesis of an RNA copy (*transcription*) of the DNA gene sequence, in the nucleus, followed by its transport mRNA to cytoplasmic ribosomes, where the encoded genetic information is *translated* into protein synthesis.

However, before moving to the cytoplasm, non-functional *introns* are snipped out and *exons* are spliced (linked) together, thus giving rise to the proper protein-encoding sequences. Once in the cell cytoplasm, the mRNA serves as a template to translate the encoded information (*codons*) into a string of individual amino acids that constitute the building blocks of protein synthesis. Codons are sequences of three DNA bases within exons that direct cells to produce a specific amino acid. For example, the sequence *ATG* codes for the amino acid methionine. There are 64 possible codons encoding 20 amino acids, thus allowing for code redundancy for all but 2 amino acids: methionine (*AUG*) and tryptophan (*UGG*). The other 18 amino acids are encoded by 2–6 codons. For example, *AAA* and *AAG* encode lysine and *UCU*, *UCC*, *UCA*, *UCG*, *AGU*, and *AGC* encode serine. In addition, there is an *initiation codon*, usually *AUG*, that initiates translation of mRNA, and a *termination codon*, usually *UAA*, *UGA* or *UAG*, that ends it. Thus, when the RNA *reads* a gene sequence it is prompted where to start and where to end the transcription process. Hence, from a logistic point of view, the genetic code is a series of codons, contained in genes in turn housed in chromosomes located in the cell nucleus, that specify which amino acids will be synthesized and in what order. The 20 amino acids, assembled in a variety of different combinations and lengths, give rise to approximately 100,000 proteins encoded in the human genome that are necessary to maintain the structural and functional integrity of human beings. Errors in DNA or RNA transcription, and in exon splicing, can result in mutations, which in turn can lead to a faulty *translation* of the gene code, including failure to synthesize the gene-encoded protein or production of an aberrant protein. The outcome of either failure will be a functional disruption of the protein-targeted cell.

3.1.2.3 Chromosomes

Chromosomes are microscopic units that house all genes. Thus, it might be expected that the number of chromosomes would increase with increasing complexity of the organism according to an evolutionary scheme. However, this is not the case. While a humble bacterium might function with a single chromosome and mosquitoes need 6, humans 46, dogs 78, and goldfish 94, the tropical plant *Ophioglossum* (snake tongue) has over 1,200. The 46 human chromosomes are organized in two sets of 23 pairs: 22 pairs of *autosomes*[4] (numbered 1 through 22) plus 1 pair of *allosomes*[5]; XX for female and XY for male. Except for sex chromosomes that determine gender and are thus distinct and different, each set of autosomal chromosomes bears identical copies of the entire human genome, and is inherited as a result of sexual reproduction; one copy from the father, the other from the mother. Indeed, germ cells or gonads (spermatozoid or sperm for short in males, ovum or egg in females) contain only 23 chromosomes: 22 autosomes plus allosome X in a female ovum, and 22 autosomes plus allosome Y or X, in a male sperm. During

---

[4] Non-sex chromosomes.
[5] Sex chromosomes.

reproduction the male sperm delivers its entire genetic load, either 22X or 22Y, into the female egg (22X) so that the fertilized egg will contain two identical and complementary pairs of 22 autosomes plus 1 pair of allosomes, either XX or XY. Women's cells contain 44XX where one X allosome is inherited from each parent, whereas in men's (44XY), the X allosome derives from the mother and the Y allosome comes from the father, who therefore is the parent that determines the gender of the offspring, whether male or female. Genetic alterations or mutations are associated with over 4,000 human diseases, including cancer, and have been mapped to specific chromosomes, as illustrated in Fig. 3.4 [145].

Alterations of any of the 22 *autosomal* chromosomes are associated with *autosomal* diseases, such as sickle cell anemia. Aberrations in *sex* chromosomes (X or Y) lead to sex-linked diseases such as hemophilia A. Genetic alterations involving major structural chromosomal abnormalities, such as multiple copies of a chromosome (as seen in Down syndrome), translocation of part of a chromosome to another (as occurs in Burkitt's lymphoma), or deletions of a chromosome or parts thereof (exemplified by the DiGeorge syndrome), are visually detectable under the microscope. This is because appropriately stained chromosomes acquire light and dark transverse bands (reflecting variations in amounts of A-T or G-C base pairs) that enable cytogeneticists to identify each individual chromosome (Fig. 3.5), and recognize structural abnormalities [147]. This test, called chromosome banding, is used routinely in the clinical setting. More subtle defects can now be detected via more sophisticated approaches, including molecular techniques.

Chromosomal analysis is of great clinical interest because many chromosomal abnormalities are linked to a number of disorders, including mental retardation, infertility, and cancer. Cancer management is impacted by chromosomal analysis because some cancers, especially hematologic malignancies, harbor structural chromosomal abnormalities that have diagnostic or prognostic significance. In fact, a small number of chromosomal abnormalities are virtually diagnostic by themselves. They include t(9;22), the so-called Philadelphia chromosome (Fig. 3.6), the hallmark of chronic myelocytic leukemia (CML) also shared by a small subset of acute lymphocytic leukemia (ALL), and t(15;17), an abnormality that is specific for acute promyelocytic leukemia. Beyond its diagnostic value, the t(9;22) translocation confers a growth advantage to CML cells that led to the development of Imatinib mesylate (Gleevec®), the first successful post-genomic molecularly targeted agent to control rather than kill malignant cells. However, most cancers exhibit either no chromosomal abnormalities detectable by current methodology, as is the case with most solid tumors, or exhibit non-specific but diagnostically and prognostically helpful abnormalities, as is the case with most hematologic malignancies. Examples of these include gene translocations, such as t(14;18) in follicular-type lymphoma, t(8;14) in Burkitt's lymphoma, trisomy 12 (three copies of chromosome 12) in CLL, and del(16)(q22) in a subset of acute myelocytic leukemia (AML). Additionally, many genetic aberrations are sub-microscopic, precluding their visual detection by chromosomal banding. Such cases can be unmasked by more powerful techniques that use DNA probes such as FISH analyses [148], comparative genomic hybridization [149], spectral karyotyping [150], recombinant DNA techniques [151], and

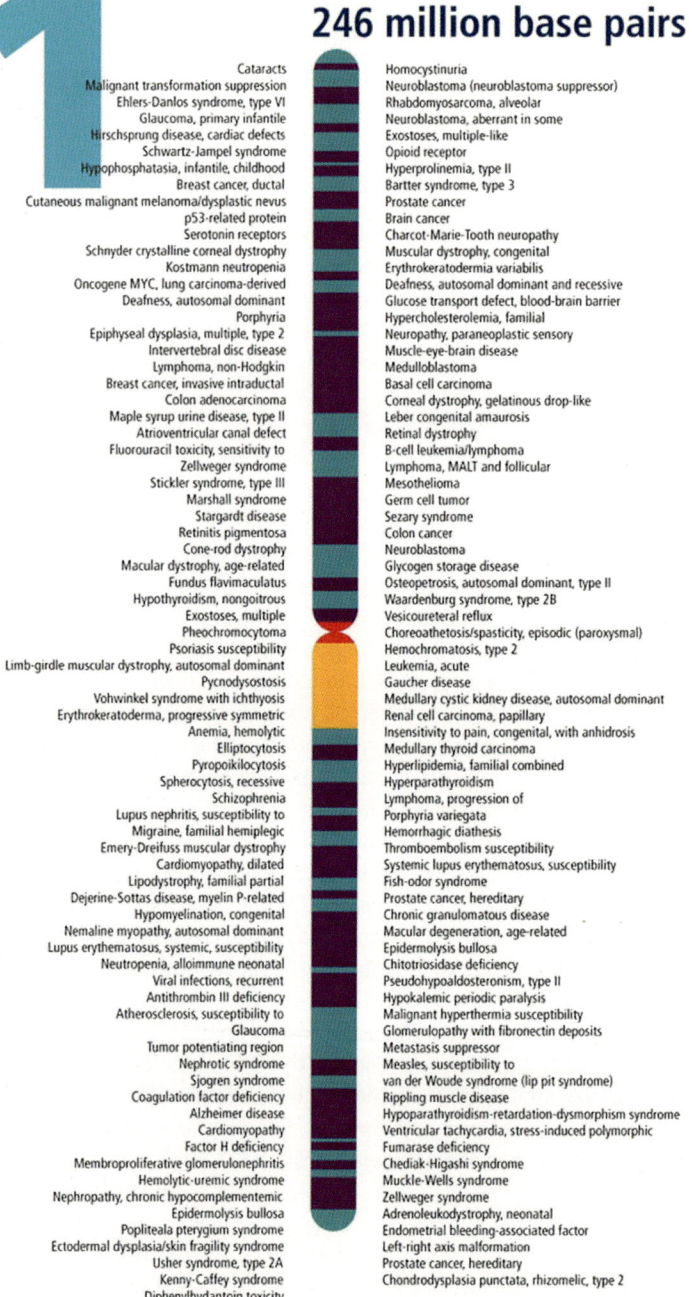

Fig. 3.4 Gene-associated disorders and traits detected on chromosome 1 (Reproduced from DOE Human Genome Project [146])

3.1 The Genetic Bases of Cancer

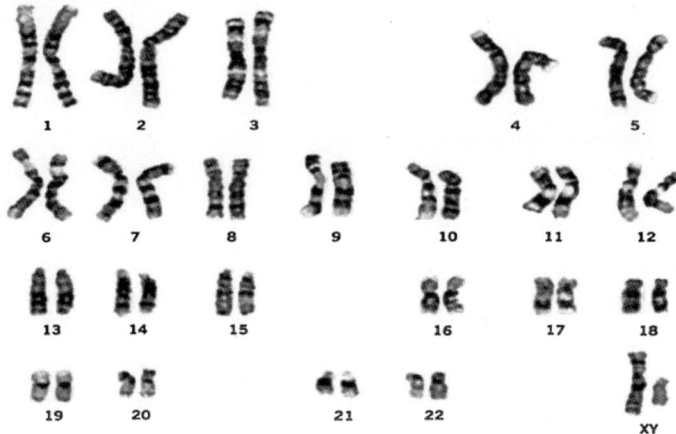

Fig. 3.5 G-banded human male chromosome (Courtesy of Dr. K. Satya-Prakash)

others [152]. One example of sub-microscopic chromosomal abnormalities is point mutations that characterize certain hemoglobinopathies, where single amino acid substitutions occur on one of the four hemoglobin chains. To illustrate, sickle cell disease and hemoglobin C, two hemoglobinopathies with different symptoms, clinical profiles, and prognoses, result when glutamic acid on position 6 of the β chain is replaced by valine or lysine, respectively.

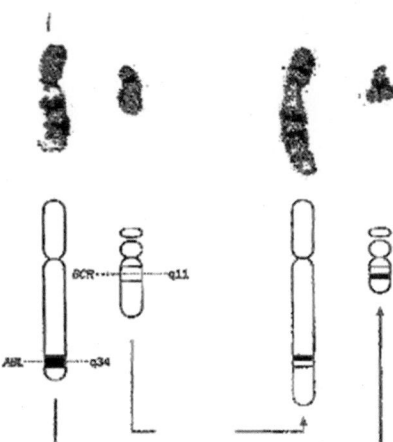

Fig. 3.6 Diagram and G-banding (L) & R-banding (R) of 9:22 translocation in CML (Courtesy of Dr. Avery A. Sandberg)

3.1.2.4 The Cell Cycle

Cells undergo two fundamentally different but complementary processes: cell cycle and cell differentiation. Cell division, which occurs via the cell cycle, ensures self-renewal of undifferentiated precursor cells, also called stem cells. In contrast, cell differentiation is designed to generate highly specialized non-dividing mature cells with distinct and varied functions. Together, these genetically controlled cellular processes sustain the structural and functional integrity of the entire organism and ensure genetic transfer to the next generation. For example, bone marrow stem cells possess the ability to divide, thus ensuring a constant pool of self-renewing precursor cells. However, stem cells also give rise to a diversity of progenitor cells that, while losing self-renewing potential, undergo differentiation into various types of cells capable of carrying out highly specialized functions. These include red cells to ensure oxygen delivery to all tissues, white cells to seek, engulf, and kill invading microorganisms, and platelets to instantly plug any vascular leak as our first line of defense against accidental blood loss. Both cell division and cell differentiation are highly regulated processes necessary to fulfill their respective functions. For instance, many more bone marrow stem cells must enter into differentiation to produce platelets, with a $T1/2$[6] of 7 days, than to produce granulocytes or red blood cells with a $T1/2$ of 36–48 h and 120 days, respectively. Such stem cells are *pre-committed* to differentiating into each cell type in contrast to *pluripotent* stem cells, which are the source of all cell lines in some tissues or organs. Some pre-committed cell lines do not cycle or differentiate until the proper conditions are met. An illustrative case is that of memory T-lymphocytes that remain in G_0 (see below) until they are *awoken* by re-exposure to the original antigen trigger, when they re-enter G_1 in order to replicate in an explosive manner so as to confer swift protection from the antigen's pathogenic effects.

The cell cycle is divided into two major phases visible under the microscope: M-phase (*mitosis* or cell division) and Interphase [153]. The M-phase comprises prophase, prometaphase, metaphase, anaphase, and telophase, whereas the Interphase includes the S-phase (DNA synthesis), G_1, and G_2 stages or gaps between M and S, and between S and M, respectively, where cells remain metabolically active in preparation for the next phase. For rapidly proliferating human somatic[7] cells that typically exhibit a total cycling time of 24 h, the M-phase lasts approximately 1 h, with most of the cell-cycling time being spent in Interphase, and G_1, S, and G_2 phases lasting approximately 11, 8, and 4 h, respectively [154]. Cells out of cycle are said to be quiescent or in G_0 and require external stimuli to move out of G_0 and into G_1 [155]. In animal cells, this step is triggered by growth factors that might include epidermal growth factor (EGF), fibroblastic growth factor (FGF), platelet-derived growth factor (PDGF), and insulin-like growth factor (IGF) or by exposure to antigens each binding to receptive cells' specific surface receptors, but also hormones entering such cells. Once in G_1, cells must pass through a *restriction point* to enter the S-phase, without which they will remain dormant, though metabolically active, until the

---

[6] Half-life.
[7] Body (non-sex) cells.

3.1 The Genetic Bases of Cancer

proper growth factor becomes available. Alternatively, many cells remain in G_0 for extended periods of time until the need arises to replace injured or dead cells as occurs in kidney, liver, and other internal organs. Other cells remain permanently in G_0, as is the case of neurons. The different events that occur in each phase of the cell cycle must be exquisitely coordinated with one another to ensure their completion in a proper sequence to prevent an aberrant cell division from transferring incomplete or defective copies of genetic material to daughter cells. Such coordination is ensured by checkpoints and feedback controls (Fig. 3.7). An important checkpoint occurs in G_2 that, upon detecting unreplicated DNA sequences, blocks cells in G_2 and prevents their progress through the M-phase, allowing both repair of DNA damage to take place and orderly completion of the S-phase. Cell cycle checkpoints are under the control of numerous genes that promote or inhibit the cell cycle depending on whether or not defective DNA-carrying cells must be repaired or eliminated. In broad terms, genes that ensure genomic integrity during the cell cycle are called *tumor suppressor genes* and include *caretakers* that prevent genomic instability and mutations from occurring, and *gatekeepers* that regulate cell cycle progression and maintain genomic stability by inducing apoptosis[8] or senescence[9] on genomically aberrant cells before they become cancer cells [156]. Of these, *RB1* and *TP53* are considered the main cell cycle gatekeepers through the activity of their encoded proteins, *pRB* and *p53*. Their role is exerted through the *E2F1*, a protein that acts as a transcription factor that promotes cell-cycle progression from G1 to S. In normal cells, E2F is inhibited by *pRB*, which in turn can be temporarily inactivated by cyclin-dependent

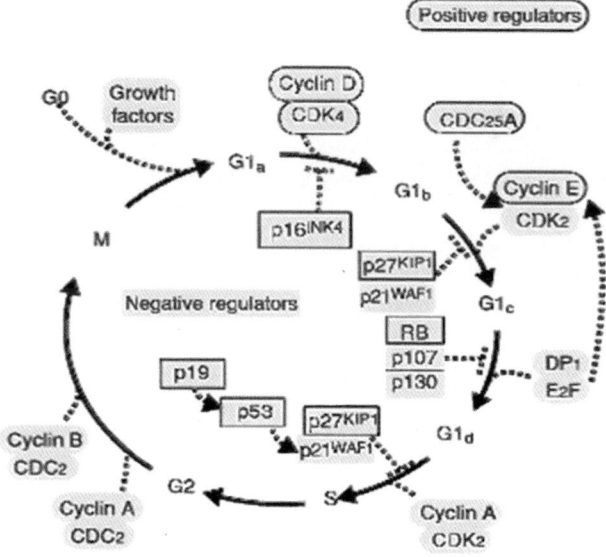

Fig. 3.7 Cell cycle regulation (Courtesy Dr. S. Collins)

---

[8] Programmed cell death.
[9] Irreversible cell cycle arrest.

kinases of the *m2m* gene product. In cancer cells, the gene encoding *TP53* is often mutated, which prevents G_1 arrest in response to DNA damage and allows damaged DNA to both replicate and be delivered to daughter cells. *pRB* is inactivated by several mechanisms, including loss of function, mutations, and by viral oncogenes, enabling *E2F*-driven excessive cancer cell proliferation. Mutated RB1 are a cause of childhood retinoblastoma, bladder cancer, and osteogenic sarcoma. *p53, a* protein encoded by tumor suppressor gene *TP53* (located at 17p13.1), is believed to have a far-reaching role, and is sometimes called the *guardian of the genome*. It includes activation of genes that control the cell cycle (*WAF1* and *CIP1/p21*), DNA damage repair (*GADD45*), G1 to S and G2 to M progression (*14-3-σ*), and apoptosis (*BAX*). Loss of the latter function is generally viewed as a common pathway in carcinogenesis. *TP53* is the most frequently mutated gene in human somatic cancers, and is responsible for the Li-Fraumeni syndrome, a rare inherited condition associated with a high risk for developing sarcomas, brain tumors, breast cancer, and leukemias [157]. Standardized nomenclature is being assigned to human genes in order to bring uniformity in scientific communications and data retrieval. This will prevent past cacophony in this field. For instance, synonyms for the cyclin-dependent kinase inhibitor 2A (CDKN2A) include ARF, CDK4I, CMM2, INK4, INK4a, MTS1, p14, p16, p16INK4a, p19, and p19Arf [158].

3.1.2.5 Programmed Cell Death

Like organisms, cells are born, live, and die. Also like organisms, cells can die of *accidental* or *natural* causes. Accidental cell death is caused by exposure to injurious stimuli, such as excessive heat, acid, radiation, or hypoxia against which cells play an entirely passive role. In contrast, natural cell death is the result of a highly complex but controlled process called *programmed cell death* that includes *apoptosis*, which is genetically induced. Cell survival is also controlled by a stretch of DNA located at the end of each chromosome, called *telomeres*. These two major pathways to cell death control cells' life span through distinct mechanisms. Apoptosis occurs when a cell commits 'suicide' in response to external signals that challenge and ultimately defeat its self-preservation mechanisms. In contrast, telomere-triggered cell death originates from within the cell as a mechanism that inherently limits its life span and by extension controls aging of the entire organism.

Apoptosis

Unless counterbalanced, cell division could result in the accumulation of so many cells that the mass of an organism could nearly double each year. The necessary counterbalance is achieved through natural cell death, mainly apoptosis that maintains cell populations at equilibrium. Cell death also occurs through necrosis, desquamation, and sloughing off of cells lining hollow organs such as the gastrointestinal, respiratory, and genitourinary tracts, and through accidental cell death, which accounts for a marginal fraction of overall cell death. Unlike natural cell death, accidental cell death is a process caused by an acute injury that destroys the cell, spills its content, and triggers an inflammatory response. On the other hand, apoptosis can be viewed as a cell implosion from within, with rapid clearing of cell debris by specialized cells called *macrophages*, without causing inflammation. "The role of apoptosis in normal physiology is as significant as that of its counterpart, mitosis. It demonstrates a complementary but opposite role to mitosis and cell proliferation in the regulation of various cell populations" [159]. Apoptotic cells are recognizable by light microscopy "as round or oval masses with dark eosinophilic cytoplasm and dense purple nuclear chromatin fragments" [160], with subcellular changes being identified by electronic microscopy. The process of apoptosis follows two main apoptotic pathways: the extrinsic or death receptor pathway and the intrinsic or mitochondrial pathway. A third pathway involves T-cell mediated cytotoxicity and perforin-granzyme-dependent cell killing, all converging at the execution pathway [161]. The extrinsic pathway involves transmembrane receptor-binding interactions where cell membrane TNF[10] or the *death* receptor is bound by death receptor ligands FasL/FasR, TNF-α/TNFR1, Apo3L/DR3, Apo2L/DR4, or Apo2L/DR5, initiating transmission from the cell surface to the intracellular *death* domain, of the signal that activates caspase-8, which in turn activates caspase-3 that triggers the final *execution pathway*. In contrast, the intrinsic pathway involves a variety of non-receptor-mediated stimuli that activate intracellular signals that cause mitochondrial events that can be positive or negative: e.g., promote or suppress apoptosis, respectively. Regulation of apoptotic mitochondrial events occurs through members of the 25 BCL-2 gene family encoding at least 14 proteins that promote apoptosis, such as Bcl-10, Bax, Bak, Bid, Bad, Bim, Bik, and Blk, or suppress it, including Bcl-2, Bcl-x, Bcl-XL, Bcl-XS, Bcl-w, BAG [162]. It has been reported that the interaction of some of these proteins bound to each other determines whether the resulting dimer promotes or blocks apoptosis. For example, the Bax/Bax and Bcl-2/Bad dimers promote cell death, whereas Bax/Bcl-2 and Bcl-2/Bcl-2 dimers protect against it. A myriad of triggers can initiate the apoptotic pathway, including chemotherapy drugs, ultraviolet and gamma irradiation, oxidative agents, certain viruses, and various cytokines.[11] In addition, cytotoxic T lymphocytes (CTLs) exert their cytotoxic activity through the extrinsic pathway via FasL/FasR interactions, but also via the secretion of *Perforin* that involves serine proteases granzyme A and granzyme B, with the latter acting directly on caspase-3 or indirectly via caspase-10 [163]. CTLs play a pivotal role in the immune surveillance mechanism said to prevent cancer from emerging by inducing tumor cell apoptosis. Regardless of the pathway taken, once initiated, the apoptotic process culminates in the

---

[10] Tumor Necrosis Factor.
[11] Cell-secreted intercellular mediator proteins.

activation of caspases, a family of cysteine proteases,[12] by cleaving a variety of cytoplasmic, nuclear, and membrane proteins, the final steps of the apoptotic pathway (Table 3.2). Abnormalities in apoptosis are thought to play an important role in a number of diseases, including cancer.

Table 3.2 Apoptotic pathways (Adapted from figure 3, ref. [164])

Extrinsic	Intrinsic	Granzyme	
↓	↓	↓	
Death ligand	Toxins, stress, hypoxia	Cytotoxic T-cells	
~~ ☉ (Death receptor) ~~~ c e l l m e m b r a n e ~~~ ☉ (Perforin) ~~~			
↓	↓	↙	↘
Adaptors	Mitochondrial changes	Granzyme B	Granzyme A
↓	↓	↓	↓
DISC formation	Apoptosome formation		SET complex
↓	↓		↓
Caspase 8 activation	Caspase 9 activation	Caspase 10 act	DNA cleavage
↘	↓	↙	
	Caspase 3 activation Execution pathway		
	↓		
	Cytomorphologic changes		
	↓		
	Apoptotic bodies		

Cancer cells can escape apoptosis through a variety of mechanisms including overexpression of BCL-2, mutated P53, down-regulation or non-functioning Fas receptors on tumor cells, among others. One example is the BCL-2, discovered in 1985 because of its involvement in chromosome translocation t(14;18), that is detected in 90 % of follicular-type non-Hodgkin's lymphomas [165]. This translocation places the BCL-2, normally located on chromosome 18, under the influence of the immunoglobulin heavy chain gene locus situated on chromosome 14, resulting in overproduction of BCL-2 protein and prolonged survival of the malignant cells. The t(14;18) was the first gene found to contribute to tumor growth by reducing cell death rather than by promoting cell division, a major breakthrough that suggests a new strategy for combating cancer. Indeed, it can be envisioned that manipulation of the pro- and anti-apoptotic forces to favor the former might restore the normal apoptotic process lost during tumorigenesis, thus removing the survival advantage of malignant cells.

Telomeres

At the end of each chromosome lies a unique stretch of repeated sequences of TTAGGG on one strand of DNA bound to AATCCC on the other strand of approximately 10,000–12,000 base pairs in length associated with a protein complex named shelterin that protects chromosome ends, called telomeres [166]. These sequences do not contain genetic codes, but are critical to the aging of normal cells and to the apparent inexhaustible ability of cancer cells to replicate [167]. Telomeres are

---

[12] Enzymes that break up proteins.

sometimes referred to as the cell *clock* or *counting mechanism* because they limit the number of divisions a normal cell can undertake. When a normal cell divides, the ends of chromosomes cannot be replicated and 50–200 telomere base pairs are lost with each division, progressively reducing the length of telomeres. Eventually, once somatic cells lose their entire telomere sequences, after multiple replication rounds, they can no longer divide and enter the phase of replicative senescence and apoptotic cell death. This is because telomerase, an enzyme that restores and maintains telomere length in undifferentiated cells, such as stem, germ line, hematopoietic, and other rapidly dividing cells, is absent or nearly absent in normal somatic cells. Yet, telomerase levels also decrease in aging normal stem cells, resulting in progressive shortening of telomeres, contrary to the persistently high levels of telomerase reported in most human malignancies [168]. While increased telomerase activity in malignant cells sustains their replicative capacity, a property that could be exploited therapeutically, it is not involved in the development, growth, or dissemination of cancer, except in rare cells that remain telomerase expression capable [169].

Telomeres and telomerase appear to play a role in human aging [170] that might be influenced by lifestyle factors [171]. The possible link between telomere length and survival is supported by *knockout mice*[13] data and by a rare human disease. Knockout mice give rise to offspring whose life span is dependent on the length of their telomeres. Likewise, dyskeratosis congenita, a fatal X-linked human disease associated with decreased RNA telomerase, decreased telomerase activity, and shorter telomeres, exhibits age-dependent chromosomal abnormalities and an increased tendency to develop malignancies. Finally, while increased telomerase activity is detected in 94 % of neuroblastomas, a mainly childhood cancer, low or undetectable telomerase levels are found in a disease subset called neuroblastoma 4S. Children afflicted by neuroblastoma 4S exhibit an astonishingly high rate of spontaneous remission, reaching 100 % in one study, a behavior not seen with any other cancer [172, 173]. Spontaneous remission in these patients is associated with a lack of telomerase expression [174]. Together, these compelling observations have led a number of research laboratories and biotechnology companies actively to study telomerase as a potential diagnostic and therapeutic target. Indeed, it is tempting to contemplate the possibility that manipulation of a single molecule, whether telomeres or telomerase, might one day prolong the lifespan of normal cells, slow the aging process, and control cancer progression by eliminating the survival advantage of malignant cells. Nevertheless, to date, most studies are based on pooled cancer cells that yield average results, which must be interpreted with caution in light of the increasingly appealing *cancer stem cell model* of tumors where a small subset of stem cells is understood to,

> constitute a reservoir of self-sustaining cells with the exclusive ability to self-renew and maintain the tumor. These cancer stem cells have the capacity to both divide and expand the cancer stem cell pool and to differentiate into the heterogeneous non tumorigenic cancer cell types that in most cases appear to constitute the bulk of the cancer cells within the tumor [175].

---

[13] Genetically telomerase-deficient mice.

In conformity with this view, gene expression profiling of single circulating tumor cells (CTC) in breast cancer patients confirmed the heterogeneity of such non-tumorigenic, non-dividing cancer cells, and demonstrated that these cells belong to subpopulations fundamentally different from pooled cells obtained from the primary tumor [176].

3.2 How Does Cancer Arise?

3.2.1 First the Basics

Cancer still is referred to as an *uncontrolled cell proliferation*. While satisfactory through the 1970s, such a definition of cancer is obsolete today in view of the prodigious advances made in the last 20 years regarding its genetic bases. It is now understood that exposure to noxious agents such as radiation, chemical, or viral mutagens throughout life can lead to alterations in DNA sequences. Cancer develops when two or more sequential DNA *hits* induce gene mutations that promote growth or confer a survival advantage to the affected cell and its descendants. Alfred Knudson proposed the two-hit hypothesis, many years before the human genome was sequenced and the *RB1*[14] was discovered, from statistical analyses of clinical and familial characteristics of 23 cases of bilateral and 25 cases of unilateral retinoblastomas [177].[15] In this regard, we published what appears to be the first prospective demonstration of the two-hit sequence of events leading to cancer by detecting the emergence of a monoclone arising in the context of a chronic Sjögren's pseudo-lymphoma that subsequently progressed to a full-blown lymphoma [178]. Gene mutations affecting a somatic cell can lead to a malignant *clone*, whereas a cancer predisposition will be the outcome in offspring of mutated germ-line cells. To date, 342 cancer genes have been linked to somatic mutations and 70 to germ line mutations. Initial mutations, called initiation events, trigger the malignant sequence but additional critical mutations are thought necessary for a cancer to become locally or distally invasive. The latter are referred to as progression events. Multiple mutational hits lead to decreased tumor suppressor gene function and/or increased oncogene function. Such multiple sequential mutagenic events give rise to cytogenetically different malignant clones that can affect response to therapy. For instance, in CML the *bcr/abl* fusion gene, discovered in 1960 [179], encodes a fusion protein with enhanced tyrosine kinase activity that confers a growth advantage to CML cells. Blocking this enzyme with imatinib mesylate (Gleevec®), a highly specific *bcr/abl* tyrosine kinase inhibitor, induces a clinical remission that lasts until a newly mutated malignant sub-clone becomes resistant. There are three major groups of normal cellular genes associated with cancer when mutated [180]: *Proto-oncogenes* (100 are currently known) and

---

[14] A tumor suppressor gene linked to retinoblastoma.
[15] A childhood form of retinal cancer.

tumor suppressor genes (over 30 are known) that regulate cell growth, and over 300 known *microRNA genes* (miRNA) that regulate gene expression.

Proto-oncogenes encode proteins that regulate the division, differentiation, and programmed cell death in normal cells. When mutated, proto-oncogenes become oncogenes that over-stimulate cell division and inhibit both cell differentiation and cell death, which are the biological hallmarks of cancer cells. Proto-oncogene mutations can occur via several mechanisms: amplification (multiple copies of the gene), as in the case of *Erb-B2* associated with breast cancer; point mutations (involving single or very few base pairs), as in the case of *RET* implicated in multiple endocrine and thyroid cancers; and gene translocation from one chromosome to another. The latter can generate a fusion (or *chimeric*) gene, as is the case with *bcr/abl* in CML, or place the gene under the hyperactive control of the immunoglobulin heavy-chain locus or the T-cell receptor genes, resulting in lymphomas or leukemias, respectively. *DNA viral oncogenes* differ from cellular oncogenes in that they derive not from *cellular proto-oncogenes* but from *DNA viruses* that transcribe into infected cells the genome signals that hijack the host DNA, triggering one or more biological hallmarks of cancer. While the Rous sarcoma virus in chickens was the first cancer-inducing virus, the best-known example of a human DNA virus-induced cancer is cervical cancer, which is caused by several HPV strains.

In contrast to the hyperactive growth-promoting effect of oncogenes, mutated tumor suppressor genes are deleted or lose their inhibitory function, thus depriving cells of the crucial brakes that normally prevent excessive cell growth. A subset of tumor suppressor genes, called DNA repair genes, were discovered studying hereditary non-polyposis colorectal cancer. Although not directly involved in the carcinogenic process, inactivation of these genes can lead to a defective DNA repair process and to genomic instability. They often are referred to as genomic caretakers in contrast to cellular caretakers that inhibit cell-cycle progression in response to DNA damage. In conclusion, mutated proto-oncogenes, tumor suppressor genes, and miRNA genes are involved in the carcinogenic process by promoting excessive cell growth, by failing to regulate cell growth, or by enabling replication of unstable genomes, respectively. Thus, regardless of the type of cancer initiation and progression events, malignant cells differ from their normal counterparts by their aberrant regulation by mutated genes, not the lack thereof. The degree of deregulation determines the biology of malignant cells, which in turn dictates the clinical course of the disease, as exemplified by the two genetic variants of CLL [181]. miRNA genes, like proto-oncogenes and tumor suppressor genes, play an important role in the life of the cell and their dysregulated expression, through amplification, deletion, or mutation, leads to the initiation and progression of most malignancies [182].

Mutations that underlie cancer development affect somatic or gonadal cells. The former, the most frequent, trigger a malignant clone and are neither inherited nor inheritable. However, a small fraction of mutations involve germ line cells and can be inherited, thus affecting all cells of an offspring. These mutant genes predispose the host to cancer and are transmitted from generation to generation by the affected gonads. Well-known examples of inherited mutant genes include *RB1*, associated with retinoblastoma of childhood, and *BRCA1*, associated with familial breast cancer in young females. As mentioned earlier, cancer results from a multi-step process that, over time, alters one or more genes. Thus, the chances that a single cell (out of 10^{14} that make up a human being) would undergo several successive mutations is negligible, were it not for the fact that some mutations affect the stability of the genome, increasing its susceptibility to additional damage. In the case of somatic mutations, genetic damage occurs over many years, which accounts for the advanced age of the vast majority of cancer patients. In contrast, in individuals born with a cancer-predisposing gene, all cells are already mutated, thus vastly expanding the cell pool susceptible to additional mutational hits, increasing the cancer risk and the likelihood that the disease will appear in childhood or early adulthood, as exemplified by *RB1* and *BRCA1* inheritance, respectively.

Oncogenes, tumor suppressor genes, and miRNA gene regulators are described in greater detail in the following pages. Readers not particularly interested in such details can bypass this segment and proceed to the section *How does cancer spread?*, starting on page 62.

3.2.2 More Details

The hallmarks of cancer include self-sufficiency in growth signals, insensitivity to antigrowth signals, evasion of apoptosis, limitless replicative potential, sustained angiogenesis, and tissue invasion and metastasis [183]. Additionally, cancer cells exhibit an increased inherent capacity to access nutrients, as demonstrated by the *Warburg effect* [184],[16] and by a selective metabolic regulation that is part of the tumorigenic process. In fact,

> Cancer cells display dramatically altered metabolic circuitry that appears to directly result from the oncogenic mutations selected during the tumorigenic process. An emerging theme in cancer biology is that many of the genes that can initiate tumorigenesis are intricately linked to metabolic regulation [185].

However, the primary cause of autonomous cancer growth is genetic dysregulation and includes oncogenes, tumor-suppressor genes, and microRNA genes [186]. They are responsible for the cancer-inducing and cancer-sustaining processes that result from concomitant or sequential genetic alterations. While their discovery launched a determined search for distinct genetic mutations responsible for specific cancers, we now know that this is not generally the case. Indeed, the same genetic defects can be found in different types of cancer. And it has recently been hypothesized that,

> ...genetically diverse cancers converge at a common and obligatory growth axis instigated by HIF-2α, an element of the oxygen-sensing machinery...that promotes autocrine growth signaling and cell cycle progression via EGF receptor (EGFR) and c-Myc-dependent mechanisms [187].

Several relevant publications of interest include [188–191]:

---

[16] Reliance on glycolysis rather than mitochondrial oxidative phosphorylation for glucose-dependent ATP production.

3.2.2.1 Oncogenes

Oncogenes were discovered through the study of retroviruses, which are RNA tumor viruses. The oncogene-containing genome of retroviruses is inserted into the DNA of infected cells, a process called *insertional mutagenesis*. This causes malignant transformation of the infected cell(s) and production of viral progeny that, by infecting adjoining cells, expands and perpetuates the process. Studies of Rous sarcoma virus (RSV) mutants revealed that the transforming gene (*v-src*) of this retrovirus was not necessary for viral replication, and that it had a counterpart gene (*c-src*) in normal cells. This surprising discovery, confirmed in all retroviruses studied to date, demonstrated that retroviral oncogenes (*v-onc*) are altered versions of normal cellular proto-oncogenes. In rare cases, weak oncogenic retroviruses initiate a mutagenic event that activates cellular proto-oncogenes. Many proto-oncogenes, also called *accelerator* genes, encode growth-promoting proteins that relay growth signals from outside the cell through a cascade pathway that begins at the level of cell membrane receptors and ends in the cell nucleus. The sequence is as follows: growth-promoting proteins attach to the extra-cellular portion of specific receptors on target cells. Attachment triggers a stimulatory signal down the intra-cellular portion of the receptor, reaching the cell nucleus through a series of complex pathways referred to as the *signal transduction cascade*. In the nucleus, another set of proteins called *transcription factors* steers the cell through its replication cycle (cell cycle). Each growth-promoting step is associated with proto-oncogenes, resulting in five classes of such genes: growth factors or external signals, growth factor receptors, signal transducers, transcription factors, and regulators of the cell cycle. Given the complexity and heterogeneity of cancer, it was predicted that each class of proto-oncogenes would have a corresponding oncogene. Indeed, such is the case. An example of growth factor oncogene is seen in dermatofibrosarcoma protuberans, a form of human skin cancer, where a fusion gene gives rise to excessive amounts of platelet-dependent growth factor-beta (*PDGF-β*), a growth signal that auto-stimulates the PDGF-receptor bearing cancer cells that produce it. Other growth factors include nerve growth factor (*NGF*), epidermal growth factor (*EGF*), and fibroblast growth factor (*FGF*). Likewise, oncogenic receptor genes have been identified. These mutated genes encode production of abnormal receptors, such as erb-B2 in breast cancer, that spontaneously fire proliferative signals down the intra-cellular cascade without the stimulus of extracellular growth factors. Signal transducer oncogenes include the prominent *ras* family, which is active in approximately 25 % of colon, lung, and pancreas cancers. While the normal *ras* proto-oncogene mediates normal growth receptor signals downstream, the mutated *ras* oncogene fires continuously and independently of any receptor gene signal, pushing cancer growth forward. Transcriptional oncogenes, such as the *myc* family, are amplified in 20–30 % of all cancers, including squamous cell carcinomas, neuroblastoma, and lung cancer, but are crucial to the development of all Burkitt's lymphoma. This aggressive lymphoma is characterized by translocation of the *c-myc* normally located at 8q24 (band 24 of the long arm of chromosome 8), to translocation partner chromosomes 14q, 22q, and 2p where it is activated by enhancer elements of the immunoglobulin heavy-chain loci, leading to enhanced proliferation of malignant cells [192]. In addition to chromosomal translocations and inversions, oncogenes can be activated by mutations, as exemplified by the RAS oncogene family (*KRAS, NRAS,* and *HRAS*). KRAS and NRAS mutations, often associated with environmental carcinogens, are common in lung, colon, and pancreas cancers, chronic myelogenous leukemia, and myelodysplastic syndrome [193]. Oncogene activation is also linked to gene amplification, as found in oncogene families MYC, cyclin D1 (or *CCND1*), EGFR, and RAS that are found in esophageal, breast, glioblastomas, and head and neck cancer, respectively, to name only a few (Table 3.3).

Table 3.3 Oncogenes. Partial list, modified from Ref. [194]

Gene (synonym)	Somatic mutation type	Cancer type
ABL1 (ABL)	Translocation	Chronic myelogenous leukemia
BAX	Inactivating codon (ICC)	Colon, stomach
BCL2/6	Translocation	Lymphomas
BRAF	Activating codon (ACC)	Melanoma, colorectal, thyroid
CCND1 (cyclin D1)	Amplification, translocation	Leukemias, breast
CTNNB1 (β-catenin)	ACC	Colon, liver, medulloblastomas
EGFR	Amplification, ACC	Glioblastomas, lung
EPHB2	ICC	Prostate
ERBB2	Amplification	Breast, ovarian
EWSR1	Translocation	Ewing's sarcomas, lymphomas, leukemias
FGFR1–3	Translocation	Lymphomas, gastric, bladder
FOXO1A, 3A	Translocation	Rhabdomyosarcomas, leukemias
GLI	Amplification, translocation	Brain, sarcomas
HOXA9/11/13 & others	Translocation	Leukemias
HPVE6/7	HPV infection	Cervical
KRAS2, N-RAS	ACC	Colorectal, pancreatic, lung
MAP2K4 (MKK4)	ICC	Pancreas, breast, colon
MDM2	Amplification	Sarcomas
MYC, MYCN, MYCL1	Amplification	Lymphomas, neuroblastomas, lung
PTNP1, 11	ACC	Leukemias, colon
RARA	Translocation	Promyelocytic leukemia
SMAD2	ICC	Colon, breast
TFE3	Translocation	Kidney, sarcomas
TGFBR1, TGFBR2	ICC	Colon, stomach, ovarian
TNFRSF6 (FAS)	ACC	Lymphomas, testicular germ cell

3.2.2.2 Tumor Suppressor Genes

An entirely different class of genes, known as tumor suppressor or "brake" genes, are involved in carcinogenesis. They normally prevent unrestrained cellular growth, promote DNA repair, and cell-cycle checkpoint activation, ultimately ensuring that normal cells possess effective breaks to balance the effect of growth promoting signals. Like oncogenes, tumor suppressor genes contribute to cancer development through structural or functional alterations that range from point mutations, insertions, duplications, inversions, and translocations to deletions of the entire chromosome where they reside. However, unlike oncogenes that are activated versions of proto-oncogenes that promote cell growth and division, mutated suppressor genes are inactivated or deleted versions of their normal counterparts that lead to a "loss of function" when both alleles (inherited one per parent) are involved. Loss of function promotes development of malignant and non-malignant diseases through several mechanisms, but mainly via releasing cells from normal proliferative breaks, or by reinforcing the over-stimulatory effect of oncogenes (Table 3.4). Retinoblastoma and breast cancer best illustrate these most clinically relevant genes. Retinoblastoma is a rare but aggressive childhood cancer of the retina caused by inactivated *RB1*, which is located at 13q14 (region 14 of long arm of chromosome 13). Approximately 60 % of retinoblastomas are sporadic,

Table 3.4 Tumor-suppressor genes (partial list)

Gene (synonym)	Syndrome	Cancer type
APC	Familial polyposis of colon	Colon, Thyroid, Gastrointestinal
AXIN2	Attenuated polyposis	Colon
BMPR1A	Juvenile polyposis	Gastrointestinal
BRCA1, BRCA2	Hereditary breast cancer	Familial Breast/Ovarian
BHD	Birt-Hogg-Dube	Renal
CDH1 (E-cadherin)	Familial gastric carcinoma	Stomach
CDK4	Familial malignant melanoma	Melanoma
CDKN2A($p16^{INK4A}$, $p14^{ARF}$)	Familial malignant melanoma	Melanoma, Pancreas
CYLD	Familial cylindromatosis	Pilotricomas
EXT1,2	Hereditary multiple exostoses	Osteosarcoma
FH	Hereditary leiomyomatosis	Leiomyomas
GPC3	Simpson-Golabi-Behmel	Embryonal
HRPT2	Hyperparathyroidism Jaw-tumor	Parathyroid, Jaw fibromas
MEN1	Multiple endocrine neoplasia	Parathyroid, Pituitary, Islet cell
NF2	Neurofibromatosis type 2	Meningioma, Acoustic neuroma
PTEN	Cowden	Hamartoma, Glioma, Endometrial
PTCH	Gorlin	Basal cell, Medulloblastoma
RB1	Hereditary retinoblastoma	Retinoblastoma & Others
SDHB, C, D	Familial paraganglioma	Paragangliomas
SMAD4 (DPC4)	Juvenile polyposis	Gastrointestinal
SUFU	Medulloblastoma predisposition	Skin, Medulloblastoma
STK11 (LKB1)	Peutz-Jeghers	Intestinal, Ovarian, Pancreatic
TP53 (p53)	Li-Fraumeni	Breast, Sarcoma, Adrenal, Brain
TSC1, TSC2	Tuberous sclerosis	Hamartoma, Renal
VHL	Von Hippel–Lindau	Renal
WT1	Familial Wilms tumor	Wilms'

occuring in individuals with no family history of the disease, and are always unilateral. The other 40 % are inherited and are frequently bilateral. In sporadic cases, both *RB1* alleles are functional in normal cells but inactive in tumor cells. In contrast, only one *RB1* allele is functional in normal cells of inherited cases, the so-called "loss of heterozygosity". Thus, while in sporadic cases, two consecutive mutations are required to inactivate the two normal *RB1* alleles, individuals who inherit only one functional *RB1* allele (*RB1-heterozygous*) will become homozygous for the mutant gene after a single mutation post-birth affecting the normal allele, greatly increasing the risk of developing retinoblastoma, and will do so at an earlier age. In fact, 80 % of inherited retinoblastomas are diagnosed before age 3. Likewise, breast cancer is usually a sporadic malignancy. However, approximately 20 % of cases occur at an earlier age, in families that inherit germline mutations of *BRCA1* and, less frequently, *BRCA2*. Inherited mutations of *BRCA1*, located at 17q21 (region 21 of long arm of chromosome 17) and *BRCA2*, located at 13q12-13 (bands 12–13 of long arm of chromosome 13) are associated with an increased risk of breast cancer and an earlier onset of the disease. *BRCA1* exhibits an approximately 85 % life-long risk of female breast cancer. *BRCA2* is associated with a 40 % and 10 % risk of female breast and ovarian cancer, respectively, and accounts for approximately 5 % of male breast cancer cases. Finally, recent evidence suggests that a third mutated tumor-suppressor, breast cancer-associated gene (*BRCA3*), also located on chromosome 13, might account for familial cases lacking *BRCA1* and *BRCA2*. In fact, a population-based analysis of breast cancer cases of high-risk families with information on BRCA1 and BRCA2 mutation status suggests that, "low penetrance genes with multiplicative effects on risk may account for the residual non-BRCA1/2 familial aggregation of breast cancer" [195].

A distinct subclass of tumor suppressor genes is normally engaged in DNA damage recognition and repair. In contrast to dominant tumor suppressor genes (such as *RB1* and *TP53*) that actively promote cancer development, mutated DNA repair genes exert a more passive role in carcinogenesis: they fail to detect and repair DNA damage ocurring during the cell cycle. Normally, most errors in DNA sequence prevent cell replication or are lethal to the cell. However, a few unrepaired DNA errors will enter the cell cycle, thus increasing the likelihood that random cancer-promoting mutations in affected daughter cells will lead to cancer. Examples of inherited cancer predisposition resulting from a defective DNA damage recognition and repair system include Ataxia-Telangiectasia, Bloom syndrome, Xeroderma pigmentosa, Fanconi's anemia, and hereditary nonpolyposis colorectal cancer. However, in these cases only homozygotes (individuals who inherit a mutated allele from each parent) appear to have a clear cancer predisposition, in contrast to the more dominant tumor suppressor genes *RB1* and *TP53* that increase cancer risk in heterozygous individuals (with only one mutated allele).

3.2.2.3 MicroRNA Gene Regulators

Discovered in 1993, miRNAs were not recognized as biological regulators until 2000 [196]. Today, approximately 1,100 miRNAs have been identified and their physiological and pathological relevance recognized. MiRNAs are non-protein-coding RNA

3.2 How Does Cancer Arise?

Table 3.5 miRNAs and associated diseases (partial list)

MiRNA name	Syndrome	Cancer type
Hsa-let-7a-1	Cardiomyopathy	Ovarian, Melanoma, Breast
Hsa-let-7b	Myopathy	AML[a], Lung, Melanoma
Hsa-let-7c	Muscular dystrophy	Lung, Breast, Liver
Hsa-let-7d	Susceptibility to stroke	Prostate, Liver, Breast
Hsa-let-7e	Systemic lupus erythematous	Ovarian, Breast, Pancreas
Hsa-let-7f-1	Susceptibility to Alzheimer's disease	Prostate, Ovarian, Breast
Hsa-let-7g	Parkinson's disease	Colorectal, Breast, Lung
Hsa-let-7i	Muscular dystrophy	Melanoma, Prostate, Breast
Hsa-mir-1-1	Supraventricular aortic stenosis	Cervical, Melanoma, Lung
Mmu-mir-16-1	Asthma	Susceptibility to CLL[b]
Hsa-mir-93	Susceptibility to stroke	Gastric, Esophageal, AML[a]
Hsa-mir-98	Cardiomyopathy	Lung, Head & Neck, Prostate
Hsa-mir-99a	Risk of Down syndrome	Breast, Ovarian, Prostate
Hsa-mir-100	Miyoshi myopathy	Leukemia, Ovarian, Breast
Hsa-mir-105-1	Idiopathic myelofibrosis	Myeloma, Lung, Pancreatic
Hsa-mir-106a	Susceptibility to psoriasis	Gastric, Ovarian, Lymphoma
Hsa-mir-125b-2	Down syndrome	Glioblastoma, Breast, Lung
Hsa-mir-128-1	Parkinson's disease	Lung, Prostate, Glioblastoma
Hsa-mir-130a	Idiopathic myelofibrosis	Breast, Colon, Lung
Mmu-mir-192	Susceptibility to diabetic nephropathy	Esophageal, AML[a]

[a]Acute Myelogenous Leukemia
[b]Chronic Lymphocytic leukemia

sequences that control the expression of most human genes at the post-transcriptional level by degrading or repressing target mRNAs [197]. They regulate diverse biological processes, including normal cell development, differentiation, cycle, and apoptosis [198]. However, altered miRNA expression via deletions, amplifications, mutations, epigenetic silencing, or deregulation of transcription factors that target specific miRNAs have been implicated in numerous disease processes and can act as potent oncogenes or tumor suppressor genes becoming involved in the initiation and progression of most human malignancies (Table 3.5) [199, 200]. They are referred to as *oncomirs*, the first of which was miRNA-21.

MiRNAs can be discovered and profiled by high-throughput sequencing methods [201], which have proven helpful in cancer prognostication. Examples include discerning early- from late-stage colorectal cancer, and distinguishing progressive from indolent CLL [202]. Likewise, in breast cancer, miRNA-21 overexpression was found correlated with advanced tumor stage, lymph node metastasis, and poor survival [203]. Hence, although the discovery of miRNA-mediated gene regulation adds another layer of complexity to cancer genetics, their taxonomy and profiling are expected to play a substantial role in the diagnosis, prognosis, and treatment of cancer.

3.2.2.4 The Epigenetics of Cancer

Simply put, epigenetics consists of heritable changes in gene expression unrelated to mutated DNA sequences [204]. Epigenetics is involved in many cellular functions by turning genes on or off. For instance, every cell of an organism contains the full complex of 46 chromosomes with exactly the same DNA. Yet, some cells become liver, pancreatic, lung, or many other types of cells with very specific and different biological functions. This is possible because different sets of genes are turned on, or expressed, and others are turned off, or inhibited. For instance, one of the two female X-chromosomes must be functionally silenced in order to preclude twice the number of X-chromosome gene-products found in males. While necessary for normal development, epigenetics is also associated with disease, including cancer, when silencing becomes dysregulated. Briefly, genes can be inhibited or silenced via three mechanisms: DNA methylation, histone modifications, and RNA-associated silencing [205]. DNA methylation, which always occurs at the Cytosine-phosphate-Guanine region (CpG), modifies gene interactions necessary for transcription. In mammals, most CpGs are normally methylated, except for non-methylated stretches of DNA, called CpG islands. However, loss of DNA methylation or excessive methylation, especially of CpG islands, permanently silences genes and is intimately involved in cancer development via overly active genes or countering the protective effect of tumor suppressor genes [206]. Methylation and acetylation are the main means that account for histone modifications, which affect the arrangement of chromatin and in turn impact DNA transcription. In addition to its role in the onset of cancer, epigenetics also plays a role in cancer progression and might be as important as genetic mutations in driving cancer development and growth. Indeed, certain hyper-methylated but not mutated genes, referred to as epigenetic *gatekeepers*, prevent infinite stem cell renewal. Aberrant silencing of these genes allows clonal expansion and cancer progression [207]. Hence, although epigenetics adds an additional layer of complexity to cancer genetics, it also provides an opportunity to explore new approaches to the diagnosis, prognosis, and especially treatment of cancer. Currently, two main therapeutic approaches are being investigated. One inhibits DNA methylation by blocking DNA methyltranferases while the other inhibits histone deacetylases, both of which lead to accumulation of acethylated histones and anti-cancer activity [208]. Other epigenetic drugs capable of regulating tumor cell biology are being developed and tested in vitro and in vivo [209].

3.3 How Does Cancer Spread?

3.3.1 First the Basics

In multicellular organisms, normal cells respond to multiple signals that enable them to discharge their functions within the anatomical confines of the organ or tissue they constitute. For example, normal liver cells remain within the liver to exert liver-specific exocrine and metabolic functions and never stray outside their anatomical or functional bounds. Even blood cells that circulate throughout the body to deliver oxygen, to seek and kill invading bacteria, and to plug vascular leaks do not disrupt the function of the tissues they serve. On the other hand, benign tumors are generally slow growing within a fibrous capsule and expand concentrically without invading surrounding tissues or distant sites. Except when located within vital organs such as brain and heart, benign tumors normally constitute no threat to the host, despite occasionally reaching enormous sizes, as occurs to careless individuals or those who have limited or no access to health services. In most cases, benign tumors can be excised without recurrences. Hence, in the US, deaths from benign tumors are less than 1 % of deaths caused by malignant tumors. Benign tumors often affect the skin (papillomas or moles), glandular tissue (adenomas), fatty tissue (lipomas), muscles (myomas), bones (osteomas), and blood vessels (angiomas). In contrast, malignant cancer cells possess the inherent ability to multiply rapidly and to trespass into the spaces of adjacent and distant tissues. The ability of cancer to aberrantly invade contiguous tissues and to spread (*metastasize*) to distant sites is the hallmark of malignancy that ultimately determines the outcome of the host. Indeed, patients' outcomes are ultimately dependent upon the invasiveness and metastatic potential of their cancer. For instance, early stage malignancies not accompanied by distant metastases are frequently curable by surgical excision. On the other hand, a single metastasis regardless of size is an indication of widespread disease no longer amenable to cure, particularly given their frequently inaccessible anatomic location in lungs, liver, bones, or brain (Table 3.6), and the limited efficacy of chemotherapy and radiation therapy.

Table 3.6 Three most frequent metastatic sites, by tumor primary [210]

Primary cancer	Main sites of metastasis
Breast	Lungs, liver, bones
Colon	Liver, peritoneum, lungs
Kidney	Lungs, liver, bones
Lungs	Adrenal gland, liver, lungs
Melanoma	Lungs, skin/muscle, liver
Ovary	Peritoneum, liver, lungs
Pancreas	Liver, lungs, peritoneum
Prostate	Bones, lungs, liver
Rectum	Liver, lungs, adrenal gland
Stomach	Liver, peritoneum, lungs
Thyroid	Lungs, liver, bones
Uterus	Liver, lungs, peritoneum

Ominously, statistics indicate that approximately 30 % of cancer patients have disseminated disease or detectable metastases at the time of diagnosis, and another 20–30 % have occult metastases or will develop them subsequently, as revealed by their subsequent clinical course. Hence, assessment of the extent (*stage*) of disease, especially the search for metastases, is crucial to patient management, as it provides the basis for treatment decisions and for assessing prognosis. For example, breast cancer surgery includes assessment of the status of axillary lymph nodes draining the affected breast: negative lymph nodes suggest a cancer restricted to the breast and a favorable prognosis. Alternatively, cancer-positive nodes indicate that cancer cells have migrated outside the breast and have likely metastasized to more distant sites, auguring a poor prognosis. Indeed, the presence of metastases plays a pivotal role on patient survival regardless of the origin and type of cancer. For example, approximately 90 % of patients with colon cancer restricted to the gut wall live 5 years after diagnosis, whereas only 65 % will live 5 years after cancer cells have invaded regional lymph nodes [211]. Likewise, 90 % of women with localized breast cancer survive 10 years, but only 15 % do so if distant metastases are present [212]. These statistics and their relevance to host survival underline early-stage detection as one of the best paths to cancer cures, as will be expanded upon in Chap. 13.

The following section describes further details on the mechanisms underlying local and distal spread of cancer. Readers not particularly interested in such details can bypass this segment and proceed directly to environmental carcinogens, starting on page 69.

3.3.2 More Details: The Invasion-Metastasis Cascade

Although the capacity of tumors to invade contiguous tissues and to metastasize distally is key to the host survival, the genetics and pathogenesis of the underlying multistep processes remain somewhat enigmatic and controversial. The multistep process, which Paget hypothesized depended on tumor-host interactions he called *seed and soil* over a century ago [213], is now known as the "cancer invasion-metastasis cascade". Anatomically, there is general agreement that the cascade involves successive steps including detachment of cancer cells from the primary tumor, invasion of (intravasation), traffic through, and eventual extravasation from lymphatic or blood vessels, implantation in the microenvironment of distant organs or tissues to form micrometastatic lesions, and growth of micrometastases (colonization) into detectable secondary tumors [214]. The process is best described as follows,

> Tumor cells must invade through a stromal tissue border and this activity is usually marked by changes in adhesion between tumor cells and proteolysis of the extracellular matrix. Intravasation involves disruption of the vascular endothelium that may also involve molecular components similar to those that drive invasion. Once in the blood, tumor cells must survive the harsh environment of the circulation. They must escape physical damage due to sheer forces, immune surveillance, and apoptosis induced by lack of a substratum or

anoikis.[17] Malignant cells are passively delivered via the circulation to distant capillary beds where they either adhere to vessel walls or arrest due to physical size constraints. The process of extravasation involves the attachment of tumor cells to blood vessel endothelial cells, followed by their invasion through the capillary wall. Finally, tumor cells in the secondary site must adjust to the foreign microenvironment and develop into metastatic colonies [215].

The invasion-metastasis cascade can occur early when the tumor is small, but it is most often associated with more advanced disease, explaining high cure rates following surgical excision of early-stage cancer and reinforcing the need for early detection. Another unexplained cancer behavior is the latency to metastases that can be short, as in the case of lung cancer, or span years to decades, as is often the case in breast cancer. However, not all cancer cells that migrate from the primary site will establish a distant colony. Indeed, the hurdles to a cancer cell in the metastatic cascade are multiple and the process is highly inefficient, as shown by the rarity of metastases given the millions of cancer cells shed by a cancer into the circulation each day [216]. This relates to seed and soil factors. Only a few cancer cells entering the invasion-metastasis cascade give rise to micrometastases while most enter apoptosis. In fact, although cancer cell homogeneity within tumors was postulated based on microarray analysis of primary and metastatic cancers with all cells having equal metastatic capacity [217], an alternate view indicates that tumors contain genotypically and phenotypically diverse subpopulations of tumor cells differing in their metastatic signatures with a few, called "cancer stem cells", having the capacity to invade and metastasize [218]. In addition, the microenvironment of the organ or tissue host to metastatic cancer cells appears to play a role in 'accepting' or 'limiting' tumor cell implantation as supported by preferential metastatic sites, which has been suggested to be linked to blood flow. Yet, other factors are at play including contiguity and the path of blood and lymphatic channels draining the primary tumor. For instance, metastases to peritoneum by adjacent ovarian, stomach, and colon cancers, and to lungs by breast and kidney cancers, are examples of the former and of the latter, respectively (Table 3.6). Moreover, some tumors exhibit a restricted metastatic kinetics as exemplified by prostate cancer that is largely confined to bone and ocular melanoma that metastasizes almost exclusively to the liver. Regardless, it is clear that the invasion-metastasis cascade involves tumor and host factors, vindicating Paget's seed and soil hypothesis.

The biological processes and genetics underlying the invasion-metastasis cascade are controversial despite intense efforts to untangle what controls and drives each step of the cascade. The following narrative summarizes some notions that have emerged in the last few years. Normal cells adhere to one another through *E-cadherins*, which are anchored to the cytoskeleton via β-*catenins*. Cadherins are part of multi-protein complexes at the cell membrane that are critical to the formation and maintenance of junctional cell-cell contacts that determine tissue architecture and integrity [219]. Hence, it is not surprising that expression of E-cadherins has been negatively corre-

---

[17] A form of programmed cell death, which is induced by anchorage-dependent cells detaching from the surrounding extracellular matrix.

lated with the invasive ability of cancer cells and that their disturbance via cell surface-associated proteolytic enzymes is an initial event in cancer development and progression [220, 221]. For example, blocking E-cadherins can turn stationary cells into invasive ones. Alternatively, restoring E-cadherins expression in cancer cells deprived of this molecule prevents these cells from forming tumors. *Integrins* on the other hand, are a large family of transmembrane glycoproteins that mediate cell adhesion to the extracellular matrix, thereby providing anchorage for cell motility and invasion [222]. Without matrix anchorage, normal cells cannot survive and undergo apoptosis. There is experimental evidence suggesting that anchorage is tissue-specific; that is, a detached normal cell cannot anchor itself in a tissue other than its own. The ubiquitous presence of integrins on tumor cells, blood components, vasculature, and stromal cells suggests their role in the different steps of the metastatic cascade. For instance, expression of $\alpha v \beta 3$, $\alpha v \beta 5$, $\alpha 5 \beta 1$, and $\alpha 6 \beta 4$ integrins by melanoma, breast, prostate, pancreatic, and lung cancer cells were found to correlate with progression of metastases [223]. Likewise, the interaction between $\alpha IIb \beta 3$ integrins on platelets and $\alpha v \beta 3$ on tumor cells via fibrinogen molecules is thought to mediate tumor cell extravasation and distal implantation [224]. Finally, $\alpha v \beta 3$ and $\alpha v \beta 5$ integrins have been detected on the vasculature of certain tumors, but not on adjacent normal vessels, suggesting their contribution to tumor angiogenesis via invasion and migration of endothelial cells [225]. *Selectins*, a three-member family (P-, E-, and L-selectins) of cell adhesion molecules expressed on platelets, endothelial cells, and leucocytes, respectively, play major physiological roles in inflammation, immune response, wound repair, and hemostasis [226]. Yet, they also are involved in the various steps of the invasion-metastatic cascade through platelet-tumor cell interactions (P-selectins), leucocyte recruitment to the micrometastatic environment (L-selectins), and via distal site colonization (E-selectins), among others.

It has been postulated that the accumulation of successive mutations occurring in a minority of cells within a tumor might be at the basis of clonal evolution that engages the multistep process that drives cancer progression towards metastases [227]. However, this has been disputed based on several lines of evidence. The most convincing relates to experiments where human cells of different origins were transformed via the introduction of identical oncogenic genes [228]. The transformed cells developed into two histo-pathologically distinct tumors: one generating metastases, the other not suggesting that the differentiation makeup of the normal cell of origin represented a strong determinant of metastatic spread rather than the subsequently introduced tumorigenic genes. Hence, it has been postulated that,

> Two key aspects of carcinoma cells point to the relevance of these embryonic programs and TFs[18] to tumor progression. First, many of the phenotypes of embryonic cells are recapitulated by aggressive carcinoma cells. Second, many of the embryonic TFs [Slug, Snail, Twist, Goosecoid, SIP-1, FOXC2 and ZEB1] that are known to play critical roles in orchestrating EMTs during embryogenesis are also found to be expressed in a variety of human tumor cells; indeed, their expression is often correlated with aggressive tumor cell-associated traits [229].

---

[18] Transcription factors.

Some TFs also repress E-cadherins expression, which, along with alterations of its gene, is key to the invasion-metastatic cascade. Another role of TFs in the invasion-metastasis cascade involves miRNAs. Indeed, *Twist* has been shown to induce miRNA-10b expression in tumor cells, which "inhibits translation of the messenger RNA encoding homeobox D10, resulting in increased expression of a well-characterized pro-metastatic gene, RHOC" [230]. However, other miRNA exert the opposite effect. For instance, while down regulated miRNA-409 in gastric cancer promotes metastases, its over-expression suppresses metastases by blocking the pro-metastatic gene *radixin* [231]. Other determinants of cancer invasion are modulators of the Hepatocyte Growth Factor (HGF)–HGF receptor (HGFR) pathway in breast cancer and the Metastasis-Associated Colon Cancer 1 (MACC1) gene in colorectal carcinoma, among others.

In the last decade, several genes have been linked to cancer progression and metastasis, including Metastasis-Promoting Genes (MPGs) WDNM-1, WDNM-2, MMP11, MTA1 and ERBB2, and 30 known Metastasis-Suppressor Genes (MSGs), the role of which is to promote or suppress metastases, respectively, at one or more stage of the metastatic process [232, 233]. For instance, expression of MSGs nm23, KAI1, and KiSS1 was found reduced in lymph node and liver metastases of gastric cancers compared to the primary tumors, suggesting their role in tumor progression to metastases [234]. Similar studies in laryngeal carcinoma and breast cancer yielded similar results [235, 236]. Taken together, these results support the view that down regulation of MSGs occurs late in tumorigenesis in accordance with the progression theory that explains the inefficiency of the metastatic process. Dormancy in metastatic cells promoted by MSGs KISS1, MKK4 and MKK7 prevent growth of micrometastases to clinically detectable, life-threatening tumors up to several years, which explains late relapses [237]. Recent experimental evidence suggests that five other MSGs, namely BRMS1, SMAD7, SSeCKS, RhoGDI2 and CTGF, might do likewise. Additionally, some mediators of the invasion-metastatic cascade appear to have prognostic significance. For instance, a decreased expression of nm23 and/or E-cadherin combined with high blood vessel count in the primary tumors of breast cancer patients might be a better negative prognostic indicator than an advanced tumor stage [238, 239]. Likewise, reduction of the KISS1 gene or overexpression of its receptor GPR54 correlates with poor prognosis and more metastases in esophageal, bladder, gastric, thyroid, and breast cancer [240]. Hence, up or down regulation of mediators of the invasion-metastasis cascade might, in the future, be exploited for prognostic and therapeutic purposes [241, 242], though the task ahead appears daunting.

Chapter 4
Environmental Carcinogens

> Scientists plan to check toenail clippings from hundreds
> of people in Garfield, New Jersey, to determine if residents
> were exposed to a toxic metal linked to lung cancer.
>
> – Reuters, March 25, 2013

4.1 First the Basics

Cancer is caused by hereditary factors and by environmental carcinogens. While the former are currently inescapable, the later are potentially preventable. A carcinogen is any substance or agent in the environment that, through genotoxic or non-genotoxic mechanisms, leads to cancer. Because ethical issues preclude prospective studies on the ill effects of agents suspected to be harmful to humans, evidence for assessing their carcinogenicity must rely on indirect studies. The most reliable are epidemiological studies (cohort, case-control, correlation, intervention studies) to which biomarkers data are included whenever available. Because these types of studies do not necessarily yield clear answers, agents studied have been classified as known, probably, or possibly carcinogenic to humans. Known carcinogens include lifestyle factors (e.g. tobacco use), exposure to non-infectious agent such as natural elements (e.g., ultraviolet light, radon gas), medical treatments (e.g. chemotherapy and radiotherapy), workplace exposure (e.g., asbestos), household exposure (e.g. formaldehyde in air fresheners), air pollution (e.g. diesel exhaust) and infectious agents (e.g. hepatitis B virus and human papilloma virus). According to the International Agency for Research on Cancer (IARC), there were 109 known (Group 1), 65 probable (Group 2A), and 275 possible (Group 2B) agents carcinogenic to humans, as of July 2013 [243]. However, because several national and international agencies study different agents at different times, lists of carcinogens, their composition, and agent carcinogenicity do not necessarily match.

The cancer-carcinogen link is highly variable, depending mostly on the intrinsic carcinogenicity of each agent, the amount and duration of exposure, and the individual's susceptibility to a particular agent. For instance, only a minority of tobacco smokers develops cancer and does so after many years of heavy exposure. In contrast, prolonged exposure to bis(chloromethyl) ether (BCME) either through inhalation or skin contact increases the risk of lung cancer up to ten-fold and the heavier the exposure the shorter the time to diagnosis. In addition, the type of cancer resulting from carcinogenic exposure depends on tissue susceptibility. For instance, while the IARC identifies 15 agents associated with lung cancer, radioactive iodide induces almost exclusively thyroid cancer. The contribution of environmental carcinogens to cancer is not negligible. Indeed, "In the industrialized nations, roughly 7 % of cancer deaths are attributable to viral infections; 4 % to occupational hazards; 2 % to sunlight; 2 % to pollutions of air, water, and soil; and less than 1 % to food additives and industrial products" [244, 245]. Indeed, it is estimated that 90–95 % of all cancers have roots in the environment, if lifestyles are included [246]. Indeed, although the National Institute for Occupational Safety and Health (NIOSH) estimates approximately 20,000 yearly deaths from occupational cancers in the US (mostly lung and bladder cancer, and mesothelioma), "the estimated percentage of cancers related to occupational and environmental carcinogens is small compared to the cancer burden from tobacco smoking (30 %) and the combination of poor nutrition, physical inactivity, and obesity (35 %)" [247]. Hence, while approximately 15 % of cancers in the US are caused by unintended daily exposure to a mixture of occupational, household, and other industrial carcinogens, the rest are caused by well-known and easier to control risky lifestyles. Yet, after highlighting asbestos and seven other chemical carcinogens, the President's Cancer Panel report (2010) advocated a new prevention-oriented chemicals policy, strongly urging the President "to use the power of your office to remove the carcinogens and other toxins from our food, water, and air that needlessly increase health care costs, cripple our Nation's productivity, and devastate American lives." Risky health behavior as the leading cause of cancer is not restricted to the US. Indeed, according to the WHO,

> About 30 % of cancer deaths are due to the five leading behavioral and dietary risks… Tobacco use is the most important risk factor for cancer causing 22 % of global cancer deaths…[and] Cancer causing viral infections such as HBV/HCV and HPV are responsible for up to 20 % of cancer deaths in low- and middle-income countries [248].

The following section briefly addresses common underlying mechanisms of carcinogens leading to cancer, but focuses on the three risky lifestyles that together account for several times more cancers in the US than all other environmental carcinogens combined and are much less challenging to prevent and control. Indeed, only a small fraction of the thousands of chemicals released into the environment by industry have been studied after several decades of efforts by the IARC, the National Institute for Occupational Safety and Health (NIOSH), and other specialized agencies in several countries. Hence, it is utterly unrealistic to expect the control of unintended and unsuspected exposure to thousands of potentially carcinogenic environmental agents, as well as the assessment of their individual carcinogenicity, especially because new untested and uncontrolled substances are released into the environment each day, and most contribute to the betterment of modern life. The most rational and efficient approach for reducing the impact of carcinogens on the population is to focus on three lifestyles that together account for approximately two thirds of all cancers in the US, as will be highlighted in the next segment.

4.2 More Details

Carcinogenicity is a highly complex and evolving field, involving epigenetic phenomena and miRNA that is still froth with uncertainties, including the recent surprising finding that "Shiftwork that involves circadian disruption is 'probably carcinogenic to humans'" [249]. Suffice it to say that while the vast majority of carcinogens exert their effects via DNA damage (e.g. are genotoxic), a substantial number are non-genotoxic, accounting for 12 % (45/371) of IARC's Groups 1, 2A and 2B carcinogens with 27 % (12/45) posing a "potential hazard" [250]. Prior to becoming genotoxic, most chemical carcinogens must be activated by cytochrome P450 enzymes. Yet, the same P450 enzymes also metabolize and inactivate chemicals. Hence, the balance between activation and deactivation will determine whether a chemical becomes carcinogenic. On the other hand, non-genotoxic carcinogens have been shown to act as,

> ...tumor promoters (e.g. 1,4-dichlorobenzene), endocrine-modifiers (e.g. 17beta-estradiol), receptor-mediators (e.g. 2,3,7,8-tetrachlorodibenzo-p-dioxin), immune suppressors (e.g. cyclosporine), or inducers of tissue-specific toxicity and inflammatory responses (e.g. arsenic and beryllium) [251].

Additionally, except for carcinogens that can easily be studied in isolation, such as tobacco, most exposures are to mixtures of very diverse agents arising from multiple sources, making it difficult to assess the carcinogenicity and assign causality of single agents. Hence, given the sheer number of potential carcinogens and the colossal task needed to remove them from the environment, I will concentrate on three lifestyles linked to cancer that, in contrast to unintended exposure to environmental carcinogens, result from individual choice and are linked to approximately 2/3 of all cancers in the US. This crucial difference in the source of exposure to carcinogens empowers involved individuals to control their own exposure via behavior modification rather than relying on governmental regulation or industry goodwill that are retro- rather than pro-active at best.

According to the Center for Disease Control and Prevention (CDC), the three leading causes of mortality in the U.S. are preventable, self-inflicted diseases. In a recent press release it reported, "The leading causes of death in 2000 were tobacco (435,000 deaths; 18.1 % of total US deaths), poor diet and physical inactivity (400,000 deaths; 16.6 %), and alcohol consumption (85,000 deaths; 3.5 %)" [252]. Additionally, ultraviolet radiation from the sun or artificial sources account for most cases of skin cancers, especially melanoma. Indeed, as the popularity of natural and artificial tanning rose through the 1980s and 1990s, incidence rates for melanoma in the US rose from 8.7/100,000 in 1975 to 28/100,000 in 2009, the fifth most frequent cancer after colorectal cancer [253]. Hence, while it is estimated that 19 % of all cancers worldwide are caused by unintended exposure to difficult to prevent or control environmental and occupational carcinogens [254], efforts at behavior modification at the national, state, and health care provider levels should focus on education designed to avoid what in essence are self-inflicted diseases caused by risky lifestyles. While lifestyle behavior modification is a long and difficult albeit overdue course of action, an incentivized healthcare payment model should be at its core [255].

4.2.1 Smoking

Since the Surgeon General's 1964 "Report on Smoking and Health" that alerted the nation to the health risk of smoking, the direct causal relationship between tobacco use and cancer has been periodically revisited and confirmed. In its 2004 report, the Surgeon General extended the tobacco-cancer link to include cancer of the lung, larynx, oral cavity and pharynx, esophagus, stomach, pancreas, kidney and renal pelvis, urinary bladder, and cervix, and AML [256]. The IARC also studied the tobacco-cancer link in 1986 and 2002 and, although the methodology used was somewhat different, its conclusions were similar [257]. In 2012, smoking accounted for approximately 85 % of 205,974 cases of lung cancers in the United States including 3,400 from secondhand exposure, which is the second leading cause of death among men and women. A recent study of mortality trends across three time periods (1959–1965, 1982–1988, and 2000–2010) among participants 55 years of age or older found a 2.73, 12.65, and 25.66 relative risks of death from lung cancer, respectively, for women current smokers and 12.22, 23.81, and 24.97 for male smokers, compared to their respective nonsmokers counterparts [258]. In 2012, lifelong male and female smokers were 23 and 13 times more likely to develop lung cancer than nonsmokers, respectively [259], despite a 54 % drop in the smoking population since 1965, as shown in Fig. 4.1. The CDC also reported 5.1 Ma of Years of Potential Life Lost (YPLL) annually linked to smoking in the United States between 2000 and 2004. The health effects of smoking are not surprising, given the more than "7,000 chemicals, including hundreds that are toxic and about 70 that can cause cancer" [260].

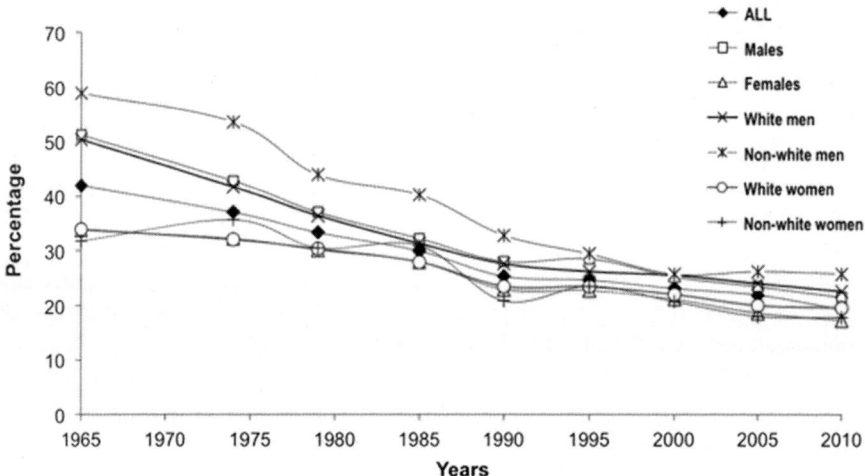

Fig. 4.1 Smoking trends by sex and race between 2005 and 2010

4.2 More Details

Lung cancer is the second leading cause of death in the US. Yet, private and public economic interests dictate our ambivalent national policy on tobacco that fails to dissuade potential smokers, as shown by the following statistics [261].

- In 2010, the cigarette industry spent $8.05 billion to promote smoking.
- In 2013, states will collect $25.7 billion from tobacco taxes and legal settlements, but will spend less than 2 % of that sum on tobacco control programs.
- In 2010, 43.8 million Americans (19.0 % of all adults) smoked.
- Nearly 20 % of young adults ages 19–28 smoke daily and 12.5 % smoke half a pack or more each day [262].
- Each day, over 3,600 persons younger than 18 years of age smoke their first cigarette.
- In 2010, cigarette smoking cost the nation more than $193 billion ($97 billion in lost productivity plus $96 billion in health care expenditures).

While the benefits of avoiding environmental carcinogens are real but difficult to assess, smoke cessation accrues enormous benefits when successful, as shown by indisputable empirical evidence. Indeed, according to the Surgeon General "when smokers quit the risk for a heart attack drops sharply after just 1 year; stroke risk can fall to about the same as a nonsmoker's after 2–5 years; risks for cancer of the mouth, throat, esophagus, and bladder are cut in half after 5 years; and the risk for dying of lung cancer drops by half after 10 years" [263].

4.2.2 Obesity

Overeating and lack of exercise have become a health problem in industrialized and underdeveloped countries alike. In the US, the prevalence of obesity[1] in adults age 20–74 rose from 15 % in the 1976–1980 period to 35 % in 2005–2006. Overweight[2] affects 15 % of children and 18 % of adolescents. More disturbingly, 11 % of infants, ages 2–5 were overweight in 2005–2006, most of whom will become obese adults [264]. The numbers of adult smokers declined by 18.5 % between 1993 and 2008, whereas the proportion of obese people increased 85 %. Between 1973 and 2008, healthy weight American adults decreased from 50 to 30 % whereas the number of obese rose from 14 to 37 % (Fig. 4.2). Like smoking, overweight and obesity lead to profound and costly health consequences in terms of human suffering and economic costs. Indeed, they are associated with an increased risk of coronary

---

[1] A Body Mass Index of 30 or greater; normal being 18.5–25.
[2] A Body Mass Index 25 or greater.

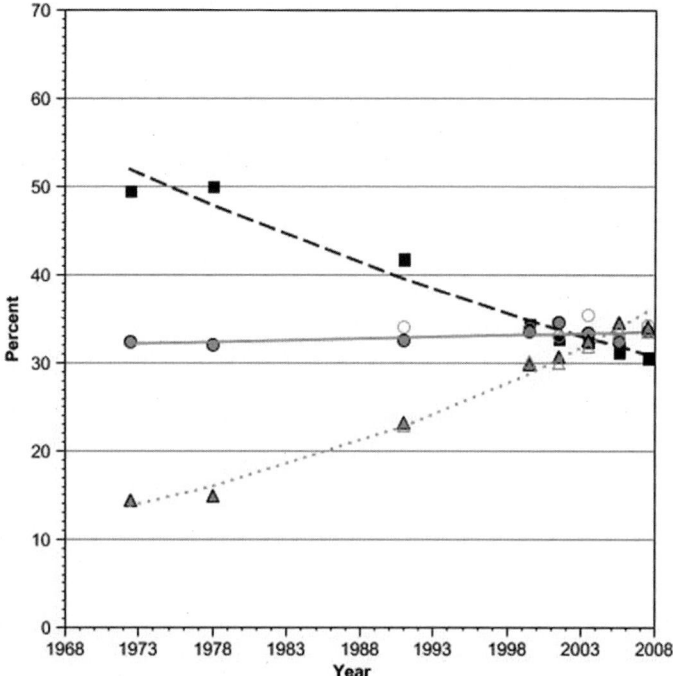

Fig. 4.2 Percentage of adults age 20–74 who were at a Healthy weight (■), Overweight (●), and Obese (▲): 1971–2008 (Reproduced from National Center for Human Statistics. National Health and Nutrition Examination Survey)

artery disease, type-II diabetes, hypertension, stroke, liver and gallbladder disease, sleep apnea, osteoarthritis, gynecological problems (e.g., infertility), and cancer (e.g., endometrial, kidney, and colon, among others) [265]. The risk of some cancers increases with increasing weight. Table 4.1 shows the relative risk of cancer in obese persons and the percentage of cancer attributable to obesity (CAO) within that population. Given the number of chronic diseases associated with obesity, its long-term effect on healthcare costs is enormous. For instance, it has been estimated that between 1987 and 2001, inflation-adjusted per capita spending for heart disease and diabetes in overweight people was 41 %, and 38 % higher, respectively, than for people of normal weight. Overall, the estimated cost of overweight and obesity was $147 billion in 2009 [266].

The definition of obesity is often filtered through a self-interest or emotional prism, within both the population and the medical community. Obesity is viewed either as a *disease* or as a *lifestyle choice* that leads to a number of diseases. Consequently, there are two major approaches for tackling obesity: one medical advocated by those who believe its cause to be biological or genetic; the other behavioral as promoted by those who consider obesity over-consumption of food akin to drug abuse leading to addiction. In contrast to smoking that is generally viewed as an addiction, obesity as a disease or as an addiction are controversial

Table 4.1 Obesity-associated cancers (Adapted from [267])

Type of cancer	Relative risk[a]	CAO (%)
Endometrial	3.5	57
Esophageal	3.0	52
Kidney	2.5	43
Gallbladder	2.0	36
Gastric	2.0	36
Colorectal men	2.0	35
Pancreatic	1.7	27
Breast (female)	1.5	23
Colorectal women	1.5	21

[a]Risk relative to populations with normal weight

models, as they imply the concepts of *victim* and *choice*, respectively. On the other hand, politically correct definitions choose the high ground, trying to stay above the fray. For instance, a panel of experts commissioned by The Obese Society examined the scientific and forensic arguments in support of obesity as a disease, and having decided that neither argument was convincing, it concluded,

> Considering obesity a disease is likely to have far more positive than negative consequences and to benefit the greater good by soliciting more resources into prevention, treatment, and research of obesity; encouraging more high-quality caring professionals to view treating the obese patient as a vocation worthy of effort and respect; and reducing the stigma and discrimination heaped on many obese persons [268].

Such a pragmatic definition of obesity, which the panel rightly called *utilitarian*, is no better that the accommodative definition of addiction by the National Institute of Drug Addiction (NIDA) as a *brain disease*. Mixing cause and effect, albeit admitting a behavioral component, NIDA experts felt justified in equating addiction to a somatic disease, arguing,

> Addiction, like heart disease, cancers, and type II diabetes, is a real and complex disease .... no one chooses to be a drug addict or to develop heart disease ... sometimes people do cated both environmental and genetic influences [269].

NIDA's seemingly rational explanatory argument is equally misguided and misrepresents the facts. It states,

> Although initial drug use might be voluntary, drugs of abuse have been shown to alter gene expression and brain circuitry, which in turn affect human behavior. Once addiction develops, these brain changes interfere with an individual's ability to make voluntary decisions, leading to compulsive drug craving, seeking and use [270].

This chemical reward theory of addiction based on gene and brain circuitry alteration by drugs of abuse as the underlying mechanism should be extended to the wide spectrum of addiction, which includes,

> Not only licit or illicit drugs, prescription medications, and chemical products, but extend to non–substance-based activities such as gambling and others that are normal, ordinary, and non-addictive for most people, such as drinking coffee, eating, and having sex. Hence, addiction is linked to the individual, not to any intrinsic addictive property of the substance or activity abused or its effect on the brain [271].

For the most ardent opponents of obesity as a disease, "The idea that addiction is a disease is the greatest medical hoax since the idea that masturbation would make you go blind" [272].

Obesity is attributed to lifestyle factors superimposed to a genetic susceptibility. The concept of obesity as behavioral rests on solid grounds as it is supported by empirical evidence drawn from socio-economic and environmental factors common to affected individuals that modulate behavioral development. Indeed,

> Most unhealthy lifestyles are deep-seeded in childhood experiences fostered by home, school, and community dynamics. For instance, high caloric diets and lack of physical activity are promoted by undisciplined home environments, sale of unhealthy food and neglect of physical education at school, lack of or difficult access to community parks or recreation centers, and by unrestrained TV watching that exposes children to hours of inactivity along with dozens of commercials promoting unhealthy snacks [273].

Nevertheless, recent data suggest that, in addition to an imbalance between calorie intake and output, a high-fat source of calories promotes the growth of a distinct microbiota[3] that is associated with increased capacity to extract energy from otherwise indigestible dietary constituents [274, 275].

4.2.3 Alcoholism

In 2011, 16.7 million Americans or 6.5 % of the population met criteria for dependence or abuse of alcohol, a 4:1 prevalence ratio compared to marijuana (4.2 million Americans) and causes four times as many deaths as all illicit drugs combined (Table 4.2). It seems ironic that, despite US government fixation on illicit drugs and after 40 years of the *War on Drugs* that "requires the incarceration of thousands of petty offenders, fosters crime resulting mainly from the criminalization of drugs, and victimizes tens of millions of American pain sufferers" [276], at an estimated annual cost of $181 billion, "American teens are less likely than European teens to use cigarettes and alcohol, but more likely to use illicit drugs" [277]. Such was the conclusion based on comparing data gathered by the *University of Michigan's Monitoring the Future* to a coordinated school survey about substance use by more than 100,000 students in 36 European countries. The National Institute on Alcohol Abuse and Alcoholism defines "low-risk" drinking as "no more than 4 drinks on any single day and no more than 14 drinks per week", for men, and "no more than 3 drinks on any single day and no more than 7 drinks per week", for women [278]. According to the same source, 18 million Americans exhibit alcohol abuse,

---

[3] Gut microbial ecology.

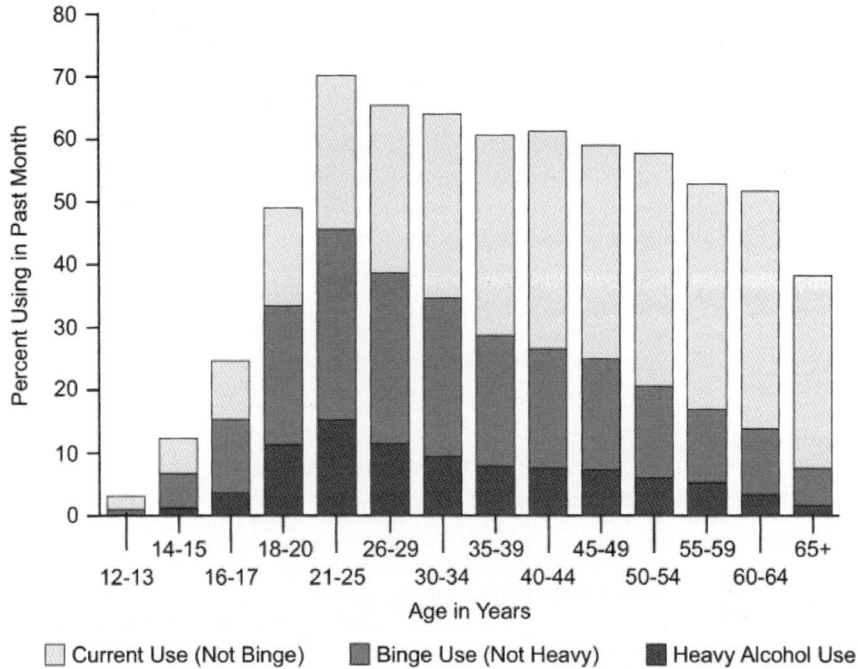

Fig. 4.3 Levels of alcohol consumption by age groups, US 2010 (Reproduced from SAMHSA [279])

alcoholism, or dependence, which it defines as being associated with craving, loss of control, and physical dependence. Alcohol accounts for approximately 85,000 annual deaths in the US, of which 21,000 are from cancer. The percentages of the US population using alcohol in 2010 and intake levels are shown in Fig. 4.3. Alcohol's major non-neoplastic health effects include disorders of the brain (e.g., depression, other mental disorders), heart (e.g., cardiomyopathy,[4] arrhythmia[5]), liver (e.g., hepatitis, cirrhosis), pancreas (e.g., acute and chronic pancreatitis), stomach (e.g., gastritis), immune system (e.g., susceptibility to infections), polyneuropathy, hypertension, hemorrhagic stroke, and cancer. A link exists between excessive long-term consumption of alcohol and an increased risk of the following cancers: oral (e.g., mouth, pharynx, and larynx); esophageal; colorectal; and liver in both men and women and breast cancer in women. The mechanisms underlying the increased risk of cancer associated with alcohol consumption are not well understood, but are thought to involve direct toxic effects, such as the genotoxic effect of acetaldehyde (ethanol's main metabolite) and indirect effects via increased estrogen levels, acting as a solvent for tobacco or other carcinogens, triggering production of reactive oxygen and nitrogen species and changes in folate metabolism. Genetic

---

[4] Heart muscle dilatation.

[5] Irregular heart rhythm.

susceptibility is suspected [280]. As in the case of illicit drug addiction and obesity, the alcoholism-as-a-disease concept has taken root within a certain segment of healthcare and of the population without solid empirical evidence to support it. By and large, efforts have been aimed at confounding dependence and addiction with diseases they cause (e.g., the *victim* model of addiction) rather than addressing the root causes that can be prevented via behavior modification (e.g., the *choice* model) [281]. In a recent review of "historical and cultural conditions under which addiction-as-disease was constructed", the author concluded,

> The ubiquity of the disease concept of addiction obscures the fact that it did not emerge from the accretion of scientific discoveries. Addiction-as-disease has been continuously redefined, mostly in the direction of conceptual elasticity, such that it now yields an embarrassment of riches: a growing range of allegedly addictive phenomena, which do not involve drugs [282].

Additionally, the claimed benefits of defining addictive behaviors as diseases in order not to "victimize" sufferers and to justify treatments other than behavior modification are illusory and misguided. Indeed,

> ...the behavioral model surpasses the disease theory of addiction in three major aspects. First, it accounts for the behavior of a majority of individuals who seek drugs and of the millions of casual users and pain patients who do not become addicted despite repeated or protracted drug exposure. Second, it provides a foundation for understanding and explaining all forms of addiction, whether substance or non-substance related. Third and most importantly, it promotes prevention, self-control, and treatment modalities aimed at restoring addicts' discipline and willpower, empowering them to develop new behavioral patterns instead of perpetuating the myth that they are powerless victims, as embodied in the disease model of addiction [283].

In summary, overuse and abuse of tobacco, foodstuffs, and alcohol, which affect a large segment of the US population, cause numerous real diseases that affect virtually every organ at an enormous human and economic cost. As shown in Table 4.2, recent estimates suggest that these three lifestyle behaviors cause nearly one million annual deaths combined, including over 300,000 from cancer (e.g., 60 % of all annual cancer deaths), and nearly ten million YPLL at a cost to the nation exceeding $500 billion annually. These statistics clearly indicate that cancer prevention through the control of these widespread lifestyle behaviors should reap enormous benefits.

Table 4.2 Prevalence and costs of smoking, obesity, and heavy drinking

	Smokers	Overweight & obesity	Heavy drinking
Prevalence[a]	27.4	68.8	6.5
Human cost			
Deaths	435,000	400,000	85,000
Cancer	205,974	84,000	21,000
YPLL	5.1	2.3	2.2
Economic cost[b]	193	147	185

[a]Percent of adult population
[b]Annual in $ billions

4.2 More Details

Mine is certainly not the first call to self-control. Indeed, the Surgeon General 1979 report emphasized personal responsibility in proper nutrition, regular physical exercise, and the elimination of other unhealthy behaviors. The 1996 report titled, "Physical Activity and Health", was another effort to motivate Americans to take responsibility for their own health. Decades later, alcohol consumption and smoking and their health effects have substantially decreased, but overweight and obesity have reached epidemic proportions. In fact, altering risky health behavior, the cause of most preventable diseases and two thirds of all cancers, is a difficult task that requires considerable human effort, substantial economic resources, persuasiveness, persistence, and most of all, compliance by the targeted population. Yet, it could be done if our nation devoted as much zeal and financial resources to achieving this potentially high-return health goal as it does to misguided policies such as the failed War on Drugs [284] that was allocated $25.59 billion for FY 2013 spread over 18 US Departments, especially because the vast majority of deaths caused by illicit drugs is linked to their prohibition (drug trade-related crime), with only a few linked to users' lack of control (overdose), rather than their pathophysiological effects [285].

Part III
Cancer Statistics

Chapter 5
Assessing the Enormity of the Problem

> *Clouds cannot cover secret places, nor denials conceal truth.*
>
> – Demosthenes

The cost of cancer in the United States, in terms of human suffering and financial resources, is enormous. Since 1990, over 6 million Americans have died of cancer, more than the combined military casualties from the Civil War (~625,000), WWI (~120,000), WWII (~400,000), and the Vietnam (~58,000) and Korean (~35,000) conflicts. Over their lifetime, about 1 out of 2 American men and 1 out of 3 American women will develop cancer [286]. The National Institutes of Health estimates the overall costs of cancer in the United States at approximately $201.5 billion in 2007, including $77.4 billion for direct medical costs and $124.0 billion for indirect mortality costs (cost of lost productivity due to premature death) [287]. The cost of cancer care has exploded over the last decade, especially the cost of drugs. For instance, "Nitrogen mustard, a drug that has been used to treat cancer since 1949, saw its price for a course of treatment increase by a factor of 13 between the beginning and the end of 2006 (from $33 to $420)" [288]. On the other hand, appropriated funds available to the NCI to support basic science and clinical research stagnated at an average $4.9 billion per year between FY 2005 and FY 2011. Yet, despite extraordinary advances in our understanding of the biology, genetics, and growth regulation of cancer, little progress has been made towards its prevention and treatment. Indeed, 1,638,910 Americans are expected to develop cancer in 2012 and an estimated 577,190 are expected to die of it [289]. Because cancer deaths shorten the average lifespan by 15.5 years per person, an estimated total of 8.8 Ma of life were lost from cancer deaths in 2009. This exceeds the years of life lost not only from heart disease (7.0 million), the leading cause of death in the US, but also from all other causes combined (8.0 million) [290]. Finally, 77 % of cancers afflict individuals 55 years of age or older and the risk of eventually being diagnosed with and dying of cancer in 2007–2009 after age 50 was 40.8 % and 21.6 %, respectively, for both sexes and all races [291].

5.1 Origin, Purpose, and Data Collection

In 1926, the Yale-New Haven Hospital set up the first cancer registry in the United States, and in 1956, the American College of Surgeons (ACoS) launched a program to encourage hospital-based cancer registries. However, based on individual card files, these data were of little use to physicians and researchers, and it would take until the advent of computerized registry systems that facilitated pooling and analyzing regional and national data for cancer statistics to become routine and useful. The purpose of cancer registries is to collect, manage, and analyze data on cancer patients in order to uncover ethnic and gender differences, and possible causal relationships to potentially hazardous agents or behaviors. There are two types of cancer registries: hospital-based and population-based, which can be administrative, research, or cancer control oriented. The Surveillance, Epidemiology and End Results (SEER), the first population-based registry, was established in 1973 by NCI. It began collecting cancer incidence and survival data on January 1, 1973 from the states of Connecticut, Iowa, New Mexico, Utah, and Hawaii and the metropolitan areas of Detroit and San Francisco-Oakland. Atlanta and the 13 Seattle-Puget Sound counties were added in 1974–1975, as were 10 predominantly black rural counties in Georgia (1978) and American Indian areas in Arizona (1980). In 1992, minority Hispanic populations living in Los Angeles County and the San Jose-Monterrey area were added. In 2001, coverage was expanded to Kentucky, New Jersey, and the previously uncovered portions of California, and in 2010, coverage was extended to the state of Georgia. Information on cancer cases is also collected by NCI from Alaska natives. Currently (2012), SEER collects and publishes cancer incidence and survival data from population-based cancer registries covering approximately 28 % of the US population. Although SEER does not cover the entire US population, validation studies based on the recorded cause of death for 17 cancer sites representing two thirds of cancer cases in the United States revealed a 90 % correlation [292]. Data collected by SEER include patient demographics, primary tumor site, morphology, stage at diagnosis, first course of treatment, and patient survival, which are essential for planning and monitoring cancer control strategies, for identifying priorities in public health, and for allocating resources for the prevention and treatment of cancer. In 1992, Congress passed the Cancer Registries Amendment Act, establishing the National Program of Cancer Registries (NPCR) to be administered by the CDC. Since 1994, "NPCR and SEER together collect cancer data for the entire U.S. population. CDC and NCI, in collaboration with the North American Association of Central Cancer Registries, have been publishing annual federal cancer statistics in the United States" [293]. Based on these databases, the ACS compiles yearly estimates of cancer incidence, mortality, and survival, standardized to the 2000 United States population. At the international level, the IARC, a non-governmental organization founded in 1966, is dedicated to fostering the aims and activities of cancer registries worldwide in cooperation with the WHO. It must be noted that some countries rely on regional rather than nationwide databases to estimate cancer incidence, which are reported to IARC via the WHO, somewhat compromising the accuracy of their cancer statistics. Nevertheless, IARC's "Cancer Incidence in Five Continents" series of monographs, updated every 5 years, has become the reference source on the global incidence of cancer. In contrast to population-based surveillance data that reflect national rates and trends, hospital registries reflect the type of practice, catchment area, and other factors peculiar to each institution.

5.2 Incidence and Mortality Statistics: Reporting and Interpretation

Cancer incidence and mortality both can be expressed as total number of cases in a population over a particular period of time and can be sorted by site, region, race, age, and other demographics. For example, 1,638,910 million Americans are expected to develop cancer in 2012; 848,170 males and 790,740 females [294]. However, total cancer cases vary with population size, age composition, and other factors, thus precluding detailed comparisons of cancer incidence or trends over time in the same country, or between countries with populations of different demographics. This problem is overcome by expressing the incidence, mortality, and other statistics for each 100,000 people in the total population surveyed, or in any segment thereof (males, whites, etc.), adjusted for age distribution in the overall population. The latter is necessary because cancer predominates in the elderly but certain types of cancer are age-dependent. For example, in the US, the median age of cancer patients at diagnosis in the 2005–2009 period was 66, but 33 for testicular cancer, 14 for ALL [295], and 80 % of inherited retinoblastomas are diagnosed before age 3. Hence, the incidence of prostate cancer in 2009, for instance, can be reported as 151.9 per 100,000 men of all-ages and all races, as 62.2 per 100,000 men of all races below age 65, or further broken down by other demographics or tumor stage [296]. These adjustments enable comparing cancer rates over time in the same country and between countries with different population size and demographics composition. There is, however, one caveat: In the US, rates per 100,000 are age-adjusted to the 2000 US population, whereas data reported by the IARC are standardized to the 1980 age-adjusted OECD population and other international reports use the Segi's or WHO's age-adjusted "world" populations[1] to remove cross-country age variations. Unless otherwise specified, in this book, all references to cancer incidence and mortality rates will be population- and age-adjusted.

5.3 Cancer Incidence and Mortality Rates, US 2013 Estimates

The American Cancer Society publishes yearly estimates of the numbers of new cancer cases and cancer deaths expected in the United States, based on last available actual rates (usually 5 years in arrears) projected onto yearly estimates of the size

---

[1] Segi's and WHO's world population standards are based on the 1950 populations of 46 countries and estimates of the average age structure of the world's population expected from 2000 to 2025, respectively.

and age distribution of the United States population. While these estimates are only projections, they have proved reasonably accurate when compared to actual data gathered and tabulated several years later, thus justifying their interim use. The American Cancer Society estimates that 1,660,290 (averaging 4,500 each day) Americans will develop cancer and 580,350 (or 1,600 each day) will die of the disease in 2013 (Table 5.1) [297]. There are well over 200 different types of cancer and the ACS reports on approximately 50. However, their relative incidence and deaths rates within a population vary greatly. Indeed, five cancers account for nearly 2/3 of

Table 5.1 Reproduced from the American Cancer Society, Cancer Facts & Figures – 2013

Estimated Number* of New Cancer Cases and Deaths by Sex, US, 2013

	Estimated New Cases			Estimated Deaths		
	Both Sexes	Male	Female	Both Sexes	Male	Female
All Sites	1,660,290	854,790	805,500	580,350	306,920	273,430
Oral cavity & pharynx	41,380	29,620	11,760	7,890	5,500	2,390
Tongue	13,590	9,900	3,690	2,070	1,380	690
Mouth	11,400	6,730	4,670	1,800	1,080	720
Pharynx	13,930	11,200	2,730	2,400	1,790	610
Other oral cavity	2,460	1,790	670	1,640	1,260	380
Digestive system	290,200	160,750	129,450	144,570	82,700	61,870
Esophagus	17,990	14,440	3,550	15,210	12,220	2,990
Stomach	21,600	13,230	8,370	10,990	6,740	4,250
Small intestine	8,810	4,670	4,140	1,170	610	560
Colon†	102,480	50,090	52,390	50,830	26,300	24,530
Rectum	40,340	23,590	16,750			
Anus, anal canal, & anorectum	7,060	2,630	4,430	880	330	550
Liver & intrahepatic bile duct	30,640	22,720	7,920	21,670	14,890	6,780
Gallbladder & other biliary	10,310	4,740	5,570	3,230	1,260	1,970
Pancreas	45,220	22,740	22,480	38,460	19,480	18,980
Other digestive organs	5,750	1,900	3,850	2,130	870	1,260
Respiratory system	246,210	131,760	114,450	163,890	90,600	73,290
Larynx	12,260	9,680	2,580	3,630	2,860	770
Lung & bronchus	228,190	118,080	110,110	159,480	87,260	72,220
Other respiratory organs	5,760	4,000	1,760	780	480	300
Bones & joints	3,010	1,680	1,330	1,440	810	630
Soft tissue (including heart)	11,410	6,290	5,120	4,390	2,500	1,890
Skin (excluding basal & squamous)	82,770	48,660	34,110	12,650	8,560	4,090
Melanoma-skin	76,690	45,060	31,630	9,480	6,280	3,200
Other nonepithelial skin	6,080	3,600	2,480	3,170	2,280	890
Breast	234,580	2,240	232,340	40,030	410	39,620
Genital system	339,810	248,080	91,730	58,480	30,400	28,080
Uterine cervix	12,340		12,340	4,030		4,030
Uterine corpus	49,560		49,560	8,190		8,190
Ovary	22,240		22,240	14,030		14,030
Vulva	4,700		4,700	990		990
Vagina & other genital, female	2,890		2,890	840		840
Prostate	238,590	238,590		29,720	29,720	
Testis	7,920	7,920		370	370	
Penis & other genital, male	1,570	1,570		310	310	
Urinary system	140,430	96,800	43,630	29,790	20,120	9,670
Urinary bladder	72,570	54,610	17,960	15,210	10,820	4,390
Kidney & renal pelvis	65,150	40,430	24,720	13,680	8,780	4,900
Ureter & other urinary organs	2,710	1,760	950	900	520	380
Eye & orbit	2,800	1,490	1,310	320	120	200
Brain & other nervous system	23,130	12,770	10,360	14,080	7,930	6,150
Endocrine system	62,710	16,210	46,500	2,770	1,270	1,500
Thyroid	60,220	14,910	45,310	1,850	810	1,040
Other endocrine	2,490	1,300	1,190	920	460	460
Lymphoma	79,030	42,670	36,360	20,200	11,250	8,950
Hodgkin lymphoma	9,290	5,070	4,220	1,180	660	520
Non-Hodgkin lymphoma	69,740	37,600	32,140	19,020	10,590	8,430
Myeloma	22,350	12,440	9,910	10,710	6,070	4,640
Leukemia	48,610	27,880	20,730	23,720	13,660	10,060
Acute lymphocytic leukemia	6,070	3,350	2,720	1,430	820	610
Chronic lymphocytic leukemia	15,680	9,720	5,960	4,580	2,750	1,830
Acute myeloid leukemia	14,590	7,820	6,770	10,370	5,930	4,440
Chronic myeloid leukemia	5,920	3,420	2,500	610	340	270
Other leukemia‡	6,350	3,570	2,780	6,730	3,820	2,910
Other & unspecified primary sites‡	31,860	15,450	16,410	45,420	25,020	20,400

*Rounded to the nearest 10; estimated new cases exclude basal cell and squamous cell skin cancers and in situ carcinomas except urinary bladder. About 64,640 carcinoma in situ of the female breast and 61,300 melanoma in situ will be newly diagnosed in 2013. †Estimated deaths for colon and rectal cancers are combined. ‡More deaths than cases may reflect lack of specificity in recording underlying cause of death on death certificates and/or an undercount in the case estimate.

Source: Estimated new cases are based on cancer incidence rates from 49 states and the District of Columbia during 1995-2009 as reported by the North American Association of Central Cancer Registries (NAACCR), representing about 98% of the US population. Estimated deaths are based on US mortality data during 1995-2009, National Center for Health Statistics, Centers for Disease Control and Prevention.

©2013, American Cancer Society, Inc., Surveillance Research

Leading New Cancer Cases and Deaths – 2013 Estimates

Estimated New Cases*		Estimated Deaths	
Male	Female	Male	Female
Prostate 238,590 (28%)	Breast 232,340 (29%)	Lung & bronchus 87,260 (28%)	Lung & bronchus 72,220 (26%)
Lung & bronchus 118,080 (14%)	Lung & bronchus 110,110 (14%)	Prostate 29,720 (10%)	Breast 39,620 (14%)
Colon & rectum 73,680 (9%)	Colon & rectum 69,140 (9%)	Colon & rectum 26,300 (9%)	Colon & rectum 24,530 (9%)
Urinary bladder 54,610 (6%)	Uterine corpus 49,560 (6%)	Pancreas 19,480 (6%)	Pancreas 18,980 (7%)
Melanoma of the skin 45,060 (5%)	Thyroid 45,310 (6%)	Liver & intrahepatic bile duct 14,890 (5%)	Ovary 14,030 (5%)
Kidney & renal pelvis 40,430 (5%)	Non-Hodgkin lymphoma 32,140 (4%)	Leukemia 13,660 (4%)	Leukemia 10,060 (4%)
Non-Hodgkin lymphoma 37,600 (4%)	Melanoma of the skin 31,630 (4%)	Esophagus 12,220 (4%)	Non-Hodgkin lymphoma 8,430 (3%)
Oral cavity & pharynx 29,620 (3%)	Kidney & renal pelvis 24,720 (3%)	Urinary bladder 10,820 (4%)	Uterine corpus 8,190 (3%)
Leukemia 27,880 (3%)	Pancreas 22,480 (3%)	Non-Hodgkin lymphoma 10,590 (3%)	Liver & intrahepatic bile duct 6,780 (2%)
Pancreas 22,740 (3%)	Ovary 22,240 (3%)	Kidney & renal pelvis 8,780 (3%)	Brain & other nervous system 6,150 (2%)
All sites 854,790 (100%)	All sites 805,500 (100%)	All sites 306,920 (100%)	All sites 273,430 (100%)

*Excludes basal and squamous cell skin cancers and in situ carcinoma except urinary bladder.

©2013, American Cancer Society, Inc., Surveillance Research

Fig. 5.1 Reproduced from the American Cancer Society, Cancer Facts & Figures – 2013

all new male and female cancers expected in 2013 and approximately 60 % of all cancer deaths in American men and women (Fig. 5.1), two of which (lung and colorectal) are lifestyle related. Interestingly, the projected two leading cancer deaths in men (prostate and lung) and in women (breast and lung) accounted for approximately the same fractions of new cases (42 and 43 %) and deaths (38 and 40 %), respectively, in 2013 and 1995 [298].

5.4 Probability of Developing and Dying of Advanced Cancer, 2007–2009

The cumulative life-long risk of developing any invasive cancer was nearly 1 in 2 (45 %) for an American male and more than 1 in 3 (38 %) for an American female in the 2007–2009 period (Table 5.2). Likewise, in the same timeframe the cumulative life-long risk of dying from cancer was nearly 1 in 4 for an American male (23 %) and 1 in 5 for an American female (19 %). However, the risk of developing and dying of cancer from any particular type of cancer is both gender and age-dependent. For example, while the male cumulative life-long risk of dying of prostate cancer (1 in 36) was identical to a woman's cumulative risk of dying of breast cancer (1 in 36) during the 2007–2009 period, only 1 in 7,964 men developed prostate cancer before age 40 whereas 1 woman in 202 developed breast cancer by the same age [299]. In the same timeframe, the leading cause of cancer death in men

Table 5.2 Reproduced from the American Cancer Society, Cancer Facts & Figures – 2013

		Probability (%) of Developing Invasive Cancers during Selected Age Intervals by Sex, US, 2007-2009*				
		Birth to 39	40 to 59	60 to 69	70 and Older	Birth to Death
All sites†	Male	1.46 (1 in 69)	8.79 (1 in 11)	16.03 (1 in 6)	38.07 (1 in 3)	44.81 (1 in 2)
	Female	2.20 (1 in 46)	9.19 (1 in 11)	10.39 (1 in 10)	26.69 (1 in 4)	38.17 (1 in 3)
Urinary bladder‡	Male	0.02 (1 in 4,924)	0.37 (1 in 272)	0.92 (1 in 109)	3.69 (1 in 27)	3.81 (1 in 26)
	Female	0.01 (1 in 12,663)	0.12 (1 in 864)	0.24 (1 in 410)	0.98 (1 in 106)	1.15 (1 in 87)
Breast	Female	0.50 (1 in 202)	3.78 (1 in 26)	3.56 (1 in 28)	6.65 (1 in 15)	12.38 (1 in 8)
Colon & rectum	Male	0.08 (1 in 1,212)	0.94 (1 in 106)	1.40 (1 in 71)	4.19 (1 in 24)	5.17 (1 in 19)
	Female	0.08 (1 in 1,236)	0.75 (1 in 134)	0.98 (1 in 102)	3.80 (1 in 26)	4.78 (1 in 21)
Leukemia	Male	0.16 (1 in 612)	0.23 (1 in 440)	0.35 (1 in 288)	1.26 (1 in 80)	1.59 (1 in 63)
	Female	0.13 (1 in 746)	0.15 (1 in 655)	0.21 (1 in 481)	0.81 (1 in 123)	1.14 (1 in 88)
Lung & bronchus	Male	0.03 (1 in 3,552)	0.92 (1 in 109)	2.27 (1 in 44)	6.82 (1 in 15)	7.77 (1 in 13)
	Female	0.03 (1 in 3,287)	0.76 (1 in 131)	1.72 (1 in 58)	4.93 (1 in 20)	6.35 (1 in 16)
Melanoma of the skin§	Male	0.15 (1 in 691)	0.63 (1 in 160)	0.77 (1 in 130)	2.02 (1 in 50)	2.87 (1 in 35)
	Female	0.26 (1 in 391)	0.55 (1 in 181)	0.40 (1 in 248)	0.84 (1 in 120)	1.85 (1 in 54)
Non-Hodgkin lymphoma	Male	0.13 (1 in 753)	0.44 (1 in 225)	0.60 (1 in 167)	1.77 (1 in 57)	2.34 (1 in 43)
	Female	0.09 (1 in 1,147)	0.31 (1 in 322)	0.44 (1 in 229)	1.40 (1 in 72)	1.93 (1 in 52)
Prostate	Male	0.01 (1 in 7,964)	2.68 (1 in 37)	6.78 (1 in 15)	12.06 (1 in 8)	16.15 (1 in 6)
Uterine cervix	Female	0.16 (1 in 641)	0.27 (1 in 374)	0.13 (1 in 795)	0.18 (1 in 551)	0.68 (1 in 147)
Uterine corpus	Female	0.07 (1 in 1,348)	0.77 (1 in 129)	0.89 (1 in 112)	1.25 (1 in 80)	2.64 (1 in 38)

*For those who are cancer-free at the beginning of each age interval. †All sites excludes basal cell and squamous cell skin cancers and in situ cancers except urinary bladder. ‡Includes invasive and in situ cancers. §Statistic is for whites only.
Source: DevCan: Probability of Developing or Dying of Cancer Software, Version 6.6.1. Statistical Research and Applications Branch, National Cancer Institute, 2012. www.srab.cancer.gov/devcan.

American Cancer Society, Surveillance Research, 2013

through age 40 was leukemia, whereas it was lung cancer after age 40. In contrast, the leading type of cancer death in women was brain before age 20, breast between ages 20 and 59, and lung after age 60 [300]. However, these statistics can change over time. For instance, as increasing numbers of smoking adolescent females come to age and breast cancer is increasingly detected in surgically curable early stages, mortality rates from lung cancer will likely shift to younger females, eventually replacing breast cancer after age 40.

5.5 Cancer Prevalence, US 2009

Cancer prevalence refers to the number of individuals with any type of cancer alive at survey time regardless of when the diagnosis was established and whether they are cured, dying of the disease, or somewhere in between. Non-melanoma skin cancers are usually excluded. In essence, prevalence includes all cases of new and preexisting cancers that are alive at a particular time regardless of cancer status. Collection of such data requires a sufficient period of time to capture all previously diagnosed cases. In the US, the Connecticut Registry is the only registry with sufficient follow-up data (cancers diagnosed after 1935) enabling calculation of cancer prevalence. Prevalence data from this regional registry is extrapolated nationwide based on the total US population. The major interest of cancer prevalence data is to policy-makers, for it identifies the level of human and financial burden imposed by cancer on the health care system and the level of support required from public and private sources. As of January 1st, 2009, 12,549,000 Americans were alive with cancer: 5,809,000 (46 %) of these were men and 6,740,000 (54 %) were women [301]. Prevalence of most cancers was gender-unrelated, fairly evenly distributed between the genders. However, some were gender-impacted, including 65 % of oropharynx, 74 % of urinary bladder, 78 % of esophageal, and 81 % of larynx, and 100 % of prostate cancers in men, and 100 % of uterine, 98 % of breast, and 78 % of thyroid cancers in women. The four most prevalent cancers accounted for 61 % of all cancer patients alive in 2009. They were: female breast (22 % of the total), prostate (19 %), colorectal (11 %), and gynecologic (9 %) cancer. This is not surprising because the most prevalent cancers are those with high incidence rates and long survivals, which in turn hinges on being more amenable to early stage diagnosis and on exhibiting relatively slow tumor growth than most. For instance, in the 2005–2008 period, female breast cancer was diagnosed while confined to the primary site in 60 % of the cases and 98 % survived 5-years [302]. In the same timeframe, 81 % of prostate cancer cases were diagnosed as localized disease and exhibited a 100 % 5-year survival [303]. In fact, "prostate cancer that is present in the prostate gland but never detected or diagnosed during a patient's life…is greater than the number of men with clinically detected disease" [304]. These usually elderly men harboring unsuspected prostate cancer die of old age or of unrelated causes. On the other hand, aggressive cancers that are less frequently diagnosed in early stages, inoperable, or unresponsive to chemo- or radiation therapy represent a very small fraction of cancers included in any prevalence report. Such is the case of pancreatic cancer that even in its earliest stage (IA) exhibits a meager 2 % 5-year survival.

5.6 Trends in Cancer Incidence and Mortality, US 1975–2009

As shown in Fig. 5.2, cancer incidence rates[2] in the US rose 28 % from 400 cases in 1975 to a peak of 511 in 1992, when they began a slow decline to 465 new cases in 2009. Cancer mortality rates[2] rose more slowly (8 %), from 199 in 1975 to 215 in 1991 after which they declined to 173 by 2009. Hence, the three and a half decades spanning between 1975 and 2009 witnessed a 16 % rise in overall cancer incidence while cancer mortality declined 15 % overall. These changes were due mostly to the rapid rise in lung cancer incidence rates, especially in women, and a four- and a nearly two-fold increase in lung cancer mortality rates[2] among women (from 10 to more than 40) and men (from 50 to 95) between the 1964 Surgeon General Report that alerted the nation to the health risk of smoking and their 2002 and 1992 respective peaks. Lung cancer mortality rates were not offset by the sharp decline in

---

[2]Rates are per 100,000, age-adjusted to the 2000 US Standard Population.

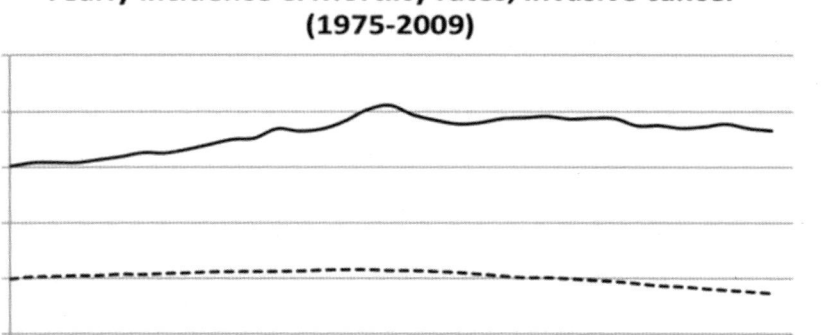

Fig. 5.2 Incidence (–)[3] and mortality (---)[4] rates for invasive cancers, US 1975–2009

stomach cancer in both men and women and other cancers with decreasing mortality rates through 2000. The drop in lung and breast cancer mortality since their respective peaks had a major impact on the overall drop in cancer mortality, though the former relates to prevention and the latter to early stage detection. Indeed, the approximately 30 % subsequent decline in lung cancer mortality is due to a 1.1 % decline in annual incidence rates linked to decreasing smoker population subsets rather than to early diagnosis or improved treatment. In contrast, the average 2.1 % annual decline in breast cancer mortality rates between 2000 and 2009 relates to increasing percentages of cases diagnosed in operable and potentially curable early stages (60 % of total cases in the 2002–2008 period with an average 98 % 5-year survival), reaching 37 % of total cases diagnosed *in situ* in 2009 [305], and to a lesser degree to improvements in the management of intermediate stages. These developments coupled to public awareness suggest that breast cancer incidence, estimated to become the leading female cancer in 2013, will continue to rise over the intermediate term while mortality should continue to decline. In contrast, the increasing number of females expected to develop lung cancer given the rise in female smoker population over the last two decades and the long latency between cause and effect, lung cancer mortality (26 % of total cancer deaths expected in 2013) is nearly twice (14 %) that of breast cancer (Fig. 5.1), and is expected to rise further in the intermediate term.

Overall cancer incidence and mortality trends often are misinterpreted, especially drops in the latter. By and large, rising incidence rates are linked to increasing numbers of people exposed to the causative agents or, more transiently, to improved accuracy of early-stage detection tools. The former is exemplified by increasing exposure to HPV by a growing segment of the population practicing oral sex that, during the 2004–2008 period, was responsible for most of the 11,726 annual cases

---

[3] Adapted from SEER 9 areas.
[4] Adapted from National Center for Health Statistics & CDC.

of oropharynx cancer. The latter is illustrated by the widespread use of Prostate Specific Antigen (PSA) that, by detecting previously unsuspected early-stage disease, nearly doubled the incidence of prostate cancer between 1987 and 1992, to 235.9 cases per 100,000 men without a corresponding rise in mortality. On the other hand, declining mortality rates are linked to decreasing incidence rates, early-stage diagnosis, improved treatment, or to combinations thereof. However, the combined impact of these and other factors often produce unexpected results or one can predominate. For instance, given their high incidence rates, cancers of the female breast, prostate, lung, and colon/rectum accounted for more than one-half of all cancer deaths in the US in 2008 [306], despite increasing detection of potentially curable early-stage cases of breast, prostate, and to a lesser extent, colorectal cancers. Yet, it is encouraging to note that in the decade of 2000–2009 (latest data available), cancers with decreasing cancer mortality trends (ovary, non-Hodgkin's lymphoma, bladder, brain, stomach, and AML) accounted for a cumulative 30.7 cancer deaths,[5] whereas mortality rates of cancers with increasing mortality trends (pancreas, liver, and uterus) were 20.5^3 [307]. Yet, it is sobering to note that, based on a 2008 death rate of 175.7^3 for all cancers, 124.5^3 (e.g., 70 % of total cancer deaths) died with cancers that were not impacted by nearly four decades of extraordinary economic and human efforts to bring cancer under control.

5.7 Historical Trends in Cancer Survival

Aside from mortality, survival is also used for a number of purposes, but mostly to assess progress in cancer control whether through early detection or treatment. For instance, female mortality trends since 1930 published by the ACS covering show a rise in lung cancer rates corresponding to increasing numbers of female smokers in the population but a precipitous decline in stomach and uterus cancer deaths between 1930 and 1975 and to a lesser degree colorectal cancer that preceded the era of rapid progress in cancer detection tools, safer anesthetic products and surgical techniques, or the advent of chemotherapy [308]. Alternative explanations include changes in dietary habits, food refrigeration, improved general medical support, and the like. However, none of these explanations adequately account for the fact that while trends in stomach mortality rates in men closely parallels women's, mortality rates for colorectal cancer in men and women went in opposite directions during the same period (Fig. 5.3) [309].

Survival also can be expressed as relative survival by time, as Annual Percentage Change (APC) for a variety of tumor and demographic variables, during specific periods of time. For instance, the overall relative survival for all sites, all ages, all races, and both sexes between 1988 and 2008 ranged from 78.7 % 1 year after diagnosis to 68 % at 3 years and 58.3 % at 10 years [310]. While these data show improved overall survival (OS) for that period, they also suggest that, on the average, cancer patients alive 3 years post-diagnosis have a nearly 80 % chance of remaining alive at ten. Likewise, APCs can be expressed for all or specific cancers

---

[5] Rates are per 100,000, age-adjusted to the 2000 US Standard Population.

Age-adjusted Cancer Death Rates*, Females by Site, US, 1930-2009

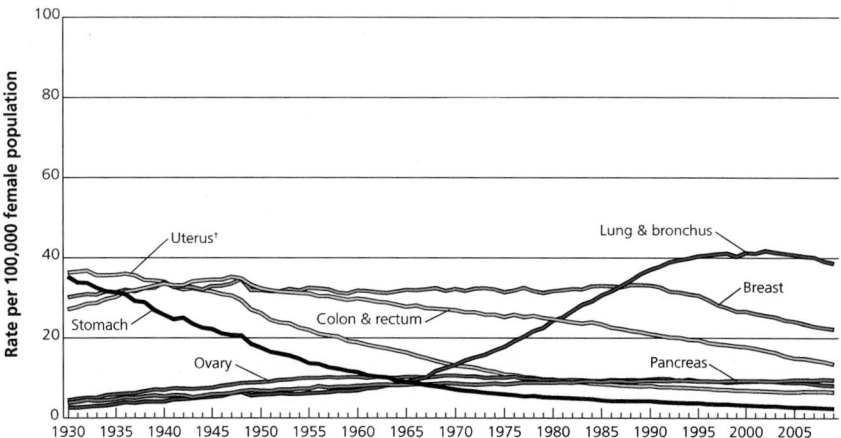

*Per 100,000, age adjusted to the 2000 US standard population. †Uterus refers to uterine cervix and uterine corpus combined.
Note: Due to changes in ICD coding, numerator information has changed over time. Rates for cancer of the lung and bronchus, colon and rectum, and ovary are affected by these coding changes.
Source: US Mortality Volumes 1930 to 1959, US Mortality Data 1960 to 2009, National Center for Health Statistics, Centers for Disease Control and Prevention.
©2013, American Cancer Society, Inc., Surveillance Research

Fig. 5.3 Reproduced from the American Cancer Society, Cancer Facts & Figures – 2013

sorted by year of diagnosis, race, sex, stage, etc. For instance, the APC for brain cancer mortality increased between 1975 and 1977, 1981 and 1991, as well as between 2007 and 2009, but decreased between 1977 and 1981, and between 1991 and 2007. While such statistics are of interest to health statisticians and economists, and to funding agencies when scrutinized prospectively, that knowledge is of little use to clinicians and clinical researchers. From a clinical standpoint, 5-year relative survival (i.e., adjusted to survival of the same age-group in the general population), sorted by different demographics and tumor criteria, is one of the most revealing and valuable. Five-year survival is useful for assessing age, sex, and racial differences for one or more tumor sites within a period of time. For instance, the relative 5-year survival for all cancers combined between 2002 and 2008 decreased progressively from 80 % below age 45–58 % by age 65. During the same time period, five cancers exhibited over 90 % 5-year survival in the white population (prostate, thyroid, testis, melanoma, and female breast cancer), but only two in black patients (prostate and thyroid), as shown in Table 5.3. The table demonstrates that stage is the single tumor variable that most affects the 5-year survival. While not shown, it must be reiterated that 5-year survival rates increase proportionally to the proportion of cases diagnosed in early-stage, for they are curable by surgical excision. Such are the cases of female breast cancer and melanoma, whereas pancreas and lung cancers exemplify tumors that are both difficult to diagnose in early stages and surgically challenging, reducing the chances of 5-year survivals. On the other hand, 5-year survival changes over several decades must be interpreted with caution, as they

Table 5.3 Reproduced from SEER program [311]

Five-year Relative Survival Rates (%) by Stage at Diagnosis, 2002–2008									
	All St	Local	Regional	Distant		All St	Local	Regional	Distant
Breast (female)	89	98	84	24	Ovary	44	92	72	27
Colon & rectum	64	90	70	12	Pancreas	6	23	9	2
Esophagus	17	38	20	3	Prostate	99	100	100	28
Kidney	71	91	64	12	Stomach	27	62	28	4
Larynx	61	76	42	35	Testis	95	99	96	73
Liver	15	28	10	3	Thyroid	98	100	97	54
Lung & bronchus	16	52	25	4	Urinary bladder	78	70	33	6
Melanoma of the skin	91	98	62	15	Uterine cervix	68	91	57	16
Oral cavity & pharynx	62	82	57	35	Uterine corpus	82	95	67	16

All St = All stages

represent the combined impact of a multitude of factors the effect of which is difficult to identify and assess individually, and at times might be meaningless. For instance, the 32 % rise in 5-year survival in prostate cancer from 66 % in 1975 to 100 % in 2008 corresponds to the advent of public awareness of effective tools to diagnose the disease in early asymptomatic stages, most of which are either surgically curable or of benign course. On the other hand, the stagnant 5-year survival (from 68 to 67 % over the same period) for cervical cancer [312] is more difficult to explain, given the excellent Papanicolaou (Pap) test to screen for early signs of cervical cancer, followed by curative conization[6] when needed [313], and more recently, the availability of a test to detect the presence of HPV on the surface of the cervix and of vaccines (Cervarix® and Gardasil®) to protect against HPV-16 and HPV-18 infections that cause 70 % of cervical cancers [314]. More importantly, while improvements in 5-year survival are frequently presented to the public and to policymakers as evidence of success in the War on Cancer, they should not be. Indeed, while progress has been made in the prevention of certain cancers, mainly cervical cancer, and the earlier detection of others, notably breast, prostate, and cervix, resulting in longer OS (called *lead-time bias*) compared to the shorter lifespan of individuals with more advanced disease diagnosed in the past, the greatest contributions to cancer survival are due to improvements in surgical techniques, anesthesia, antibiotics, and general medical support.

---

[6]The excision of a cone-shaped sample of the cervix for diagnostic or therapeutic purposes.

Chapter 6
An Uncontrolled Problem

> *Turn your face to the sun and the shadows fall behind you.*
>
> – Maori Proverb

In the US, cancer deaths and death rates increased year after year since records have been kept, reaching peaks in the early 1990s. Indeed, while 12,769 Americans were reported to have died of cancer in 1900 or 3.7 % of total 343,217 deaths, 158,335 cancer deaths were recorded in 1940, 553,768 in 2001, and 597,689 in 2010, or 11.2 %, 23 %, and 24 % of total deaths (1,417,269, 2,416,425, and 2,468,435, respectively). Although older statistics lack accuracy, they reveal that, while cancer was the eighth cause of death (64/100,000) in 1900, it has risen to be second only to heart disease since 1940, reaching a rate of 186/1000,000 in 2010 [315]. This progressive rise in cancer deaths is linked to four major factors: increasing population (Fig. 6.1), increasing longevity, and a shift to an older population (Fig. 6.2), placing more individuals at risk of exposure to carcinogens for longer periods, and hence, an increased probability of developing cancer.

As reported by the US Bureau of the Census, the US population expanded by 104 % between 1950 and 2010 (from 151.3 to 308.7 million). Moreover, during the same period, the over-65 population subset more than trebled: from 12.4 to 40.2 million (e.g., from approximately 7.9–13 % of the total US population, respectively), as shown in Fig. 6.2. As a result of the aging population, the average life expectancy in the US rose from 62.9 years in 1950 to 78.7 years in 2010. In addition, 76 million American children born between 1945 and 1964, the so-called *baby boomers*, will reach the age of retirement in the late 2000s, further increasing the size of the aging population. Aging increases the risk of developing cancer, as approximately 75 % of cancers occur in individuals 55 years of age and older. Moreover, the risk rises exponentially with increasing age in both men and women. For example, the average age-specific cancer death rates during the 2000–2010 for both sexes were 11.7[1] for the 30–34 age group, but rose to 153.8[1] for ages 50–54, 870.2[1] for ages 70–74, and peaked at 1,759.2[1] for individuals age 85 and over (Fig. 6.3) [316].

Substantial gains in life expectancy also have occurred in other regions of the world, except Sub-Saharan Africa, which accounted for 66 % of the 1.8 million

---

[1] Per 100,000.

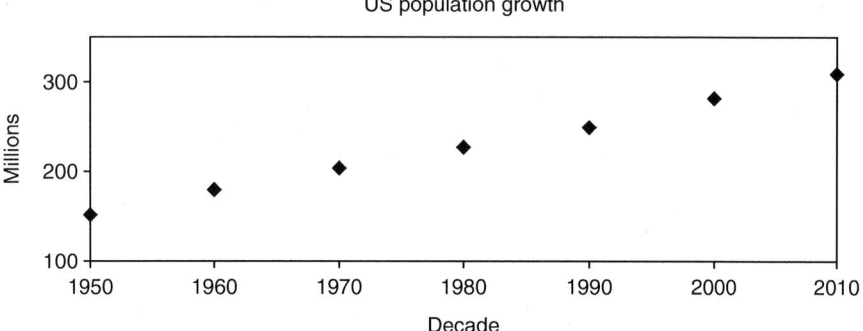

Fig. 6.1 US population, 1950–2010

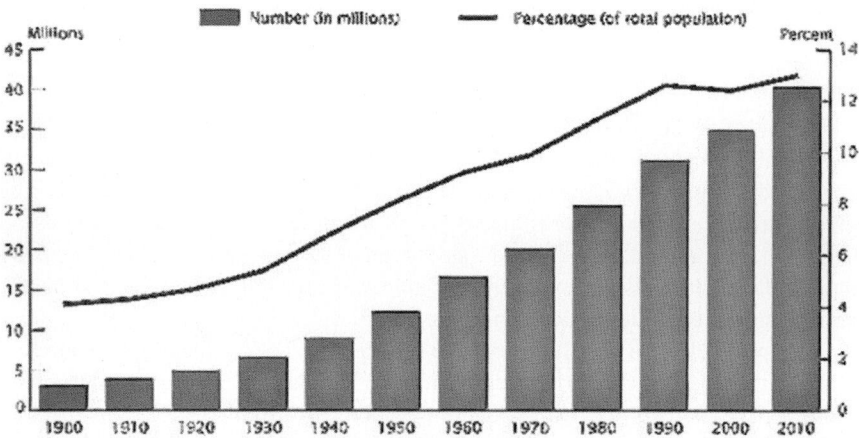

Fig. 6.2 Population 65 and over by size & percentage of the total population (Reproduced from Census Bureau decennial census of population, 1900–2010)

worldwide deaths from AIDS in 2010, the Russian Federation affected by the collapse of the socio-economic order where the average life expectancy has stagnated at 68.7 years since 1960, and some parts of Central Africa plagued by famine or convulsed by wholesale genocide. Whether such population aging trends are sustainable long term is questionable. While some believe biological factors will cap average life expectancy at approximately 85 years, others view improved nutrition, judicious behavioral and life-style changes, and broad-based access to ever improving health care as extending average life expectancy well beyond the 100-years mark. The latter scenario, though unlikely, is supported by rising rather than plateauing life expectancy in Western Europe and in Japan. In some of these countries, life expectancy is rising at a faster rate now than it did in

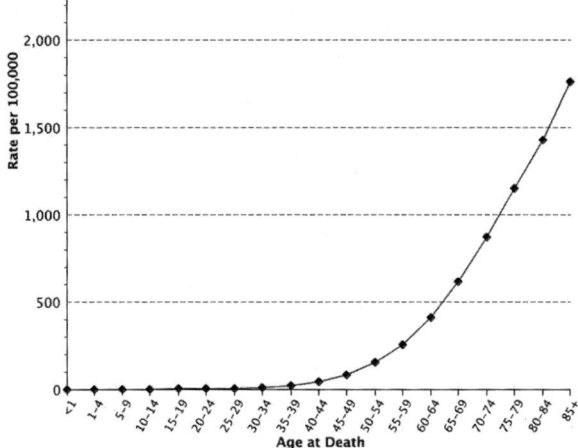

Fig. 6.3 Age range-specific cancer mortality rates, US 2000–2010 (Reproduced from National Center for Health Statistics, CDC)

the early 1900s. For instance, Japan enjoys the longest survival worldwide (83.0 years in 2009) after having soared 15.2 years since 1960 [317]. In the meantime, barring catastrophic events such as global wars or uncontrollable epidemics, the US and world populations will continue to increase and age for the foreseeable future. As a result, increasing numbers of individuals will be at risk of developing cancer and dying of their disease unless drastic changes are made in the way the *War on Cancer* is conducted.

Part IV
How Is Advanced Cancer Treated?

> *We physicians are creatures of habit. Surgeons operate whenever they can gain the use of the operating rooms, radiotherapists, for the most part, treat patients 5 days out of each week, not because we know it is the best schedule but because of interposing weekends, and medical oncologists treat patients on 'days 1 and 8' because of succeeding weekly clinics.*
>
> – Vincent T De Vita, Jr.

Chapter 7
The Cancer Cell-Kill Paradigm and Beyond

7.1 An Historical Overview

According to NCI, "Cancer is a term used for diseases in which abnormal cells divide without control and are able to invade other tissues" [318]. In fact, most definitions use "uncontrolled" proliferation or growth at their core. More generic terms include tumors and neoplasms, though they can be benign, pre-malignant, or malignant. Implicit in the terms tumor (*abnormal mass*) and neoplasm (*new growth*) is the notion that these processes, particularly in their malignant variety, like invading bacteria, are inherently different from the host and must be thoroughly eradicated in order to prevent metastases and death. The application of the infectious disease model to cancer steered cancer research, diagnosis, treatment, and outcome assessment strategies towards both surgical excision of early-stage disease and the cancer cell-killing paradigm to eradicate advanced cancer, which is the focus of this chapter. From this basis, two major practical corollaries followed. The first is that cancer research has been oriented towards the search for therapeutically exploitable differences between cancer and normal cells, guided by successive hypotheses ranging from excessive cancer cell proliferation [319], a misconceived generalization that drove drug use for decades, to tumor-specific antigens targetable for therapy [320], an illusion not yet abandoned. As decried in a recent article, "It could be argued that medical treatment of cancer for most of the past century was like trying to fix an automobile without any knowledge of the internal combustion engines or, for that matter, even the ability to look under the hood" [321]. The second corollary is the concept of *"cytotoxicity"* (e.g., cell killing) of rapidly dividing cells introduced to describe the quintessential property that drugs must exhibit in order to be successful in the treatment of disseminated cancer. However, how these drugs were to kill cancer cells preferentially while sparing normal cells was never adequately explored nor fully explained. The notion of cell-killing as the cornerstone of cancer treatment became untenable when the carcinogenic process was shown to involve oncogenes that promote cell growth, mutated tumor suppressor genes that fail to counteract cancer-promoting oncogenes, defective DNA repair genes that enable replication and propagation of unstable genomes, microRNA that control the expression of most human genes, or defective cell death pathways that confer a survival advantage to cancer cells. From this flawed concept about cancer treatment, an entire lexicon emerged in attempts to explain empirical clinical observations. For example, the tendency of some tumors to outgrow adjacent normal tissues, a phenomenon that can be slowed and sometimes stopped by anti-cancer drugs, suggested a pivotal role for the cell cycle in tumor growth and anti-cancer drug activity. Thus, cancer drugs were classified as *cell cycle dependent* if they acted upon one of the phases of the cell cycle, and *cell cycle independent* if their anti-tumor activity was independent of the cell cycle. The former, in turn, were classified as S-specific (drugs such as the antimetabolites and anti-purines that inhibit DNA synthesis), M-phase dependent (drugs that arrest mitosis, such as Vinca alkaloids, Podophyllotoxins and Taxanes), or G_1- and G_2-phase dependent, such as Corticosteroids and Asparaginase, and Bleomycin and Topotecan, respectively. Cell-cycle independent drugs included the alkylating agents, such as Busulfan, Melphalan, and Chlorambucil that, by crosslinking guanine nucleobases on the DNA, prevent uncoiling and replication of the double helix, hence the cell division. Mechanism of action to a large degree determined the type of toxicity. Likewise, it was quickly discovered that anti-tumor activity was dose-dependent, but, given its non-specificity, dose escalation was limited by type and severity of toxicity resulting from drug effect on normal cells. Thus, in order to enhance anti-tumor activity while reducing toxicity, drugs with different mechanisms of action were combined and administered intermittently to reduce toxicity on normal tissues, especially the high turnover bone marrow, and enable time to recover from toxicity between treatment cycles. Perhaps the most successful example of this approach was the MOPP (Nitrogen mustard, Vincristine, Prednisone, and Procarbazine) chemotherapy regimen for Hodgkin's disease that proved curative in most cases [322]. However, this early success was seldom replicated despite a myriad of clinical trials launched to test a variety of intermittent combination chemotherapy regimens in many types of cancers over the ensuing four decades.

In response to the marginal success achieved by cytotoxic chemotherapy in the management of most advanced malignancies, cancer researchers explored new treatment modalities with renewed enthusiasm and unrealistic expectations. One such direction was based on the *immune surveillance* hypothesis that emerged from observations made in the 1960s of an increased cancer risk in patients with severe congenital or acquired immunodeficiencies [323]. According to this hypothesis, cancer cells emerge from time to time but are eliminated by a sort of search-and-destroy defense mechanism before they can develop into full-blown tumors. Defects in immune surveillance were believed not only to contribute to cancer development but also to prevent the elimination of the few cancer cells remaining after successful chemotherapy, thus precluding relapses. This conceptually attractive hypothesis found widespread following. For example, at the *International Conference on Immune Surveillance* held at Brook Lodge, MI in May 1970, the Chairman opened the meeting declaring,

> Everyone here surely accepts the reality of tumor-specific immunity and would also favor the proposition that cell-mediated immune mechanisms have something to do with recognition and attack on tumor-specific antigens [324].

7.1 An Historical Overview

Proponents of the immune surveillance theory, supported by rare cases of "spontaneous" regressions of several human solid tumors [325], suggested that immune defects could be overcome and anti-tumor activity might be enhanced by immune stimulants. Experimental attempts to potentiate the anti-cancer properties of the immune system begun in the mid-1960s using BCG (Bacillus de Calmette Guérin), an attenuated strain of Mycobacterium bovis for the treatment of childhood leukemia [326], were followed in the 1970s and 1980s by the introduction of the Interferons [327], Levamisole [328], and the highly toxic Interleukins [329]. As the concept of cancer immunotherapy gathered momentum, new agents such as colony-stimulating factors and monoclonal antibodies [330] were added to the list under the evocative name *Biological Response Modifiers,* which are at the core of *Biological Therapy,* or *Biotherapy* for short. Their mechanism of action is said to "alter the interactions between the body's immune defenses and cancer, to boost, direct, or restore the body's ability to fight the disease" [331] and to,

- Stop, control, or suppress processes that permit cancer growth.
- Make cancer cells more recognizable and, therefore, more susceptible to destruction by the immune system.
- Boost the killing power of immune system cells, such as T cells, NK cells, and macrophages.
- Alter the growth patterns of cancer cells to promote behavior like that of healthy cells.
- Block or reverse the process that changes a normal cell or a precancerous cell into a cancerous cell.
- Enhance the body's ability to repair or replace normal cells damaged or destroyed by other forms of cancer treatment, such as chemotherapy or radiation.
- Prevent cancer cells from spreading to other parts of the body [332].

Each immune enhancer rode a wave of enthusiasm in the medical community and in the press. For example, Interferon, discovered in the early 1950s by Nagano and Kojima [333] (but attributed to Isaacs and Lindenmann in the English-language literature [334]) and produced in large scale from human white blood cells in the 1970s [335] or from cultures of genetically modified bacteria in the 1980s [336], and later from yeast and from recombinant mammalian cells [337], was greeted with a deluge of global media coverage thanks to astute promoters. It was touted as a "magic bullet", a "miracle cure", or "the genie in a fairy tale" that was equally effective for curing the common cold and cancer. Business media touted Interferon as a "*gold mine for patients and for companies.*" General enthusiasm about Interferon led the American Cancer Society to award, in the late 1970s, a $2 million grant, the largest in its history, to conduct clinical trials, and biotechnology firms Burroughs-Wellcome, Hoffmann-La Roche, and Schering-Plough to allocate large portions of their research and development (R&D) budget to Interferon. However, 2 months after *Time* Magazine heralded on its cover "Interferon: The IF drug for cancer", a May 1980 New York Times article raised doubts about the anti-cancer efficacy of Interferon based on unpublished clinical trial results. In response to the article, four scientists from the Sloan Kettering Institute for Cancer Research wrote a letter to the newspaper expressing concern that such reporting might undermine public support for interferon research. Eventually, as results of clinical trials became known, the public mood switched from premature enthusiasm to hasty pessimism, especially when four patients treated with interferon in France died as a result of the treatment. An historical analysis of the impact of the media on public perception of science [338] made the following observations using Interferon as an example. "First, imagery often replaced content...Second, the press covered Interferon research as a series of dramatic events. Readers were treated to hyperbole, to promotional coverage designed to raise their expectations and whet their interest." The role of scientists was described as follows: "Far from being neutral sources of information, scientists themselves actively sought a favorable press, equating public interest with research support." Nothing original here, for politicians most often claim their personal views to reflect their constituents'. Interleukin-2 (IL-2) was another darling of the media through the early 2000s, as typified by the premature enthusiasm of its main promoter, who wrote, "The demonstration that even bulky invasive tumours can undergo complete regression under appropriate immune stimulation by IL-2 has shown that it is indeed possible to treat cancer successfully by immune manipulation" [339], and his numerous guest appearances on ABC's "*World News Tonight with Peter Jennings*". Today, BCG is used for treating *in situ* bladder cancer, Interferons are active in Hairy cell leukemia, an extremely rare form of leukemia (fewer than 700 yearly cases in the US), and only marginally beneficial to 15 % of patients with disseminated skin melanoma and kidney cancer. Likewise, despite encouraging early reports [340] of IL-2 as part of a triad involving chemotherapy and "tumor-infiltrating" T-lymphocytes, its use is limited by severe adverse effects often requiring intensive care management when treating the only two types of cancer (e.g., skin melanoma and kidney cancer) for which it has shown relative efficacy. Indeed, the approximate 15 % long-term complete and partial responses in patients receiving high-dose IL-2 must be balanced by a concomitant 4 % death rate from complications [341].

A variant of immunotherapy was based on searching for antigens that could be used as therapeutic targets or for generating immune-enhancing vaccines. A dual strategy has been pursued: to attempt inducing antigen-specific immune responses in cancer patients or prevent its development. The former has used whole cancer cells or single-antigen peptides derived from cancer cells used alone or as complex cocktails combined with cytokines or other adjuvants[1] as an immune enhancer [342]. These approaches have been largely unsuccessful. Indeed, Provenge® was the first and thus far only FDA-approved (29 Apr 2010) therapeutic cancer vaccine. It is used for the treatment of hormone-refractory metastatic prostate cancer [343]. Although initially hailed as a breakthrough immunotherapy for prostate cancer, Provenge® has shown only a modest 4-month survival advantage compared to a placebo [344], despite an approximate $31,000 per infusion cost. In its second full year of marketing, Provenge® generated $325 million. In the meantime, another

---

[1] A secondary treatment modality, such as hormones, radiation, etc., added to the primary treatment.

7.1 An Historical Overview

direction of the *War on Cancer* that generated enormous enthusiasm and consumed large resources was the virus link. The old hypothesis that viruses caused most cancers was revived with renewed interest following the 1981 discovery of HTLV-1,[2] the first retrovirus [345], and of HIV[3] 2 years later [346]. Given the high stakes involved, the latter was marred by controversy and legal action [347], accentuated by the 1988 Nobel Prize in Physiology or Medicine awarded to two scientists of only one of two laboratories involved [348] that eventually ended in a sanitized version of the events written by the main participants [349]. The new push to find cancer-causing viruses, vigorously promoted and generously funded by NCI, helped establish a cancer link to eight viruses, listed in Table 7.1.

Table 7.1 Human cancer viruses (Adapted from ref. [350])

Virus	Cancer types	Year/references
Epstein–Barr virus (EBV)	Burkitt's, pharyngeal, some Hodgkin's	1964 – [351, 352]
Hepatitis B-virus (HBV)	Hepatocellular carcinoma.	1965 – [353]
T-cell Leukemia Virus (HTLV-1)	T-cell leukemia	1980 – [354]
Human Papilloma Virus (HPV-16/18)	Cervical, Penile, Oropharynx, Anogenital	1983/1984 – [355, 356]
Human Immunodeficiency Virus (HIV)	AIDS	1987 – [357]
Hepatitis C-virus (HCV)	Hepatocellular carcinoma.	1989 – [358]
Kaposi's sarcoma virus (KHSV)	Kaposi's sarcoma & Castleman's disease	1994 – [359]
Merkel-cell polyomavirus (MCV)	Merkel cell carcinoma.	2008 – [360]

However, by the mid-1990s, it became clear that the notion that most cancers were caused by viruses was a false lead, and the idea was largely discarded. Nevertheless, a successful strategy has emerged to use vaccines against known cancer-causing or promoting viruses responsible for approximately 15 % of all cancers. To date, the FDA has approved Cervarix® (16 Oct 2009) and Gardasil® (22 Dec 2010), two highly efficacious cancer-preventive vaccines that protect against the HPV-16 and HPV-18 infections that cause approximately 70 % of all cases of cervical cancer worldwide. While Gardasil® and Cervarix® are highly effective in cervical cancer prevention, our inability to develop effective bio-therapeutic agents and the very modest survival outcome gain associated with the use of Provenge® suggest that therapeutic immunotherapy is unlikely to play a prominent role in the future management of most cancers. On the other hand, die-hard supporters of immunodeficiency as a cause of cancer extend the scope of what they consider immune enhancers to products with very different mechanisms of action, including nonspecific inflammatory inducers, cytokines, monoclonal antibodies, and immunotoxins [361]. Regardless, after decades of clinical trials, at great human and financial cost, therapeutic immunotherapy of any type has shown marginal usefulness in the adjuvant setting and essentially none as primary treatment of advanced disease

---

[2] Human T-cell Leukemia Virus, the cause of a rare human leukemia.
[3] Human Immunodeficiency Virus.

[362]. This is not surprising given our current knowledge of cancer genetics and epigenetics, which suggests that most cancers develop and progress not as a result of immune deficiencies or by escaping immune detection, but driven by factors and mechanisms independent of any distinct cancer cell feature recognizable by the host's immune system.

While the search for anti-cancer agents progressed at a snail's pace, giant strides were being made in the development of both technologies and assays designed to detect internal and intra-cavitary tumors in early stages. The former include imaging techniques such as computerized axial tomography (CAT- or CT-scan), magnetic resonance imaging (MRI), and ultrasound, all suited to detect cancer at the multi-cellular level. The latter include cellular and molecular methods, such as cytogenetics, fluorescence in-situ hybridization, comparative genomic hybridization, spectral karyotype, microarrays, flow cytometry, genomic analysis, and polymerase chain reaction (PCR), all capable of detecting specific abnormalities at the subcellular or molecular levels [363, 364]. For example, PCR, a powerful molecular tool applicable to hematologic malignancies, enables detection of as few as one leukemia or lymphoma cell out of one million normal cells [365]. To these must be added more ordinary laboratory testing for cell products that, although produced by normal cells often are produced in excess by cancer cells, such as PSA and Chorioembrionic Antigen, which are associated with prostate and colon cancer, respectively. Such remarkable discriminant diagnostic power has thrust the definition and notion of complete remission from the clinical and pathologic domains to the molecular realm and to detection of increasing numbers of surgically resectable and potentially curable early stage cases. However, this has had two unintended consequences: one, fostering more aggressive and prolonged chemotherapy in attempts to eradicate the very last detectable cancer cell and achieve complete molecular remissions, inevitably resulting in greater toxicity; the other, in diagnosing and treating early non-progressive disease with little impact on the bearer's survival. Regardless of its definition, complete remissions are rarely achieved and true cures remain elusive, forcing the coinage of an entire lexicon of terms designed to characterize and quantify intermediate treatment outcomes. These fall under two general categories: tumor outcomes and patient outcomes. The former includes an array of terms that often complicate direct comparison of clinical trials results, such as partial and complete remission, response duration, and time to progression. The latter is measured by survival prolongation and Quality of Life (QOL) or health-related QOL (HRQOL) to be further discussed in Chap. 9. Tumor outcome assessment is useful as an early indication of the effectiveness of a particular therapy, but not for predicting patient survival, despite the fact that meaningful survival prolongation is generally preceded by complete remissions. On the other hand, patient survival constitutes the gold standard for gauging the success or failure of cancer treatment, as advocated by ASCO's Health Services Research Committee [366]. Survival rates are said to be *relative* when describing survival rates in cancer patients compared to those for persons in the general population matched for age, gender, race, and calendar year of observation. Relative survival also adjusts for life expectancy in the population at large. Unless qualified (such as disease-free or relapse-free), relative survival rates include persons who are living after diagnosis, whether disease-free or not. From a practical standpoint, 5-year survival is the preferred benchmark as a meaningful and achievable indicator of treatment outcome. Yet, while most patients achieve some degree of tumor response, 5-year survival rates remain unsatisfactory for most patients with advanced cancer, as discussed in Chap. 9. While all these terms were designed to assess, compare, and communicate outcomes of clinical cancer research, tumor response has become entrenched in the clinical setting as an indication of treatment success or failure. This is because, while patient survival is judged in retrospect, tumor response is attractive to both physicians and patients, for it allows assessment of tumor status at each step, including marking the first step towards a complete remission and, it is hoped, prolonged survival or a need to change direction. However, focusing on tumor responses rather than on patient survival is an implicit acknowledgment of the ineffectiveness of anti-cancer agents and of the unresponsiveness of most cancers to such agents, and detracts clinicians from their primary raison d'être, mainly designing management plans to optimize patient welfare rather than relying on mostly ineffective drugs in attempts to maximize tumor shrinkage at any cost. This latter approach also misleads patients, given the promises implied in evocative words such as *response* and *remission* that permeate Oncologist-patient interactions, as further discussed in Chap. 12. More on this under the section, *The New Targeted Therapeutics* at the end of this chapter.

7.2 Nitrogen Mustard: Cytotoxic Chemotherapy Is Born

While surgery is most adept and successful at managing early stage cancer, Medical Oncology is the discipline that uses FDA-approved agents for treating advanced, inoperable cancer. Today, the vast majority of patients with disseminated or metastatic cancer are treated with chemotherapeutic drugs either alone or with surgery, radiotherapy, or biological agents as adjuvants. Cancer chemotherapy is a recent development, with its historical origins in observations of the toxic effects of mustard gas (sulfur mustard) in WWI servicemen, in soldiers and civilians accidentally exposed during the Bari raid during WWII, and in animal and human experimental studies preceding and during WWII, respectively. Mustard gas is the common name for 1,1-thiobis(2-chloroethane), a vesicant chemical warfare agent synthesized in 1860 by Frederick Guthrie (1833–1886) [367] and first used on July 12, 1917 near Ypres (Flanders). Thus, its alternate name: Yperite. Because it could penetrate masks and other protective equipment available during WWI, and given its widespread use by both sides of the conflict, its effects were particularly horrific and deadly. Out of 1,205,655 soldiers and civilians exposed to Mustard gas during WWI, 91,198 died [368]. In 1919, a captain in the US Medical Corps reported decreased white blood cell counts and depletion of the bone marrow and of lymphoid tissues in survivors of mustard gas exposure he treated in France [369]. Shortly thereafter, military researchers from the US Chemical Warfare Service reported similar effects in rabbits injected intravenously with dichloroethylsulfide contaminated with mustard gas [370]. Other reports between 1919 and 1921 described various properties of dichloroethylsulfide in vitro and in laboratory animals [371–373], previously developed for screening thousands of potential anti-cancer compounds [374, 375]. Fifteen years later, the anti-cancer activity of mustard gas in experimental animal models was reported for the first time [376]. At the beginning of WWII, the Office of Scientific Research and Development (OSRD), an agency of the US War Department, funded Milton Winternitz of Yale University to conduct secret chemical warfare research in search of antidotes [377]. Winternitz asked Alfred Gilman and Louis Goodman to assess these agents' therapeutic potential. Their initial studies confirmed the toxicity of nitrogen mustard (where the sulfur atom on the mustard gas is substituted by a nitrogen atom) on rabbits' blood cells, and later documented anti-tumor activity in mice xenotransplanted with a lymphoid tumor. These encouraging results led to the first experimental use of nitrogen mustard on JD, a 48 year-old Polish immigrant with refractory lymphosarcoma. Given the secrecy surrounding mustard gas studies, which remained in place well after the war had ended, JD's records were lost until May 2010, when two Yale surgeons found their off-site location through persistence and luck and revealed their content at the a Yale Bicentennial Lecture on January 19, 2011 [378]. Unsurprisingly, nowhere in JD's record was nitrogen mustard mentioned, with references instead to a "lymphocidal" agent or "substance X." Given its historical significance and interest to our readers, a synopsis of JD's clinical case is included.

In August 1940, JD developed rapidly enlarging tonsillar, submandibular, and neck lymph nodes that revealed lymphosarcoma when biopsied. Referred to Yale Medical Center in February 1941,

> He underwent external beam radiation for 16 consecutive days with considerable reduction in tumor size and amelioration of his symptoms. However, his improvement was short lived, and by June 1941, he required additional surgery to remove cervical tumors. He underwent several more cycles of radiation to reduce the size of the tumors, but by the end of the year they became unresponsive and had spread to the axilla. By August 1942, two years after the initial onset of symptoms, he suffered from respiratory distress, dysphagia, and weight loss, and his prognosis appeared hopeless [379].

Having exhausted standard lymphoma treatment, Drs. Gillman, Goodman, and Gustaf Lindskog, a Yale surgeon, offered JD Nitrogen Mustard as an experimental treatment.

> At 10 a.m. on August 27, 1942, JD received his first dose of chemotherapy recorded as 0.1 mg/kg of synthetic lymphocidal chemical. This dosage was based on toxicology studies performed in rabbits. He received 10 daily intravenous injections, with symptomatic improvement noted after the fifth treatment. Biopsy following completion of the treatment course remarkably revealed no tumor tissue, and he was able to eat and move his head without difficulty. However, by the following week, his white blood cell count and platelet count began to decrease, resulting in gingival bleeding and requiring blood transfusions. One week later, he was noted to have considerable sputum production with

recurrence of petechiae,[4] necessitating an additional transfusion. By day 49, his tumors had recurred, and chemotherapy was resumed with a 3-day course of "lymphocidin". The response was short-lived, and he was administered another 6-day course of substance "X". Unfortunately, he began experiencing intraoral bleeding and multiple peripheral hematomas and died peacefully on December 1, 1942 (day 96). Autopsy revealed erosion and hemorrhage of the buccal mucosa, emaciation, and extreme aplasia of the bone marrow with replacement by fat [380].

Given the secrecy surrounding research involving war gas, all experimental studies were kept secret until 1946 when the Yale researchers were allowed to begin publishing their wartime clinical experiments, the first of which included the following disclosure:

> This paper was prepared as a background for forthcoming articles on the clinical application of the 3-chloroethyl amines with the approval of the following agencies: Medical Division, Chemical Warfare Service, United States Army; Division 9, NDRC, and Division 5, Committee on Medical Research, OSRD; Committee on Treatment of Gas Casualties, Division of Medical Sciences, NRC; and Chemical Warfare Representative, British Commonwealth Scientific Office [381].

In the meantime, mustard gas was brought to the medical community's attention by a WWII incident when servicemen and civilians were accidentally exposed to the agent released during the bombardment of the Italian town of Bari by Hitler's Luftwaffe, on December 2, 1943, launching the era of cancer chemotherapy [382].

Bari was a usually sleepy town of approximately 65,000 people, capital city of the Apulia region on the Adriatic coast of the Italian "boot". Old Bari, perched on a promontory around its medieval fortified Castello Normanno Svevo, built in 1132 by Norman King Roger II, and the Basilica di San Nicola, built between 1087 and 1187, along with new Bari were transformed in late 1943 by the arrival of approximately 30 allied ships in its small harbor. Under British jurisdiction, Bari was the main supply center for British General Montgomery's Army, and had just been designated headquarters of the American Fifteenth Air Force division. Occasionally, German reconnaissance planes would fly over Bari undisturbed by the Allies who believed the Luftwaffe was spread too thin to mount a successful attack on the city. In the early afternoon of December 2, 1943, Werner Hahn, flying his Messerschmitt Me-210 reconnaissance plane, made two undisturbed high altitude passes over the city, reporting to his headquarters, led by Marshal's Albert Kesselring and Wolfram von Richthofen, two of the best and most underrated German tacticians of the war, the suitability of Bari as a target for an air strike. Later that day, British Air Vice-Marshall Sir Arthur Conningham held a press conference. Answering war correspondents' pointed questions regarding lax security, he declared, with characteristic British self-confidence, "I would consider it a personal insult if the enemy should send so much as one plane over the city" [383], despite knowing the town had no meaningful air or port defenses. A few hours later, a squadron of 105 twin-engine Junkers Ju-88 A-4 bombers led by Lieutenant Gustav Teuber left their base in northern Italy and, flying low to evade Allied radar, descended on Bari in a

---

[4] Tiny, flat, red, and round spots caused by intradermal bleeding.

surprise air raid that would become known as the "second Pearl Harbor". When the squadron arrived, the German pilots could hardly believe their eyes and their luck: The entire harbor was brightly lit, highlighting ships and personnel unloading cargo! A few rounds fired by the sole, antiquated anti-aircraft battery in the city were futile. By 19:50, 20 min after the raid began, 28 merchant ships and 8 allied ships were sunk or destroyed, including the U.S.S. *John Harvey*, a 7,176-ton Liberty-type American ship, carrying a secret load of 2,000 M47A1 60–70 lb sulfur mustard (mustard gas) bombs [384, 385]. Some of the mustard bombs were damaged,

> …causing liquid mustard to spill out into water already heavily contaminated with an oily slick from other damaged ships. Men who abandoned their ships for the safety of the water became covered with this oily mixture that provided an ideal solvent for sulfur mustard. The casualties were pulled from the water and sent to medical facilities unaware of what they carried with them on their clothes and skin. Equally unaware were the medical personnel who treated these casualties. Before a day passed, symptoms of mustard poisoning appeared in both the casualties and the medics. This disturbing and puzzling development was further compounded by the arrival of hundreds of civilians for treatment; they had been poisoned by a cloud of sulfur mustard vapor that blew over the city from some of the bombs that had exploded when the ship sank [386].

A witness of that evening's pandemonium later reported,

> Some mustard gas sank to the bottom of the harbour, but a lot floated on the oil. Many of the survivors – as well as rescuers, some of whom dived into the water to rescue others – were covered in mustard gas. The gas, oil, and phosphorus caused frightening burns. Also when the men reached the hospital in Bari, the heat in the operating theatres evaporated the mustard gas, allowing it to get into the surgeon's eyes, creating dreadful results [387].

At first, casualties seemed relatively modest compared to the extent of materiel losses. However, the symptoms exhibited by many survivors were not usually seen among war casualties. Moreover,

> The destroyer U.S.S. *Bistera,* well outside the harbor and undamaged by the raid, had pulled 30 men from the water in a rescue effort. By the next day, the officers and crew of the *Bistera* were blinded from the effects of the sulfur mustard carried onto the ship by those rescued [388].

Informed of the mysterious malady, Deputy Surgeon General Fred Blesse dispatched Lt. Col. Stewart Francis Alexander, a military physician. From his experience treating mustard gas victims during WWI, Dr. Alexander quickly suspected mustard gas. Carefully tallying the location of the victims at the time of the attack, he was able to trace the epicenter to the John Harvey, confirming mustard gas as the culprit when he located a fragment of an M47A1 bomb, which he knew carried the agent. By the end of the month, 83 of the 628 hospitalized military mustard gas victims had died. The number of civilian casualties, thought to have been much greater, could not be ascertained accurately, because most had sought refuge with relatives out of town. This would be the only episode of exposure to a chemical warfare agent during WWII. Allied Supreme Commander General Dwight D. Eisenhower approved Dr. Alexander's full report, though details of the episode were not declassified until 1959 [389]. British Prime Minister Winston S. Churchill ordered all British documents to be purged, listing mustard gas deaths as "burns due to enemy action". It was not until 1986 that the British Government finally acknowledged that British servicemen had been exposed to mustard gas during the Bari raid and amended survivors' pensions accordingly.

7.3 Drug Discovery: Five Decades of Trial & Error

While therapeutic exploitation of the cytotoxic effect of mustard gas on bone marrow and lymphoid tissues was suggested in 1935 [390], it would take another 15 years before awareness of the 1943 Bari incident and of the Yale group's 1946 publication would prompt an intense search for anti-cancer agents. Of the thousands of compounds generated and tested in animal models, nitrogen mustard, or NH_2, emerged as the first agent with anti-cancer activity similar to its parent compound but with less toxicity. Nitrogen mustard is still available today under the brand name Mustargen®. With the lifting of the US OSRD publication ban in 1946, a series of clinical trial reports demonstrating the therapeutic activity of nitrogen mustard in a variety of human malignancies [391–394], accelerated development of numerous derivatives with anti-cancer activity. Many are still in use today, including chlorambucil or Leukeran®, cyclophosphamide or Cytoxan®, Iphosphamide or Ifex®, and melphalan or Alkeran®. However, initial enthusiasm was tempered by the transient nature of tumor responses and the inescapable relapses. It would take 25 years of trial and error to discover the optimal utilization of nitrogen mustard derivatives that, combined with other drugs (vincristine, procarbazine, and prednisone), would prove capable of inducing prolonged, disease-free survival in most patients with Hodgkin's disease [395]. However, the drug screening approach can be traced back to Murray Shear of the Office of Cancer Investigations at the PHS, who, in 1935, organized a model drug screening program [396] that ultimately would test over 3,000 compounds in the murine S37 mouse model with the collaboration of US and international colleagues. However, only two compounds progressed to clinical trials but proven too toxic, and the program was abandoned in 1953. In the meantime, the success of penicillin in the treatment of WWII-related wound infections led to a large-scale screening program of potential antibiotics agents, and recognition of the role of p-aminobenzoic acid in the anti-streptococcal activity of sulfa drugs [397] led to a rational proposal for a new direction in drug development [398]. In the same timeframe, folic acid deficiency was found to produce a nitrogen mustard-like effect on the bone marrow, which led to the synthesis of anti-folic acid antagonists Aminopterin [399] that, in 1948, induced the first remissions in acute childhood leukemia [400] and the first cure of widespread gestational choriocarcinoma a few years later [401], and Amethopterin (today's Methotrexate) [402]. These successes stimulated the synthesis of numerous purines and pyrimidines antagonists, including 6-mercaptopurine [403] and 6-thioguanine [404], both still in use today. While such successes vindicated cogent and organized research, serendipity played a pivotal role in the discovery of numerous cancer drugs, including Vinca alkaloids, epipodophyllotoxins, and platinum, as well as X-rays, penicillin, and many other discoveries [405]. In fact, cancer drug development via mass screening of thousands of natural and synthetic compounds is a process pioneered by Paul Ehrlich at the turn of the twentieth century in his 7-year quest to discover anti-microbial agents. Such a step-by-step approach had its critics in prominent researchers as the National Cancer Act of 1971 was being debated. Sidney Farber, its main detractor, stated at a congressional House Health Subcommittee hearing,

> It is not necessary for us to make great progress in the cure of cancer, for us to have the full solution of all the problems of basic research. The history of Medicine is replete with examples of cures obtained years, decades and even centuries before the mechanism of action was understood for these cures [406].

Four decades later, the process of anti-cancer drug development remains mostly anchored on this century-old, conceptually antiquated, technically inefficient, labor intensive, costly, and low-yield "hit-and-miss" screening approach engineered and sponsored by the NCI. Indeed, in a massive, highly complex, and far-reaching undertaking, the NCI's Developmental Therapeutics Program (DTP) has operated a repository of natural and synthetic products that have been evaluated as potential anticancer agents for over 30 years. The repository, run by a private contractor, has accumulated over 600,000 compounds gathered from the world over. Additionally, since 1986 over 50,000 samples of plants and over 10,000 samples of marine invertebrates and algae from tropical and subtropical waters were added to the repository. The potential anti-cancer activity of each sample is assessed according to its capacity to inhibit the growth of 60 cancer cell-lines (NCI-60) representing leukemia, melanoma, and cancers of the lung, colon, brain, ovary, breast, prostate, and kidney as part of NCI's "In vitro Cell Line Screening Project" [407]. This project, fully implemented in 1990, has screened approximately 2,500 compounds per year using sequential steps, as follows: New compounds are first pre-screened for *in vitro* activity against 3 human cancer cell lines. If the growth of at least one cell line is inhibited, the compound is tested against each of the cell lines included in NCI-60. If one or more cell lines are killed, or their growth inhibited at very low concentrations, or if the compound has a unique mechanism of action, it progresses to the next step. At this point, the compound is tested against a standard panel of 12 tumor cell lines placed in individual "hollow-fibers" (small tubes that retain cells but are permeable to the compounds tested) and implanted in mice. Implanted mice are then administered the compound at two different doses, and 4 days later, the hollow-fibers are retrieved and analyzed for cell density. Agents that retard cell growth in implanted hollow-fibers are tested in mice transplanted with specific human cancers. Compounds that kill or inhibit tumor growth after approximately 30 days with minimal animal toxicity become eligible for pharmacology and toxicology studies in animal models and in humans, and, if successful, become eligible for clinical trials (described in the section *Clinical trials* in Chap. 10).

NCI's DTP was expected to expose growth inhibition patterns that would unveil groups of agents with distinct mechanisms of actions that in turn might reveal their molecular targets. However, no existing laboratory method can accurately predict the anti-cancer efficacy of a particular chemical and, despite high hopes and years of labor-intensive and costly search, relatively few clinically useful new cancer drugs emerged from NCI's DTP. Indeed, of 70,702 compounds screened between 1990 and 1998, 6,452 showed potential *in vitro* activity, 1,546 were chosen for testing in mice, 79 revealed some activity against human tumor cells, of which 10 (or 1.4 per 10,000 screened agents) were eligible for toxicity trials in animals and humans. Yet, according to NCI, "DTP has played an intimate role in the discovery or development of more than 40 U.S.-licensed chemotherapeutic agents, with the rest coming directly from the pharmaceutical industry" [408]. At this writing (May 2013), drugs still in use that can be partly traced to this trial-and-error drug discovery process range from Chlorambucil (1957), to Vincristine (1963), to Hydroxyurea (1967), to Cytosine arabinoside (1969), to BCNU (1977), to Etoposide (1983), to Mitoxantrone (1987), to Carboplatin (1989), to Fludarabine (1991), to Taxol (1992), to Erbitux (2004), and Erbulin (2010) [409]. Cytosine arabinoside, inspired by C-nucleoside derived compounds isolated from the Caribbean sponge *Cryototheca crypta*, and its fluorinated derivative Gemcitabine are the only cancer drugs rising from the sea. This extremely expensive, labor-intensive, and low-yield drug development approach gives additional meaning to the view, expressed at the turn of the century, that,

> The fields and forests, the apothecary shop and temple have been ransacked for some successful means of relief from this intractable malady. Hardly any animal has escaped making its contribution in hide or hair, tooth or toenail, thymus or thyroid, liver or spleen, in the vain search for means of relief [410].

More importantly, all drugs generated by this discovery process are cancer non-specific, cytotoxic agents toxic both to cancer and normal cells. Additionally, they exhibit a narrow "therapeutic window"[5] that renders them largely inefficacious against cancer. Attempts to enhance anti-cancer activity while minimizing toxicity have achieved neither, as described below.

7.4 Attempts to Surmount Cancer Drug Inefficacy: Five Decades Lost

When I published the *War on Cancer* in 2005, there were 76 FDA-approved anti-cancer (or anti-neoplastic) drugs. Seventeen of these had been classified by the WHO as "*essential*" for the treatment of "*curable cancers and those cancers where the cost-benefit ratio clearly favors drug treatment*" [411]. All 17, developed between 1953 and 1996, are now generic drugs available at low cost. Missing fromced expensive proprietary drugs, notably Imatinib Mesylate and Trastuxumab. Drugs included in a second and third groups, including most of the newer, more expensive drugs, were described as having "*some advantages in certain clinical situations*" and "*not essential for the effective delivery of*

---

[5] The margin between therapeutic and toxic effects.

cancer care", respectively [412]. Likewise, the WHO has included 5 new drugs in its 2011-updated list of "essential antineoplastic" drugs [413], but, once again, all are cytotoxic agents discovered between 1953 (Methotrexate) and 1996 (Docetaxel). Whether old or new, most cancer drugs in clinical use have anti-proliferative rather than anti-cancer activity, affecting proliferative cancer cells but also normal tissues with high rates of cell turnover. As a result, their therapeutic window is modest and side effects are the norm. With very few exceptions, most of these drugs were discovered by trial and error (i.e., synthetic analogs of the anthracycline antibiotic Daunorubicin), inference (i.e., Nitrogen mustard, a by-product of mustard gas), or serendipity (i.e., Mitoxantrone, a derivative of Ametantrone, a coal-tar derivative originally intended as an ink). For decades, agents initially developed to treat infections but discarded because of excessive toxicity, especially to highly proliferative bone marrow and intestinal lining cells, became prime candidates for screening for anti-cancer activity. Early examples of this strategy include Dactinomycin [414], the second antibiotic discovered after Penicillin, and other so-called anti-tumor antibiotics still in use today, such as Mitomycin-C, Daunorubicin, Mithramycin, Doxorubicin, Bleomycin, Mitoxantrone, and Idarubicin.

By 1951, thiopurines 6-thioquanine and 6-mercaptopurine had shown activity not only against acute leukemia but also in a variety of disorders, including herpes, gout, and as immunosuppressive agents in organ transplantation [415]. Based on observation of greater uracil uptake by rat hepatoma cells than by normal tissue, researchers at the University of Wisconsin synthesized 5-fluorouracil (5-FU) by fluorination of a uracil pyrimidine base [416]. This agent proved active against a range of solid tumors and remains the cornerstone for treating colon cancer today. Shortly thereafter, choriocarcinoma became the first curable invasive cancer and the future of chemotherapy seemed assured [417]. However, failure to replicate these successes in other cancers led researchers to search for exploitable differences between normal and cancer cell biology for therapeutic gain, focusing attention on the cell cycle. This, despite admonitions by a pioneer cancer researcher who warned,

> Those who have not been trained in chemistry or medicine may not realize how difficult the problem of cancer treatment really is. It is almost, not quite, but almost as hard as finding some agent that will dissolve away the left ear, say, yet leave the right ear unharmed: so slight is the difference between the cancer cell and its normal ancestors [418].

Nevertheless, it was discovered that while all cancer drugs seemed to block cell replication, they did so via inhibiting specific phases of the cell cycle (phase-specific drugs), or acting directly or indirectly on DNA, RNA or the cell membrane (not phase-specific drugs). Phase-specific drugs exert their effect either during the S or DNA synthesis phase, the M or mitotic phase, or during the G1 or G2 phases of the cell cycle. Hence, anti-tumor drugs are sub-classified into several distinct categories according to their mechanism of action. Alkylating agents, such as the nitrogen mustards, nitrosoureas, and the platinum subgroups, are not phase-specific drugs but impair cell replication by forming bonds with DNA, RNA and certain proteins. Anti-tumor antibiotics, such as Dactinomycin, Doxorubicin, and Bleomycin are non-phase-specific agents with a complex mechanism of action. These agents, best

7.4 Attempts to Surmount Cancer Drug Inefficacy: Five Decades Lost

exemplified by the Anthracyclin subgroup, can intercalate between base-pairs of DNA, disrupting DNA replication and RNA transcription, produce single- and double-stranded DNA splits, damage DNA through creation of free radicals, and possibly disrupt cell membranes; Antimetabolites, such as Methotrexate, Cytarabine, and 5-fluorouracil, are S-phase specific agents that are structural analogs to normally occurring metabolites involved in DNA synthesis. They exert their cytotoxic activity by competing with metabolites involved in key RNA or DNA regulatory enzymes or by directly substituting metabolites normally incorporated in the RNA or DNA molecules themselves; Mitotic inhibitors, best represented by the Vinca alkaloids (Vincristine and Vinblastine), bind tubulin, a cell protein that polymerizes to form the microtubular filaments along which chromosomes migrate during mitosis (cell division). Vinca alkaloids prevent tubulin polymerization, resulting in arrest of cell division in metaphase, followed by lysis; finally, a number of older drugs, such as L-asparaginase, and many of the newer ones, such as the monoclonal antibody and the immunotoxins groups, not to mention cancer-active hormones, have mechanisms of action that do not fit into any of these categories. Furthermore, as in any biologic process, the factors and steps involved in cytotoxic cell death are multifaceted and the result of a multitude of contributing intra- and extra-cellular signals, and other factors peculiar to a particular cancer and a given host. For example, one would expect that an antimetabolite purine analogue that blocks DNA synthesis via inhibiting DNA polymerase alpha, ribonucleotide reductase, and DNA primase, Fludarabine would be very active against cancers with high growth rates. Instead, it is active against and FDA-approved for the treatment of adult patients with B-CLL, a human malignancy characterized by one of the lowest growth rates where the main defect is impaired apoptosis that causes the accumulation of long-lived malignant cells. Additionally, cell cycle kinetics alone fail adequately to describe tumor growth or to explain unexpected tumor response patterns to anti-tumor drugs. Indeed, the cell cycle time for normal cells is 1–2 days versus 2–3 days in most cancers [419], and the proliferative cell pool in CML is up to tenfold greater than in AML, despite its much less aggressive course amenable to much longer survival. The explanation for this apparent incongruity rests on the fact that CML myeloblasts differentiate into mature, functional, and short-lived granulocytes, whereas AML myeloblasts do not, and, given their high proliferative rate and longer life span, accumulate rapidly [420, 421].

Thus, as clinical trial results often failed to confirm anti-tumor drug efficacy predicted by their presumed mechanisms of action and by cell kinetics data, new hypotheses were postulated to explain the observed discrepancies. H.E. Skipper and colleagues of the Southern Research Institute proposed an early and influential hypothesis based on the L1210 mouse leukemia model, a versatile animal tumor screening system adopted by NCI. The hypothesis included two laws widely regarded as ground-breaking [422]. The first law established that the doubling time of proliferating cancer cells is constant and exponential. The second law postulated that anti-tumor drugs follow "first-order kinetics"; that is, the fraction of cells killed by a given drug at a given dose in a given tumor is constant regardless of the size or state of the cancer. According to this view, a drug that kills 90 % of cells of a tumor will do so each time it is administered, whether the tumor is very large or microscopic. However, clinical observations were at variance with Skipper's laws, leading to the Mendelsohn's concept of growth fraction [423] and the Goldie-Coldman hypothesis on drug resistance, which is based on a mathematical model that predicts that tumor cells mutate to a resistant phenotype at a rate dependent on their intrinsic genetic instability [424]. Indeed, most human tumors do not expand exponentially and respond to chemotherapy, following patterns far more complex than suggested by a simplistic first order kinetics model.

According to Mendelsohn's concept of growth fraction, tumors are composed of proliferative and non-proliferative cell pools, with the former dictating the growth of the entire tumor and its response to chemotherapy [425]. Mendelsohn's concept of growth fraction provided the kinetic basis for the non-exponential growth pattern of human cancers first proposed by Gompertz in 1825. The Gompertzian tumor growth curve follows a sigmoid pattern, with the fastest growth occurring when tumors reach about one third of their final size, and slower growth at both ends of the curve when absolute and relative numbers of proliferative cells, respectively, are few. In theory, the growth rate and response to therapy of a tumor depends on where it lies on the Gompertzian curve, with small tumors and micro-metastases being more sensitive to chemotherapy and easier to eradicate than large tumors. However, clinical observations regarding metastatic recurrences after chemotherapy-induced complete remissions seemed to contradict this postulate, triggering several clinical trials designed to examine the issue scientifically. Of these, perhaps the most convincing was conducted in women with operable breast cancer given adjuvant chemotherapy in attempts to eradicate metastases [426]. After a 10-year follow-up, this study demonstrated that chemotherapy failed to eradicate most metastases, thus supporting the Goldie-Coldman hypothesis on drug resistance. According to this hypothesis, cancer cells mutate with a probability that increases exponentially with tumor size, with mutants-laden tumors larger than 0.1 cm^3 in size being incurable with any single anti-cancer drug.

None of these hypotheses led to more efficacious cancer management, and today, the outcome of most cancer patients remains grim, as illustrated by lung cancer, the most lethal malignancy in the US, accounting for 28 % of all cancer deaths estimated in 2013 and one of the few cancers for which numerous randomized clinical trials have compared best available care with numerous drug types in various combinations and permutations, enabling assessment of the evolution of lung cancer therapy over time and, by extension, of the evolving status of cancer management as a whole. This is illustrated by a meta-analysis[6] of 33 eligible randomized Phase III clinical trials conducted in North America between 1973 and 1994 on a total of 8,434 patients with advanced (stage III and IV) NSCLC.[7] Only 5 of the 33 trials showed a 2-month survival advantage of patients receiving the experimental drugs compared to controls, with median survivals edging up from 5.2 months in the

---

[6] A quantitative statistical analysis of combined studies to uncover patterns not obvious in any single study.

[7] Non-Small Cell Lung Cancer.

first decade (1973–1983) to 5.8 months in the second (1984–1994), with one outlier at 11 months. A previous meta-analysis of 21 Phase III clinical trials including 5,746 patients with advanced SCLC[8] conducted between 1970 and 1990 had reported a median survival advantage of 2 months or longer in 2 of 21 trials, but longer survival in 4 of 21 [427]. For comparison, patients with advanced-stage NSCLC in the SEER database exhibited no significant improvement in median survival between 1973 and 1974 (6.9 months) and 1993–1994 (7.3 months). These results from a total of 54 clinical trials conducted over a 22-year span involving 24 anti-cancer drugs used singly or in combination are not only sobering in themselves but, as the authors of one study correctly pointed out,

> Factors that may also have contributed to prolonged survival include improvements in supportive care and general medical management of these patients, in addition to more selective inclusion criteria for trials in more recent years. Improved surgical and imaging staging techniques may have also resulted in the identification and treatment with less extensive 'advanced-stage' disease in more recent years [428].

Since then, no breakthroughs have occurred. Indeed, in a 1998 article commemorating the 50th anniversary of Karnofsky's 1948 lung cancer trial, which achieved a 49 % response rate lasting 3 weeks and a median survival of 5 months in 35 patients treated with Nitrogen mustard [429], the author titled his essay, "The snail's pace of lung cancer therapy", and concluded, "in the past 50 years, the progress in controlling advanced or metastatic lung carcinoma has been slow, but minor improvements have been made" [430]. In 2002, a Cochrane Review reported on a meta-analysis performed on 52 randomized trials that included 9,387 patients with NSCLC, treated with surgery, radiation, or supportive care alone or with adjuvant chemotherapy. The addition of chemotherapy appeared to confer a marginal survival benefit, leading the authors to conclude very cautiously, "These results offer hope of progress and suggest that chemotherapy may have a role in treating this disease". The same year, a large phase III trial that randomized 1,207 patients with NSCLC to one of four chemotherapy regimens reported 16–21 % response rates, lasting 3.5–4.5 months, and median survivals ranging from 7.4 to 8.3 months [431]. Such discouraging results have led to instituting longer periods of treatment. For instance, a meta-analysis of 13 randomized controlled studies involving 3,027 patients with advanced NSCLC compared a standard number of chemotherapy cycles, to more cycles, to the standard number of cycles followed by additional cycles of an alternative chemotherapy, to treatment until disease progression. Outcomes studied included, not the seldom-achieved 5-year survival, but OS, PFS, adverse events (AE), and HRQL. Extending chemotherapy improved PFS "substantially", OS "modestly", and AE in all trials, but impaired HRQL in two of seven trials [432]. On the other hand, in another recent meta-analysis of seven randomized trials that included 1,559 patients with advanced NSCLC designed to ascertain the impact of prolonged chemotherapy on survival concluded that 4 cycles of chemotherapy or more increased PFS but not OS, and was associated with higher incidence

---

[8] Small Cell Lung Cancer.

of AE [433]. Today, and according to SEER, only 2.8 % of patients with advanced SCLC and 3.8 % of patients with advanced NSCLC achieved 5-year relative survivals in the 2002–2008 period [434]. Thus, the number one cancer killer in the US remains essentially unaffected after four decades of searching by means of hundreds of clinical trials assessing the efficacy of many anti-cancer drugs administered as single agents or in combination over varying periods of time. Given these sobering facts, it is astonishing that a review on the cost of NSCLC treatment by a prominent clinical researcher concluded,

> The available literature suggests that combined modality therapies for locally advanced NSCLC and most chemotherapeutic approaches used in the treatment of metastatic NSCLC fall within the generally accepted definitions of cost-effectiveness [435].

Attempts to increase the effectiveness of chemotherapeutic drugs and reduce toxicity followed three main paths: combination of drugs, dose intensity, and high-dose chemotherapy with stem cell rescue. Multi-drug regimens, modeled after the treatment of tuberculosis with combinations of antibiotics with different mechanisms of action and different side effects, were developed based on the premise that administration of drugs with non-overlapping mechanisms of action and different dose-limiting toxicities might reduce the emergence of drug-resistant mutants, exhibit greater therapeutic efficacy, and be less toxic [436, 437]. The first successful combination regimen was developed to treat childhood leukemia and became known by its acronym VAMP (vincristine, amethopterin, 6-mercaptopurine, prednisone) [438]. This well-designed regimen incorporated the potential advantages cited above, plus intensive, short, intermittent treatment cycles in attempts to achieve high leukemia-cell kill while allowing bone marrow recovery between treatment cycles. The increased rate and duration of remissions achieved caught researchers' attention, leading to large-scale studies testing the precept of the curability in childhood leukemia [439]. The success of this regimen influenced the design of the MOPP protocol (nitrogen mustard with vincristine, methotrexate, and prednisone) for advanced-stage Hodgkin's disease [440]. In a large study including 198 patients with mostly advanced stages III and IV Hodgkin's disease, MOPP induced unprecedented 80 % complete remission rates, and 68 % of patients remained disease-free beyond 10 years from the end of the treatment [441]. However, although the concept of combining drugs with different mechanisms of action and non-overlapping toxicities was quickly incorporated into almost all chemotherapy regimens to treat a variety of cancers, only one potentially curative regimen, named PVB (platinum, vinblastine, and bleomycin), this time for testicular cancer, was added to the list of highly successful regimens [442]. These isolated successes led researchers not to question the appropriateness of this approach or the efficacy of cytotoxic drugs, but to test escalation of drug delivery through "dose intensity" and "high-dose chemotherapy" as solutions for achieving higher cure rates.

Dose intensity refers to the cumulative dose administered over a prescribed period of time. It was based on the observation that reductions in the cumulative dose resulting from dose adjustments or treatment delays led to falling cure rates in Hodgkin's disease [443], and decreased tumor response rates in breast and colon cancers [444]. The concept of dose intensity was not espoused in the clinical setting, perhaps because it implied that chemotherapy regimens as initially designed were somehow therapeutically optimal, and attention quickly turned to dose intensification, an age-old notion that drugs are likely to be more effective if administered in very high doses. For instance, arsenic, the most widely used anti-cancer agent through the centuries, "could be given in large, heroic doses for variable periods… (and that)…timid doses were only homeopathic and not worthy of consideration" [445]. Under this scenario, the dose was escalated as permitted by the degree of "epithelial, neurologic or gastrointestinal toxicity." A gruesome example of arsenic balm toxicity reported in 1803 described, "In less than a month, it ate away the breast, the pectoral muscles, the ribs, and the pericardium so that one could see the heart beat for 3 days, after which she died" [446]. Two centuries later, the belief that potentially lethal doses of chemotherapy would cure cancer took hold when technological advances enabled administration of bone marrow or peripheral blood stem cells (BMSC and PBSC, respectively), the purpose of which was to "rescue" the most vulnerable tissue – the bone marrow – after patients received very high doses of chemo- and/or radiation-therapy. Patients treated according to this approach first receive high-dose chemotherapy, sometimes complemented by radiation therapy, which, although directed against cancer cells, also destroys the highly susceptible, fast dividing bone marrow cells. Then, the patient's damaged bone marrow, no longer able to make sufficient red blood cells to carry oxygen to tissues, white cells to fight infection, and platelets to prevent bleeding, can be "rescued" by intravenous infusion of stem cells contained in bone marrow or in peripheral blood. Cord blood is also used, though less frequently. Stem cells for transplantation can be preserved from the patient prior to treatment or obtained from a matched related or unrelated donor. In the first case, the transplant is called "autologous", in the latter, "allogeneic." In rare cases where donor cells derive from a patient's identical twin, the transplant is called "syngeneic". In allogeneic transplants, a graft-versus-tumor effect that occurs when donor lymphocytes recognize and attack cancer cells can play a crucial role in certain types of leukemia. On the other hand, when the number of matched HLA antigens is not ideal, a complication known as graft-versus-host disease (GVHD) can develop. During GVHD, engrafted immune T-lymphocytes identify host cells as foreign and damage them, especially skin, liver, and intestines. Several tools developed to take advantage of the former and treat the latter are beyond the scope and intent of this book, as is the discussion of other complications of stem cell transplantation.

The bone marrow rescue procedure, made possible by advances in histocompatibility typing methods in the 1960s, evolved from a majority of allogeneic bone marrow transplants in the 1970s and 1980s, to the technically easier and better tolerated autologous peripheral stem cell procedure that predominates today. Yet, high dose chemotherapy with BMSC and PBSC rescue has enjoyed phenomenal growth since the 1980s. For example, in 2010, 634 transplant teams in 45 countries performed a total of 30,012 first time transplants [447]. Of these, 41 % were allogeneic and 59 % were autologous. Indications included lymphoid neoplasia (59 %), leukemias (31 %), solid tumors (5 %), non-malignant disorders (3 %), bone marrow failure (2 %), and others (0.03 %). The source of donor cells was 40 % allogeneic, of which 71 % were PBSC, 22 % BMSC, and 6 % Cord blood, and 60 % were autologous, of which 99 % were PBSC, 0.9 % BMSC, and only 3 cases received cord blood. Hence, 88 % of all transplants performed in 2010 by the 634 teams were of PBSC [448]. While certain subsets of leukemias, lymphomas, and neuroblastoma of childhood often benefit from this approach, its impact on solid tumors has been deceiving. For example, after preliminary encouraging reports in the early 1990s, breast cancer patients and advocates began demanding this type of treatment, leading some US courts to mandate that insurance companies cover the costs of this expensive procedure. Many drives were organized in local communities to raise funds for uninsured breast cancer victims. As a result of public pressure, by the mid-1990s, most women with breast cancer were receiving the then-experimental treatment. Eventually, several randomized studies were begun in the late 1990s. Results from four of five breast cancer studies in America, Europe, and South Africa have shown that high-dose chemotherapy plus BMSC rescue conferred no survival advantage over conventional chemotherapy. In the largest of these studies, conducted by the Cancer and Leukemia Group B, 784 women with metastatic breast cancer were first treated with four cycles of conventional chemotherapy, and then randomized to either high dose chemotherapy plus PBSC rescue, or to intermediate dose chemotherapy. Women with hormone-receptor positive or unknown tumors received radiation therapy to the chest and Tamoxifen. DFS and OS at 3 years was comparable in both groups. There was a slight reduction in relapses (20 % vs. 28 %), but a higher death rate (7.4 % vs. 0 %) in women receiving high dose chemotherapy with PBSC rescue [449]. In another two trials involving 533 and 525 women with breast cancer, one conducted by the Eastern Cooperative Oncology Group, the other in Scandinavia, no survival advantage was demonstrated for women treated with high-dose chemotherapy plus autologous PBSC when compared to women receiving conventional-dose chemotherapy [450]. Likewise, a French study showed no difference in the two groups of women in terms of PFS or OS. The only contrasting study was conducted at the University of Witwatersrand in South Africa. However, inconsistencies in the records led to a formal audit at the request of the South African Medical Research Council and the University of Witwatersrand that found unequivocal evidence of scientific misconduct and data falsification that led to a formal retraction of the published data [451]. A meta-analysis of nine randomized trials involving 3,525 breast cancer patients, published in 2004, concluded that high-dose chemotherapy plus BMSC or PBSC transplantation offer no substantial survival advantage at 3 or 5 years over conventional chemotherapy [452]. This, despite more frequent and more severe side effects and impaired QOL during treatment. Thus, cumulative evidence has shown that, while valuable in acute leukemia, lymphoid neoplasia, and neuroblastoma, high-dose chemotherapy plus BMSC or PBSC transplantation is of little value in the management of breast cancer and of most other solid tumors. Hence, breast cancer is rarely an indication for transplantation. Indeed, only 66 cases of breast cancer or 0.2 % of 30,012 overall transplants were performed in 2010 by the European Blood and Marrow Transplantation Group [453]. Likewise, only 1 case of breast cancer was transplanted in the US out of 17,938 transplants performed between 2008 and 2011, which included 31 % of multiple myeloma and 19 % each of non-Hodgkin's lymphoma and acute myeloid leukemia [454]. The 5-year survival of these three most frequently transplanted conditions in ranged from 15 to 70 % depending on type of disease, status, age, Karnofsky performance status, and source of transplanted cells [455]. In multiple myeloma, seven randomized trials comparing autologous stem cell transplantation (ASCT) to conventional chemotherapy showed a survival advantage in three. Yet,

> a systematic review and meta-analysis of these randomized trials reported improved overall median progression-free survival with no significant improvement in OS following ASCT when compared to conventional chemotherapy" [hardly justifying declaring ASCT as the] "standard of care for multiple myeloma patients under the age of 65 with normal renal function [456].

Moreover, in a retrospective analysis of 1,036 patients who had undergone bone marrow transplantation for leukemia, lymphoma, and genetic disorders, the long-term incidence of second malignancies was 3.8-fold higher than in age-matched controls [457]. Thus, high dose chemotherapy followed by BMSC or PBSC rescue has yet to deliver on the high expectations of its proponents and is often associated with unforeseen long-term complications.

Nevertheless, allogeneic stem cell transplantation has proven valuable in hematologic malignancies where it can be curative to certain subsets of patients despite the potential for life-threatening complications. This is demonstrated by a review of 10,632 records reported to the CIBMTR[9] of patients who exhibited a 2-year DFS after completion of the first allogeneic hematopoietic cell transplantation (HCT) for AML and other hematologic diseases [458]. Median follow up was 9 years, and 3,788 patients were observed for at least 10 years. The review included 4,017 cases of AML, 85 % of whom received BMSC, with many receiving a conditioning regimen mostly without T-cell depletion or GVHD prophylaxis. The risk of mortality peaked at approximately 3 years after HCT, with most deaths being caused by relapsing or progressing disease, GVHD, infections, organ failure, and second malignancies, in that order [459]. Thirty-seven percent of AML and 35 % ALL patients were observed for 10 years or longer after transplantation. The probabilities for survival at 10 years after HCT were 84 % for both AML and ALL [460]. However, these excellent results are mitigated by the fact that most transplanted AML and ALL patients exhibited prognostic indicators predictive of favorable outcome, including age (94 % and 99 % below 50 years, respectively), status (Karnofsky score greater than 90 in 79 % and 81 %, respectively), and in 75 % and 65 %, the donor was an HLA[10]-identical sibling. Other prognostic indicators are paramount to data interpretation. Indeed,

> The value of allogeneic HSCT needs to be reassessed based on the identification of AML-related genetic changes that profoundly impact on prognosis, on the availability of different transplant sources (bone marrow, blood) and donor types (matched related, unrelated and haploidentical donors, umbilical cord stem cell grafts), and in light of the use of reduced-intensity conditioning (RIC) regimens [461].

---

[9] Center for International Blood and Marrow Transplant Research.
[10] Human Leukocyte Antigen system.

Nevertheless, these results must be assessed in view of chemotherapy-induced cure rates of approximately 80 % in childhood ALL [462] and 30–40 % AML [463]. Although dose intensity, multi-drug regimens, and high-dose chemotherapy with or without SCT proved largely unsuccessful strategies for overcoming drug resistance and for enhancing anti-tumor activity, especially in solid tumor management, their foundations were cogent. However, some proposals were highly imaginative if fanciful, as exemplified by "chronotherapy". This hypothesis theorized that the efficacy and toxicity of cancer drugs vary with human circadian rhythms. This idea led adhering oncologists to administer chemotherapy at odd hours of the day and night and at various infusion rates, expecting enhanced efficacy and reduced toxicity. Mathematical models were developed to match "chronotolerance" with "chronoefficacy" to take advantage of,

> ...differences in the circadian and cell cycle dynamics of host and cancer cells, especially with regard circadian entrainment and cell cycle variability...[leading to] Model-based personalized circadian drug delivery aimed at jointly improving tolerability and efficacy of anticancer drugs based on the circadian timing system of individual patients, using dedicated circadian biomarker and drug delivery technologies [464].

This was accomplished through electronic pumps and devices capable of delivering drugs at preset times, rates, and following certain infusion patterns designed to harmonize drug delivery with each patient's "biorhythm" [465] At the time, a chemotherapy textbook addressed "Circadian timing and toxicity", concluding, "This medical movement toward temporal considerations will abolish the separate science of chronobiology and ultimately make all biologists and physicians chronobiologists" [466]. Sections of Medical Chronobiology were instituted at several US medical schools to accommodate these new developments. Enthusiasm for this unusual approach to cancer treatment persists. In a review on the impact of biorhythms in cancer management, the author concluded, in part,

> [chronotherapy is a] logical therapy in which anti-cancer drugs are administered with optimal timing according to circadian rhythms of anti-cancer action and those of adverse effects on normal cells. Advances in chronobiology have identified the suprachiasmatic nucleus (SCN) as the center of biological rhythms and the area in which clock genes such as PER1, PER2, PER3, CLOCK, BMAL1, TIM, CRY1, CRY2, to generate and coordinate biological rhythms [467].

Interestingly, the issue of biorhythms-guided chemotherapy administration has spilled over non-medical disciplines, as revealed in a thesis by a student in Writing and Humanistic Studies who passionately denounced a presumed conspiracy of silence, writing,

> Circadian rhythms govern almost every process in our bodies. Chronotherapy is the practice of giving medications in synchrony with these rhythms. For cancer chemotherapy, study after study has shown that paying attention timing makes a big difference. Patients receiving chemotherapy at the specified times had their tumors shrink faster and suffered from fewer side effects. In a few studies, patients receiving chemotherapy linked to circadian rhythms survived longer than those who received their drugs at any random time of day. Yet some 25 years after the first human trials, most oncologists still have never heard of chronotherapy. This is the story of why. From money to attitude problems, logistics to dogma, the tale of chronotherapy's dance around the fringes of oncology has almost nothing to do with the science. Instead it is a story of a promising new therapeutic concept and how it

must contend with the interests of drug companies, insurance providers and an overburdened medical system steeped in a culture famously resistant to change [468].

Despite some dedicated and enthusiastic advocates, chronotherapy failed to become mainstream for the treatment of cancer, and is seldom practiced today but for notable exceptions [469]. In order to achieve that position, cancer chronotherapy must empirically address a pivotal question: how is the therapeutic exploitation of biorhythms expected to convert inefficacious cancer drugs of marginal benefit into efficacious agents?

This brief discussion of the evolution of cytotoxic chemotherapy demonstrates that, given its non-specificity and narrow therapeutic window, the anticancer activity of these drugs reached a low efficacy plateau that could not be breached by dose escalation, drug combination, SCT, timing or schedule of administration, or by other manipulations. As a result, and despite the most assiduous and lengthy efforts by the largest number of researchers ever assembled to conquer a disease, most advance-stage cancers respond only marginally to cytotoxic chemotherapy drugs.

7.5 The New Targeted Therapeutics

At the other extreme of the cancer drug development spectrum, in time and sophistication, are current attempts to design drugs to alter molecular targets pivotal to the proliferative or survival advantage of cancer cells, as exemplified by Gleevec®. This agent, the first of its kind, is a tyrosine kinase inhibitor that blocks the *bcr/abl* fusion gene-encoded product, and in so doing, removes the proliferative advantage of chronic myelogenous leukemia cells [470], without cell kill and with little toxicity. Our increasing understanding of genetic, epigenetic, and other phenomena that control normal cell biology and survival but also cancer development, progression, and metastasis has led to the era of targeted cancer therapeutics. In part due to the surging activity in this area, we now (May 2013) have 121 FDA-approved anti-cancer drugs (Fig. 7.1).

In this section, I will highlight some basic concepts and developments that illustrate the advantages, but also the limitations, of this novel cancer treatment modality, rather than engage in a detailed description of a vastly complex and rapidly evolving field. In contrast to non-specific cytotoxic drugs and radiation therapy, targeted cancer therapy involves agents that block or interfere with a variety of cellular processes that promote tumor development, growth, and progression [471]. Some examples are listed in Table 7.2. The most frequently chosen target is the group of tyrosine kinases, a large family of approximately 90 enzymes that regulate both tumorigenesis and tumor angiogenesis. Tyrosine kinases are of two classes: Receptor Tyrosine Kinases (RTKs) that are embedded in the cell membrane and Non-Receptor Tyrosine Kinases (NRTKs) that are located within the cell [472]. Hence, two main types of tyrosine kinase inhibitors have been developed: small tyrosine kinase inhibitor molecules (TKIs) that target both RTKs and NRTKs, and MoAbs that, too large to penetrate cells, target growth factor receptor tyrosine kinases and other cell surface receptors.

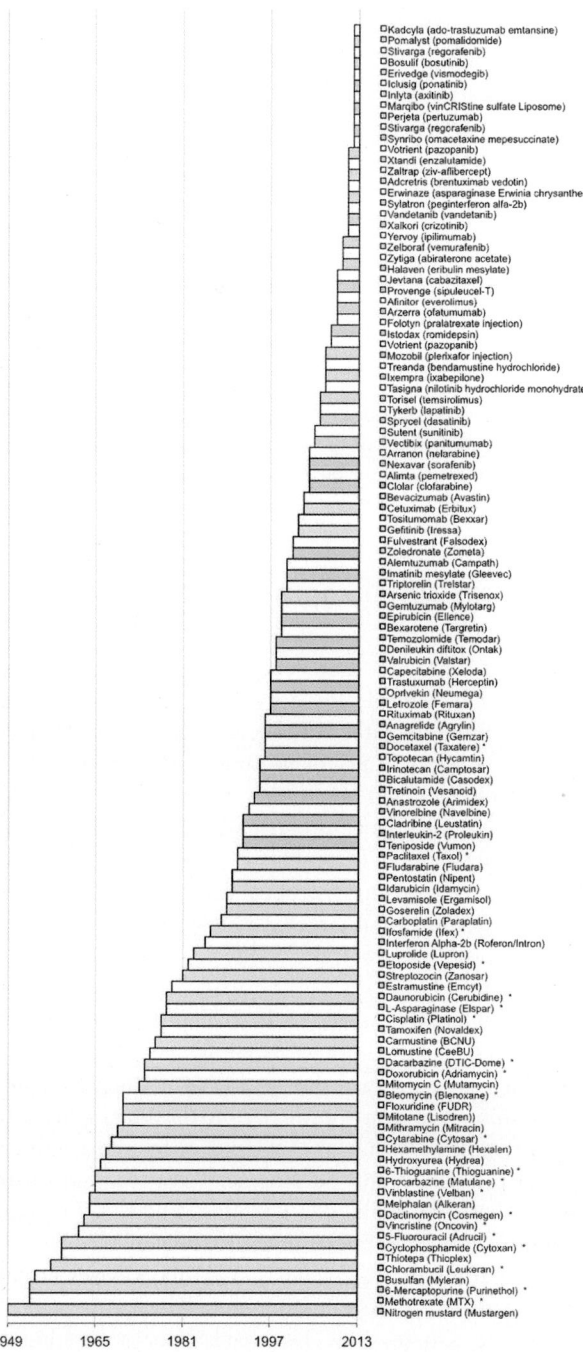

Fig. 7.1 FDA-approved anti-cancers drugs through February 2013

7.5 The New Targeted Therapeutics

Gleevec®, the first approved such agent, effectively blocks the activity of the mutant kinase fusion protein Bcr–Abl that drives CML and the c-Kit or PDGFR[11]-kinases that drive Gastrointestinal Stromal Tumors (GIST), inducing dramatic clinical responses. However, most responsive patients exhibit residual disease as determined by quantitative PCR for the Bcr–Abl fusion breakpoint and new mutations occuring in the targeted enzyme despite continued therapy, leading to drug-resistant tumor subclones and clinical relapses [473]. Gleevec® is also efficacious against chronic myelomonocytic leukemia and rare cases of dermatofibrosarcoma protuberans. Its efficacy in other types of cancers depends on the extent to which

Table 7.2 Major types of FDA-approved targeted agents and their main tumor targets [474]

Type	Name	Tumor target
Signal transduction inhibitors	Imatinib mesylate – Gleevec®	CML, GIST
	Trastuzumab – Herceptin®	Breast cancer
	Gefitinib – Iressa®	Non-small cell lung cancer
Gene expression regulators	Vorinostat – Zolinza®	Cutaneous T-cell lymphoma
	Tretinoid – Vesanoid®	Acute promyelocytic leukemia
	Romidespin Istodax®	Cutaneous T-cell lymphoma
Apoptosis inducers	Bortezomib – Velcade®	Multiple myeloma
	Carfitzomid Kiprolis®	Multiple myeloma
	Pralatrexate – Folotyn®	Peripheral T-cell lymphoma
Anti-angiogenesis[a]	Bevacizumab – Avastin®	Glioblastoma
	Pazopanib – Votrient®	Renal cell carcinoma
	Zlf-Aflibercept Zalprap®	Metastatic colorectal cancer
Immune stimulators	Ipilimuab – Yervoy®	Metastatic melanoma
	Rituximab – Rituxan®	Non-Hodgkin's lymphoma
	Alemtuzumab – Campath®	B-cell CLL
Immunotoxins[b]	Denileukin diftitox – Ontak®	Cutaneous T-cell lymphoma
	Brentuximab – Adcetris®	Lymphoma and Hodgkin's disease
	Tositumomab & Tositumomab-I[131]	B-cell non-Hodgkin lymphoma

[a]Block growth of blood vessels to tumors
[b]Monoclonal antibodies carrying a lethal payload (toxin, radioisotope, of IL2) to cancer cells

such cancers exhibit kinase-pathway abnormalities that drive tumor progression and whether such abnormalities occur early or late in the tumor progression [475]. Other examples of TKIs that interfere with the intracellular signaling of tyrosine kinases include EGFR, HER2/neu, and VEGF, which promote cell growth, proliferation, migration, and angiogenesis of both cancer and normal tissues. These molecular pathways are the most frequently targeted for the treatment of colorectal, lung, and breast cancer.

---

[11] Platelet derived growth factor receptor.

At the other end of the spectrum of targeting agents are monoclonal antibodies, with Orthoclone OKT3® being the first to receive FDA approval for human use in 1986. This MoAb targets the membrane protein CD3 receptor on T-lymphocytes interfering with immune processes, including acute rejection of transplanted organs, its main clinical indication [476]. MoAbs were greeted as the first true "magic bullets", an idea popularized by Paul Ehrlich, discoverer of Arsphenamine, the first efficacious agent against syphilis, and winner of the 1908 Nobel Prize in Physiology or Medicine for his work in immunology. Yet, it would take the advent of the hybridoma technology, described by Georges Köhler and César Milstein in 1975, for "designer" MoAbs to be developed against a wide range of targeted molecules from many laboratories, including my own in 1987 [477]. A major drawback of these large protein agents[12] is the need for intravenous administration to bypass the proteolytic function of the stomach, triggering anti-mouse antibody formation in patients so treated. This obstacle was overcome by the generation of human-mouse chimeric and humanized antibodies through genetic engineering that, by reaching their designated specific targets without triggering a host immune response, proved clinically valuable. Early MoAbs targeted differentiation markers on the cell surface, including CD20 (e.g., Rituxan®), CD33 (e.g., Myelotarg®), and CD52 (e.g., Campath®) that are over expressed or mutated on CLL, acute myeloid leukemia, and lymphoma cells, but are present on their normal counterparts. For instance, Rituxan®, the first such antibody, which received FDA-approval in 1997 for the treatment of refractory CLL and small cell lymphoma also has shown efficacy for the treatment of certain autoimmune diseases, such as rheumatoid arthritis [478]. The efficacy of targeted therapy has limits. For instance, Herceptin®, a MoAb efficacious in approximately 25 % of patients with breast cancers that overexpress the targeted HER2 receptor, shows no activity against the other 75 % of breast cancers that do not express it [479]. Likewise, cancer cells that are not or are less dependent on molecules being targeted will remain unaffected, as will the clinical outcome of patients so treated. In addition to attacking cancer cells via recruiting the host immune function, other approaches attempt to block intracellular signaling pathway inducing apoptosis or reducing angiogenesis, or to deliver a lethal payload directly to targeted cancer cells via MoAbs and other carrier molecules conjugated to radioisotopes or to toxins [480, 481]. Some of the earliest immunotoxins were developed in my lab in 1993 [482]. Immunotoxins bind to the targeted cell surface molecule, are subsequently internalized by endocytosis, and the toxin's enzymatic fragment translocates to the cytosol, killing the cell on a 1:1 ratio (e.g., one toxin kills one cell), making this approach theoretically the most efficient. Ontak® (IL-2 conjugated to diphtheria toxin) was the first (1999) and still only FDA-approved immunotoxin for human use. Its administration to persistent or recurrent CD-25 positive cutaneous T-cell lymphoma (CTCL) has induced modest prolongation in DFS. Currently (July 2013), a recombinant anti-CD3 immunotoxin (A-dmDT(390)-bisFv[UCHT1]) conjugate is undergoing phase I/II clinical trials in several CD3-positive malignant T-Cell tumors, including CTCL, Sézari syndrome, and Mycosis

---

[12] Approximately 150,000 Da *vs*. 500 Da for small-molecule inhibitors.

fungoides [483]. MoAbs-drug conjugates also have been developed. For instance, Adcetris®, a conjugate of anti-CD30 MoAb and monomethyl auristatin E, is designed to bind the cell surface CD30 where the monomethyl auristatin E is internalized to induce apoptosis. Clinical experience to date suggests that smaller toxin conjugates of either growth factor or Fv fragments of MoAbs are the most useful, especially for hematologic malignancies. Another targeted approach is exemplified by Provenge®, approved for the treatment of refractory metastatic prostate cancer. This agent, which consists of prostatic acid phosphatase (PAP) linked to granulocyte-macrophage (GM-CSF), is incubated with each patient's antigen-presenting cells to induce an immune response to the PAP, an antigen found on most prostate cancer cells. Despite the effort and cost involved in generating this therapeutic vaccine, its impact on patient survival has been marginal.

Speculating that molecules that control cancer cell biology and survival were not present on normal cells or were substantially different, it was initially hoped that targeted therapy would demonstrate high anti-tumor efficacy with minimal side effects. However, as in the case of non-specific cytotoxic chemotherapy, targeted therapy also can trigger side effects. In contrast to the former, which affects mostly rapidly dividing normal cells regardless of lineage, the latter affects all normal cells that express the targeted molecule. For instance, Gleevec® administered to CML or GIST patients also inhibits the kinase activity of c-Kit expressed on interstitial cells of Cajal[13] and on hematopoietic cells, inducing diarrhea and myelosuppression,[14] respectively. Musculoskeletal pain is another Gleevec® toxicity caused by inhibition of PDGFR expressed in muscle cells. Likewise, patients receiving Erbitux® for the treatment of colorectal or head and neck cancer often experience dermatologic and gastrointestinal side effects, for the targeted EGFR is present in normal skin and mucosal cells. In other instances, toxicity results from the combined effect of a targeted agent co-administered along with a cytotoxic drug. For instance, the concomitant administration of Herceptin® and anthracyclines for breast cancer has shown modestly to improve patient survival in approximately 25 % of women, but also to induce cardiomyopathies ranging from QT prolongation to heart failure, which is related to the apparent role of HER2 in cardiomyocyte development [484]. Targeting VEGF reduces tumor neo-vascularization, a critical factor for tumor growth, but can also affect VEGF-expressing normal blood vessels, thereby inducing toxicities, including bleeding, thrombosis, and hypertension.

Despite major advances in decoding the molecular pathways that drive cancer development, growth, and dissemination, targeting these pathways has produced mixed results. Gleevec®, Rituxan®, Sutent®, and Herceptin® have proven efficacious in the treatment of CML, CLL and non-Hodgkin's lymphoma, renal cell carcinoma, and subsets of breast cancer, respectively. Others have proven less effective than cytotoxic drugs in certain types of cancer. For instance, while 5-fluorouracil and Oxiliplatin improve patient outcomes in colon cancer, Camptosar®, Avastin®, and Erbitux® have shown no benefit. In other cases, tumor response appears medi-

---

[13] Gut cells that control the peristalsis of the small intestine.
[14] Depressed bone marrow capacity to produce blood cells.

ated through mechanisms other than the targeted receptor, calling into question the specificity of targeted therapy. For instance, it has been suggested that proteasome inhibitor Velcade® might owe its activity in multiple myeloma and mantle cell lymphoma to mechanisms other than apoptosis induction [485]. Likewise, clinical trial results failed to confirm the mechanism of action of Avastin®, an FDA-approved recombinant humanized MoAb, against VEGF for metastatic colorectal cancer, and of Iressa®, an agent that blocks the tyrosine kinase activity of EGFR that is overexpressed on NSCL cancer cells. Indeed, although a modest survival advantage was reported for patients receiving Avastin®, there was no correlation between pretreatment VEGF blood levels and treatment outcome, and Iressa® exhibits no activity against several types of cancer that express high levels of EGFR receptors [486, 487]. If specific targeting of cellular molecules presumed responsible for cancer development and progression has produced mixed results, indirect targeting is unlikely to be more successful, as illustrated by (Provenge®), the only FDA-approved immune-enhancing vaccine that, despite the enormous enthusiasm surrounding the concept of cancer immunotherapy, has not met expectations. Hence, given the long list of shortcomings of targeted therapeutics, it seems unlikely that targeting a single promoter of cancer development or progression will be sufficient to eradicate or control most cancers, contrary to the concept of "oncogene addiction" that theorizes that cancer hinges on one or a few genes to maintain the malignant phenotype [488]. Yet, the current practice of combining one or more cytotoxic drugs with a targeting agent seeking enhanced therapeutic effects suggests that we have not learned the lesson that a trial-and-error approach involving non-specific cancer agents, whatever their hypothetical target, has failed. Pursuing such an approach in attempts to vindicate new hypotheses is likely to suffer the same fate. Those who have witnessed the many thousands of clinical trials using a myriad of drug combinations and permutations in hopes of discovering the Holy Grail must be horrified at the prospect of re-cycling through another five decades of failure.

Chapter 8
Complementary and Alternative Medicine

> *Man is a credulous animal, and must believe something;*
> *in the absence of good ground for belief, he will be satisfied*
> *with bad ones.*
>
> – Bertrand Russell

The lure of non-traditional remedies for all sorts of ailments has been with us for centuries ranging from herbs, to fruits, to plants, to salts of several heavy metals. As described in the previous Chapter, NCI tested tens of thousands of compounds, including plants, marine invertebrates, and algae, in a vast and expensive but low yield effort to uncover anti-cancer agents. Yet, a number of clinically useful agents emerged from the search, including Irinotecan (Camptosar®), extracted from the Camptotheca Acuminata, a fern-like deciduous tree; Paclitaxel (Taxol®), extracted from the Pacific Yew tree; Etoposide (VePesid®), extracted from Podophyllum Peltatum, a North American herb; and Vincristine (Vincasar PFS®), extracted from the periwinkle plant. Such a powerful endorsement of the medicinal properties of plants is often used to justify the promotion of many empirically unproven "natural" means to treat ailments ranging from backaches to cancer. On the other hand, despite recent progress understanding the nature and causes of cancer, its standard treatment remains inefficacious at best and harmful at worst, and the lives of patients with disseminated cancer continue to be wretched and short. In such an environment, the stage was set for the proliferation of new alternate cancer treatment approaches, often promoted by self-serving healthcare providers or charlatans making farfetched claims. For historical perspective, I will cite only some of the most outlandish cancer remedies of the eighteenth, nineteenth, and twentieth centuries that captured the public imagination, including the *"Storck"* and *"lagartija"* cures, the *"cura famis"* and *"treatment by cold"*, and the *Gerson diet*, respectively.

In the eighteenth century, Anton Storck (1731–1803), a Viennese physician and Rector of the University of Vienna, claimed that a concoction of his based on hemlock (the highly toxic plant that caused Socrates death) was highly effective against breast and uterine cancers when administered in sufficiently high doses to cause faintness (his version of today's *toxicity-limiting* approach to chemotherapy dosing), though he had few followers and the method was abandoned. A colorful example of the extraordinary gullibility of physicians and of the public followed publication of a 14-page booklet, in 1783, by José Felipe Flores (1751–1824), a physician and professor at the Real University of Guatemala, praising the curative properties of a Central American *lagartija* (lizard) [489]. This particular lizard could cure many illnesses, including venereal diseases, leprosy, and cancer. The lizards had to be beheaded, skinned, disemboweled, and swallowed whole "while the flesh is still warm" [490]. One lizard per day was generally sufficient, but the dose could be increased to three lizards daily, which, according to Mexican Indian tradition, was always effective. To make the remedy more palatable and patients more compliant, animals could be sliced into small pieces and made into wafers or pellets "slightly smaller than a bullet"[491]. The exotic nature of this treatment, its peculiar formulation and dosing schedule, and the fact that it was shrouded in the mystique of an old American Indian remedy contributed to its immediate success and enthusiastic acceptance throughout Europe, where Flores' booklet was translated into French, German, English, and Italian. The lagartija cure was the subject of innumerable testimonials, several books and reports, and of at least one doctoral thesis before it finally vanished into oblivion half a century later.

In the nineteenth century, two of the most interesting cancer cures were the *cura famis* and *treatment by cold*. These are of interest to us because, although they rallied few patrons at the time, they resurfaced mutated in the late twentieth century, inspired by advances in molecular biology and biotechnology. The *cura famis,* or cure by starvation, consisted of starving the cancer through a water diet that could last up to 40 or 50 days. However, patient non-compliance and its ineffectiveness led to a more radical variant: the severing of the cancer's blood supply. The idea is attributed to William Harvey, who observed that ligation of afferent testicular arteries, to deprive the testis of nutrients, resulted in testicular atrophy and necrosis [492]. However, testicular cancer was the only natural target for such an approach given its anatomy that facilitated access to feeding vessels, and the procedure never caught on, despite its well-founded if simplistic rationale. One and a half centuries later, a variant of *cura famis* reappeared under the name of *angiogenesis inhibition*, or the starving of tumors using biological agents that inhibit new vessel formation necessary for cancer growth [493]. The *treatment by cold*, proposed by British surgeon John Hughes Bennett (1821–1875) consisted of applying cold, which he described as "one of the most powerful means we have to slow the progress of cancer" [494]. Bennett's method entailed applying a mixture of two parts of chopped ice and one part of sea salt to the tumor for 15–20 min each week [495]. Although this treatment had no effect on cancer progression, it seemed to alleviate pain. Bennett is better known for his emphasis on the use of the microscope in medical pathology, and is credited for first describing leukemia, though the credit should rightfully go to French physician Alfred Donné (1801–1878), inventor of the photoelectron microscope, also known as photoemission electron microscopy. Ironically, Bennett questioned the validity of Pasteur's pivotal experiments refuting spontaneous generation. It is worth mentioning that, although Bennett's treatment by cold method never achieved any degree of success, the concept resurfaced at the end of the twentieth century in the form of heat and hypoxia used as an adjunct to chemotherapy in futile attempts to enhance the susceptibility of cancer cells to the cytotoxicity of cancer drugs [496]. Heat or cold have been delivered during surgery ("thermo- or cryosurgery"), under magnetic resonance imaging guidance, to treat drug-resistant cancers, especially in anatomically inaccessible sites such as liver metastases, with limited success [497, 498]. The recycling of old ideas about cancer treatment is a reminder of the biblical admonition,

> The thing that hath been, it is that which shall be; and that which is done is that which shall be done: and there is no new thing under the sun [499].

In the twentieth century, it was the turn of the Gerson diet, among others, which was forcefully brought to my attention after publication of my 2005 book titled *The War on Cancer* [500]. In it, I exposed the poor outcomes of cytotoxic chemotherapy for treating advanced cancer, but did not include CAM approaches to cancer management as a potential solution, for my focus was on traditional medicine, and I was unaware of any convincing empirical evidence of their usefulness, despite their widespread use over decades, and in some cases, centuries. Interestingly, many of my statements and views expressed in that book were used or quoted by practitioners and promoters of CAM methods to bolsters their claim that their favorite alternate method succeeds where chemotherapy fails. To illustrate, a review of my book – published in the *Journal of Medical Truth*, no less – stated,

> What Faguet doesn't know – having spent all his life in the Cancer Establishment club – is that this technique already exists and has a documented *real* [original emphasis] cure rate of more than 40 %; it even cures pancreatic cancer. It's known as nutritional medicine or the Gerson Therapy. Therapeutic doses of nutrients combined with detoxification restores those molecular genetic pathways perfectly, predictably, and measurably. The dream of standard oncology is daily reality with this therapy [501].

Hence, while I have no intention of engaging in a pointless debate with promoters of non-traditional medicine, I decided to fill my knowledge void on the *Gerson diet*, arguably the best known non-traditional cancer cure method. My main source of information was gathered in April 2013 from the Gerson Institute website, which I assume to be current and the most reliable coverage of the Gerson diet. The following represents the essence of what I learned. Max Gerson (1881–1959), a German physician, developed the Gerson diet in the 1920s. According to the Gerson Institute, founded by his daughter in 1977,

> The Therapy activates the body's extraordinary ability to heal itself through an organic, vegetarian diet, raw juices, coffee enemas and natural supplements. The Gerson Therapy treats the underlying causes of disease: toxicity and nutritional deficiency…rather than selectively targeting a specific condition or symptom. Over the past 60 years, thousands of people have used the Gerson Therapy to recover from so-called "incurable" diseases, including: Cancer (including melanoma, breast cancer, prostate cancer, colon cancer, lymphoma, pancreatic cancer and many others)… [502].

While the Gerson diet includes supplements such as vitamin B-12, thyroid hormone, lugol's solution, pancreatic enzymes, and potassium, its curative power appears to rest on,

> ... flooding the body with nutrients from about 15–20 pounds of organically grown fruits and vegetables daily...[to] boost the body's own immune system to heal cancer, arthritis, heart disease, allergies, and many other degenerative diseases...[and on] Coffee enemas [up to 5 each day for cancer patients that] are the primary method of detoxification of the tissues and blood... [503].

No one will argue with the tenet that fresh fruits and vegetables must be part of a balanced diet or that certain unhealthy diets increase the risk of developing cancer, as documented in this book and elsewhere. However, reliance on any diet as the exclusive or primary approach to treating cancer is a farfetched proposition supported not by rigorous empirical evidence but by well-chosen testimonials. Likewise, I am not aware of any scientific study supporting the therapeutic value of coffee enemas in any disease, let alone cancer. In my judgment, this is another classic case of an *alternate method* supported by an *alternate proof* of concept, an approach that is broadly applicable to all CAM[1] methods. One wonders whether Gerson diet patients share the same cheerfulness after eating such voluminous amounts of fruits and vegetables day after day and after having submitted to 5 enemas each day, unless cured of their disease or having attained the 5-year survival benchmark. While such discomfort is justifiable for the occasional outlier long-term survivor, adhering to the Gerson diet or to any other CAM method as exclusive treatment enables the progression and dissemination of early-stage cancers, rendering such tumors incurable and fatal. Nevertheless, having gone through previous Chapters condemning traditional cancer management, readers will understand that critiquing CAM methods is not an indictment of CAM promoters, but of the lack of evidence-based proof of the efficacy of their methods. Indeed, most promoters of CAM methods, like practitioners of traditional medicine, believe in their approaches to cancer management despite repeated failures on both sides. Moreover, patients are free to make an informed choice of whatever treatment method they prefer, whether traditional or alternate. Yet, a rational resolution to the entrenched views on both sides must be guided by the evidence. Hence, I urge – better yet, challenge – promoters of non-traditional cancer treatment methods to conduct credible clinical trials on their own or assisted by clinical researchers at reputable cancer research centers of their choice. Such trials would generate the database necessary to assess the comparative advantages and disadvantages of each CAM method against each other and against traditional approaches to be disclosed to patients faced with a difficult choice. Should the outcome of any CAM trial match either pre-clinical claims or results from established traditional approaches, it could convert skeptics and become mainstream, but, more importantly, potentially benefit hundreds of thousands of cancer patients each year. In the meantime, I will continue to call for a paradigm shift in traditional cancer management to eventually conquer this large group of diseases that continue to frustrate

---

[1] Complementary and Alternative Medicine.

the scientific community, or at least ensure that treatment does not reduce QOL in patients unlikely to benefit, as proposed in the last Chapter.

Public and political pressure led NCI to establish the Office of Cancer Complementary and Alternative Medicine (OCCAM) in 1998. Its mission is "to acquire and develop high-quality information about cancer and CAM for NCI and for dissemination to the health care community, researchers, patients, and the general public," which it ensures through intramural and extramural research programs at a cost exceeding $100 million in 2011. In its latest report (2011), OCCAM listed the following CAM categories and subcategories under its radar [504],

- Alternative Medical Systems: Ayurveda, Homeopathy, Traditional Chinese Medicine, Tibetan Medicine.
- Energy therapies: Electromagnetic-based therapies, Biofield therapies.
- Exercise therapies: T'ai chi, Yoga asanas
- Manipulative and body-based methods: Chiropractic, Therapeutic massage, Osteopathy, Reflexology.
- Mind-body interventions: Meditation, Hypnosis, Art therapy, Biofeedback, Imagery, Relaxation therapy, Music therapy, Cognitive-behavioral therapy, Aromatherapy
- Nutritional therapeutics: Macrobiotic diet, Vegetarianism, Gerson therapy, Kelley/Gonzalez regimen, Vitamins, Soy.
- Pharmacological and biologic treatments: Antineoplastons, Low-dose naltrexone, Immunoaugmentative therapy, Laetrile.
- Spiritual therapies: Intercessory prayer, Spiritual healing.

Although exploring any realistic avenue that might lead to improving cancer management by evidence-based methods, as I advocate private CAM promoters should do, the breath and scope of CAM categories and subcategories under OCCAM's politically-correct radar is likely to take several decades without leading to the desired outcome. Instead of NCI's bewildering and self-defeating mandate, perhaps the best approach would be to encourage and sponsor clinical trials of the most popular CAM methods in each OCCAM category, a strategy that would prove cost-effective and conclusive.

Chapter 9
The Cell-Kill Paradigm: Bleak Outcomes

> *Insanity: doing the same thing over and over again and expecting different results.*
>
> – Albert Einstein

What has the cell-kill paradigm and its dominance of cancer research, diagnosis, treatment, and outcome assessment achieved in the context of the "War on Cancer" since the enactment of the National Cancer Act of 1971? The answer will vary depending on how achievement is measured and who does the assessment. For example, in a 1996 review article titled *The war on cancer* [505] marking the 25th birthday of the National Cancer Act of 1971, the author used a quote from Charles Dickens to dramatize its failure: "Dead, your Majesty. Dead, my lords and gentlemen. Dead, right reverends and wrong reverends of every order. Dead, men and women, born with Heavenly compassion in your hearts. And dying thus around us every day". Less than a year later, an editorial written by a former Director of the NCI rejoiced "Happy birthday 'War', you deserve a pat on the back" [506]. Both authors converged on crediting major scientific advances made during this period, especially the breathtaking advances in molecular biology and molecular genetics, including the genome project, that have revolutionized our knowledge about cancer. Yet, while both see a brighter future after these advances are applied to the practice of medicine, the former author concluded, "We must develop new approaches to control this plague of deaths, adopting an ethic of prevention ....to prevent disease before it becomes invasive and metastatic" [507].

Such drastically contrasting perceptions of the War on Cancer achievements seem surprising, for a dispassionate analysis of the facts should provide a clear and objective answer. However, selection and interpretation of some statistical endpoints can support different points of view. For instance, in a recent article, ACS staffers examined "trends in death rates for all cancers combined and 19 common cancers from 1970 to 2006 and review the contribution of prevention, early detection, and treatment to reducing cancer death rates", concluding,

> Progress in reducing cancer death rates is evident whether measured against baseline rates in 1970 or in 1990. Downturns in overall cancer death rates since the early 1990s are largely a result of tobacco control efforts beginning in the 1960s, screening and early detection for several cancers disseminated in the 1980s and 1990s, and modest to large improvements in treatment and survival for specific cancers [508].

While such a conclusion places prevention, early detection, and treatment on an equal footing, the authors correctly noted, "Lung, female breast, prostate, [and] colorectum [cancer] accounted for about 60–80 % of the total decrease in all-cancer death rates since 1990/91", which they attributed, also correctly, to smoking cessation and to screening for surgically resectable breast, colorectal, and prostate cancer. This implies a rather modest contribution by advanced cancer treatment to patient survival, despite the rhetoric and high cost of new cancer drugs in recent years, especially with the introduction of targeted therapeutics. For instance, the monthly Medicare price for Proleukin® was $13,503 at approval time (1992), $19,925 for Campath® (2001), and $19,425 for Arranon® (2005). Moreover, the high initial cost of some agents has increased over time, as exemplified by Gleevec® that cost Medicare $3,401 per month in 2001 but more than doubled to $92,000 annually to become a blockbuster drug for its manufacturer Novartis, with sales of $4.7 billion in 2012 [509]. The price escalation of 101 cancer drugs between the 1970s and 2008 has been compiled recently, comparing, on an interactive graph, monthly prices on approval to those in 2007 [510]. In a recent joint communication, 100 CML experts lamented, "Of the 12 drugs approved by the FDA for various cancer indications in 2012, 11 were priced above $100,000 per year" [511]. In addition to blockbuster drugs, "orphan" drugs[1] can be equally profitable, not because of their wide distribution but because of their unit price. For instance, Kalydeco®, a drug for first cystic fibrosis, costs $290,000 annually, while at $410,000 per patient per year, Soliris®, a drug used to treat paroxysmal nocturnal hemoglobinuria, is the world's priciest. It is to be noted that the essential "carte blanche" that pharmaceutical companies enjoy in pricing the new crop of targeted drugs will escalate cancer treatment costs so that only the well-off or the well-insured can afford them, marginalizing large populations in both rich and poor countries.

Other cancer experts, after years of clinical and research experience and a detailed multifactorial analysis of the facts, have pointed out that decreased cancer mortality reflects lower incidence and increased early detection with minor improvements in cancer treatment [512], and that,

> Factors other than treatment have contributed to lower mortality rates after 1992, and to increased survival over several decades. While the latter is due mostly to improvements in overall health care over time, the former resulted from public education campaigns that foster prevention via reduction in environmental and behavioral risk exposure, and early stage diagnosis via screening programs. Overall, fifty years of cytotoxic chemotherapy contributed minimally to the modest improvements in mortality rates or survival. This is because the faulty cell-kill paradigm, that views cancer as a *"new growth"* distinct from the host that must be eradicated at any cost, has misguided drug development and patient care for decades [513].

More recently (October 2012), the status of the war against cancer was reviewed by leading epidemiologists, researchers, clinicians, policy makers, cancer advocates, and industry representatives, who gathered in Lugano, Switzerland at the World Oncology Forum (WOF). Their consensus conclusion was even harsher:

---

[1] Drugs targeting rare diseases.

> Current strategies for controlling cancer are clearly not working: preventable cancers are not being prevented; patients are suffering and dying unnecessarily from cancers that are detectable and treatable; and the model for developing effective new curative therapies is not fit for purpose and needs a radical rethink [514].

At the final session, participants issued an appeal to world leaders to fulfill commitments made at the World Health Assembly in May 2012 to cut preventable deaths from non-communicable diseases by 25 % by 2025. *The Stop Cancer Now!* appeal was published in major newspapers on World Cancer Day (4 February 2013) followed by a subsequent editorial in The Lancet [515]. WOF participants' broad-based, if somewhat diffuse, 10-point plan rests mainly on waging a worldwide war against tobacco, developing early detection of cancers that are the most detectable, treatable, and have the greatest social impact, providing optimal pain control by removing bureaucratic, legal, and logistical barriers to the medical use of morphine, and accelerating delivery of affordable therapies to benefit patients across the world [516].

It is clear that in order to make progress in the War on Cancer, we must identify where progress has been made and where it has not, how progress is measured, and what confounding factors might impact data analysis. Only then will we be in a position to advocate and implement changes necessary to impact cancer patients' lives, to which the concept of value is central. Yet, while perception of what constitutes value in cancer care varies among stakeholders, patients' perception must predominate over all others, as pointed out at a recent conference convened by the drug industry,

> …value is 'in the eye of the beholder' and to which perceptions of value (both clinical and economic) vary among stakeholders, including patients, industry, insurers, politicians, physicians, advocacy and interest groups…the patient's concept of value must be given a primary role at the center of the cancer care ecosystem [517].

In that context, most patients agree that disease prevention, survival, and QOL epitomize the most meaningful issues they care about. Yet, interpretation of the latter two must take into account a host of impacting factors that, while tangential, are decisive for guiding and formulating cancer policy. Some of the most obvious confounding factors include recent shifts towards early-stage and slow-growing tumors and overall improvements in general medical care over time. For example, increasing numbers of early-stage and slow-growing tumors fostered by better screening tools contributed to rising incidence and survival rates, at least temporarily, while new screening tests are being implemented nationwide, as in the case of breast and prostate cancer. Likewise, refinements in cancer staging techniques have contributed to "stage migration" over time. That is, patients with occult metastases undetected in the era preceding CAT scans and MRI were classified as having local or regional disease, whereas they are now included in the advanced stage category. As a result of their removal from the former group and their inclusion in the latter, the average survival for both groups has risen. This is because fewer poor prognosis patients are included in the former group and the latter now includes patients with "early" advanced disease (based on CT or MRI staging), whereas in the past it was populated by patients with clinically far-advanced disease. An obvious contribution to declining incidence and death rates is linked to prevention and early-stage detection. The classic example is lung cancer where an approximately 30 % decline in lung cancer mortality after reaching a peak in 1991 is due to a 1.1 % decline in annual incidence rates linked to decreasing smoker populations rather than to early diagnosis or improved treatment. On the other hand, the average 2.1 % annual decline in breast cancer mortality rates between 2000 and 2009 was caused by increasing percentages of cases diagnosed in operable and potentially curable early stages [518], and to a lesser degree, to improvements in the management of intermediate stages. Less obvious is the impact of improvements in general medical support measures, such as potent antibiotics for treating chemotherapy-associated infections, easier access to blood product transfusions, and other life-sustaining measures that contribute to survival of previously fatal treatment complications. Efforts to control cancer necessarily must rest on three stools: prevention, early-stage diagnosis through screening, and treatment of patients who, for one reason or another, exhibit advanced-stage cancer at diagnosis. Hence, benchmarks to monitor must include trends in incidence rates to assess the effectiveness of preventive measures, survival and mortality rates to assess screening and treatment efficacy, and QOL to judge the impact of all cancer management efforts combined, but most particularly treatment of advanced-stage cancer [519].

In the next few pages, I will examine progress made thus far in the War on Cancer with a focus on 5-year survival and QOL of patients with invasive and metastatic cancers treated with cytotoxic chemotherapy. Experience with targeted therapeutics is limited and still evolving, though results to date seem to parallel those achieved with cytotoxic chemotherapy. Indeed, whereas "molecularly targeted therapeutics" evokes the notion of absolute cancer specificity and heralds therapeutic achievement,

> It is important to keep in mind that some older, empirically discovered agents are actually quite targeted – e.g., camptothecin derivatives that target topoisomerase I. On the other hand, some 'targeted therapies' that were designed to be directed against a specific target have been shown to have clinical utility for unrelated reasons (e.g., sorafenib [Nexavar] was not effective as a BRAF inhibitor; its utility likely stemmed instead from effects on the vascular endothelial growth factor [VEGF] receptor [VEGFR]). Finally, recent successes in cancer treatment may yet come from empirically derived chemical entities (e.g., bendamustine, which is active against a number of hematologic malignancies) [520].

Cure rates as a treatment outcome benchmark will not be addressed for lack of statistics and uncertainties on the meaning of the term, given the occurrence of minimal residual or slowly recurrent disease that can remain asymptomatic and undetected for years. Indeed, tests available for assessing the status of most cancers are non-specific and insufficiently sensitive to detect minimal residual disease in the absence of symptoms or signs of recurrence, and cancer-specific detection tools only exist for a few cancers and are not widely available. For example, while leukemias can be assessed at the cellular and molecular levels on easily accessible blood and bone marrow specimens, such highly discriminant detection tools are not available for most cancers. Furthermore, residual and early recurrent asymptomatic cancers other than leukemias are often deeply seated and must rely on cruder techniques, such as CT-scans and MRIs, for their detection as a prelude to obtaining a tissue specimen for pathologic confirmation, all subject to interpretation. Given these limitations, the consensus is that, for most patients and in most circumstances, a continuous DFS lasting 5 years or longer after completion of treatment is a strong indication that a recurrence is unlikely to occur. On the other hand, the 5-year survival benchmark is probably the best available, if imperfect, indication of therapeutic success.

The lack of meaningful progress in cancer treatment outcomes is shown by meager improvements in 5-year survival between 1975 and 2008 for the 10 most prevalent cancer sites that together accounted for 1.2 million cases in 2008 (e.g., 71 % of new cases) and 65.5 % of all cancer deaths. Indeed, 5-year survival gains between 1975 and 2008 for all patients regardless of demographics and disease stage exceeded 15 % in only four cancers (e.g., breast 15 %, kidney 22 %, non-Hodgkin's lymphoma 24 %, and prostate 32 %), were below 10 % in another four (e.g., pancreas 4 %, lung 5 %, thyroid 6 %, and bladder 7 %), and declined in two (e.g., larynx −3 % and uterus −4 %). For all cancer sites, the average 5-year survival improved by a modest 19 % between 1975 and 2008 (Fig. 9.1) [521]. As could be expected, these figures

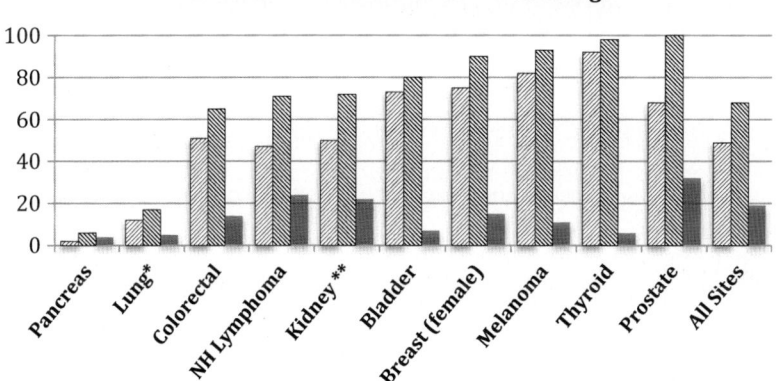

Fig. 9.1 Five-year survival rates for the ten most prevalent cancers and for all sites: 1975–1977 vs. 2002–2008 (* & bronchus, ** & renal pelvis)

are even worse for the subset of patients with advanced stage disease. Indeed, patients with advanced cancer within the subset of the ten most prevalent sites (approximately 45 % of total cases) exhibited the worst 5-year survival in the 2002–2008 period, averaging 2–16 % (Fig. 9.2) [522].

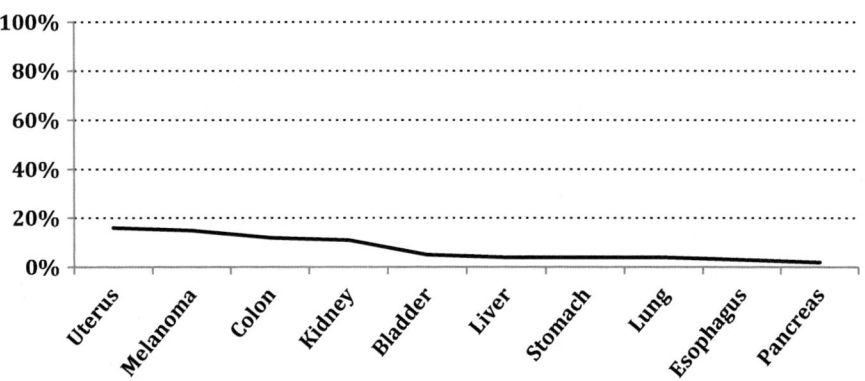

Fig. 9.2 The ten advanced cancers with the worst 5-year survival

In this context, the NCI's Cancer Trends Progress Report: 2011/2012 Update warns, "The nation is losing ground in other important areas that demand attention", listing, among others,

- Incidence rates of some cancers are rising, including melanoma of the skin, non-Hodgkin lymphoma, childhood cancer, cancers of the kidney and renal pelvis, leukemia, thyroid, pancreas, liver and intrahepatic bile duct, testis, myeloma, and esophagus.
- Lung cancer incidence rates in women continue to rise, but not as rapidly as before.
- Death rates for cancer of the pancreas, liver, intrahepatic bile duct, and corpus and unspecified uterus are increasing.
- More people are overweight and obese.
- Alcohol consumption has risen slightly since the mid-1990s. Fruit and vegetable intake is not increasing. Red meat and fat consumption are not decreasing.
- Pap test use peaked in 2000 at 81 %. Since then, it has fallen. Rates were 74 % in 2010. Mammography rates peaked in 2000 at 69 %. Rates dropped slightly between 2003 and 2005. Between 2008 and 2010, mammography rates stabilized at 67 %; screening for colorectal cancer remains lower than Pap testing and mammography, despite its proven effectiveness. However, use of colorectal cancer tests is increasing [523].

The notion that trends in incidence rates for approximately 40 % of cancers continue to rise is sobering and doesn't augur well for the future, and neither does the increasing death rates of another group of cancers. However, of greater concern are the future consequences of unabating unhealthy lifestyles and of non-adherence to screening recommendations that enable surgically resectable early-stage cancer to progress to fatal disease.

Finally, given the meager impact of chemotherapy and targeted therapeutics on mortality and survival rates, the attention of researchers and clinicians has recently turned to QOL as a desirable complementary or alternative goal of cancer management [524]. QOL is defined by the WHO as *"not only the lack of infirmity but also a state of physical, mental, and social well being."* While QOL is an intuitively easy notion to grasp and define in broad terms, as the WHO does, it is a multidimensional, dynamic, and subjective concept, impacted by psychological, spiritual, personal, familial, and social issues that, being unique to an individual, impact each differently [525]. Additionally, the attitudes of healthy individuals, nurses, and physicians towards chemotherapy *vis a vis* QOL differ substantially from those of cancer patients who, facing issues of life and death, are likely to perceive treatment benefits through a prism of hope and high expectations and to embrace any treatment that offers some respite, however slight, even to the detriment of QOL [526]. Hence, no consensus has been reached on how objectively to assess and quantify QOL or how to design treatment protocols with QOL outcome goals [527]. As a result, clinical trials focused on QOL remain limited in scope, uneven in quality, and more importantly, unable to provide concrete answers. Ideally, the pursuit of a cure, survival prolongation, or improved QOL should not be viewed as mutually exclusive but as concurrent goals in the context of treatment outcome. That is, a temporary assault of the patient's QOL by cytotoxic chemotherapy expected to cure or meaningfully prolong survival is amply justified. In contrast, this is not the case for most patients with advanced cancer where the inescapable negative impact of chemotherapy on QOL is not counterbalanced by a potentially favorable clinical outcome. Notwithstanding this self-evident principle, in practice, QOL is often invoked by tumor-focused physicians to justify to themselves and their despondent patients the use of inefficacious chemotherapy, oblivious to the fact that such decisions usually lead to more suffering without mitigating benefits. More on this later.

In conclusion, an objective analysis of cancer chemotherapy outcomes since President Nixon signed the National Cancer Act on December 23, 1971 reveals that, despite vast human and financial expenditures, the cell-kill paradigm has failed to achieve its objectives, the former rallying slogan *War on Cancer* has been abandoned by the NCI, and the conquest of cancer remains a distant and elusive goal. Moreover, as long as the use of inefficacious but toxic drugs is justified by the exigencies of the cell-kill paradigm, a model based on flawed premises with an unattainable goal, cytotoxic chemotherapy alone or as adjunct will neither eradicate cancer nor alleviate suffering. On the other hand, while targeted therapy has acquired an aura of being the next generation of therapeutic strategies in the management of cancer, reality on the field lags far behind theory and expectations. Hence, given the failure of both cytotoxic and targeted therapy to control advanced cancer but in a few cases and the success of surgical eradication of early-stage disease, prevention and screening should become the pillars of any national policy designed to control cancer, as will be discussed in the final Chapter.

Part V
Stakeholders' Role in the Status Quo

In the previous Chapter, I presented evidence that most advanced cancers remain incurable and progress in the War on Cancer measured by patient survival and QOL have improved little since the National Cancer Act was enacted in 1971. I have also shown that, in large measure, the stagnation results from an unbalanced focus on the efficacious treatment of advanced cancer to the detriment of prevention and early-stage detection, and to adherence to the infectious disease model that has driven drug development towards the cancer cell-kill paradigm, the hallmark of cytotoxic chemotherapy. The era of molecularly-targeted therapeutics, heralded by the advent of drugs that interfere with specific molecular events that promote cancer development and progression, remains largely unfulfilled. Indeed, despite therapeutic successes of some agents such as Gleveec®, broad-based results to date do not match early enthusiasm for this therapeutic modality. Hence, given the non-specificity and narrow therapeutic window of largely inefficacious cytotoxic drugs and our current inability to block complex molecular events that drive cancer development and progression effectively, it is unlikely that drugs available today in either category will succeed in controlling cancer. While others have previously questioned the status or direction of the War on Cancer, they have done so mostly within the confines of the scientific community [528–530], or have publicly denounced or implied a conspiracy among players in the cancer field [531], an unfounded position that merits little credibility. The questions we must ask are, why does such a system persist year after year, decade after decade, and why have so few voices decried this state of affairs? The answers to these questions can be found in an analysis of the entrenched views, perceptions, and motivations of the major stakeholders that directly or indirectly impact cancer drug development, clinical cancer research, and patient management, as described in the next two Chapters.

Chapter 10
The Role of the National Cancer Institute

> *The National Cancer Institute coordinates the National Cancer Program, which conducts and supports research, training, health information dissemination, and other programs with respect to the cause, diagnosis, prevention, and treatment of cancer, rehabilitation from cancer, and the continuing care of cancer patients and the families of cancer patients.*
>
> – NCI Mission Statement [532]

10.1 Current Organization, Role, and Influence

As one of the National Institutes of Health's 27 Institutes and Centers, NCI's broad mandate is exercised via its two key programs: the *Extramural Research Program* and the *Intramural Research Program*. The former links the NCI to a myriad of off-site investigators at academic institutions, research centers, and other sites throughout the country and overseas, whereas the latter encompasses the work of "almost 5,000 principal investigators, from basic scientists to clinical researchers [that] conduct earliest phase cancer clinical investigations of new agents and drugs." The NCI's Extramural Research Program includes five divisions:

- Division of Cancer Biology (DCB) that supports and facilitates basic research in all areas of cancer biology at academic institutions and research foundations across the United States and abroad.
- Division of Cancer Control and Population Sciences (DCCPS) that supports a comprehensive program of genetic, epidemiologic, behavioral, social, and surveillance cancer research.
- Division of Cancer Prevention (DCP) that supports research to determine and reduce a person's risk of developing cancer, as well as research to develop and evaluate cancer screening procedures.
- Division of Cancer Treatment and Diagnosis (DCTD) that supports the translation of promising research areas into improved diagnostic and therapeutic treatments for cancer patients.

- Division of Extramural Activities (DEA) that coordinates the scientific review of extramural research before funding, and provides systematic surveillance of that research after awards are made.

The NCI's Intramural Research Program includes:

- Center for Cancer Research (CCR), the basic and clinical intramural research program of NCI, which conducts research with the goal of improving the lives of people affected by cancer and HIV/AIDS.
- Division of Cancer Epidemiology and Genetics (DCEG), which conducts population and multidisciplinary research to discover the genetic and environmental determinants of cancer and the means of prevention [533].

Hence, given its large budget ($5.1 billion requested by the President for FY 2014) and reach, the NCI has the financial resources to, and does in fact, fund most of the nation's non-private cancer research at any given time. This financial muscle, backed by an excellent and far-reaching organizational infrastructure, gives the NCI the power to plan, prioritize, direct, coordinate, evaluate, administer, and serve as the focal point for most of the nation's basic and applied cancer research. It is ironic that the country that stands the tallest among nations for the free flow of ideas leads its War on Cancer through a central bureaucracy whose mandate is to control the type and direction of nearly all publicly funded cancer research. Thus, given its extraordinary influence on the direction of basic and applied cancer research, the NCI must be credited for the nation's advances in molecular biology and genetics of cancer, but should also be held accountable for four decades of near-stagnation in cancer management and control.

10.2 NCI's Cancer Centers Program Network

In 1961, the NIH established three new grant programs aimed at fostering cancer research in the United States. They included the Cancer Research Facilities Grant (CRFG), the Program Project Grants (PPG), and the Cancer Clinical Research Center Grant (CCRCG). These funding mechanisms were intended to support broad-based institutional and individual basic and applied cancer research. But it was the National Cancer Act of 1971 that broadened the center's mandate and scope to include research, patient care, training and education, and cancer control within the same institution. The intended multidisciplinary approach to Cancer Centers was patterned after well-established models, such as Roswell Park Cancer Institute in Buffalo, NY, M.D. Anderson Cancer Center in Houston, Texas, and Memorial Sloan-Kettering Cancer Center in New York City. Evolution of the model led to three types of cancer centers in the 1980s: Basic, Clinical, and Comprehensive, but the classification of NCI-designated Cancer Centers was simplified in 2004 to include Cancer Centers and Comprehensive Cancer Centers, based on the center's depth and breadth of research activities in laboratory, clinical, and population-based research. Together, they are the centerpieces of the nation's efforts to reduce morbidity and mortality from cancer. In 2012, the NCI Cancer Center Program supported a total of 67 Cancer Centers, including 41 Comprehensive Cancer Centers in 34 states, plus the District of Columbia, at a cost of $278.3 million in 2011, or 5.5 % of NCI's total budget [534]. With 10 Cancer Centers, California had the most, followed by New York State with 6 and Pennsylvania with 5. It is noteworthy that, in contrast, NCI's Intramural Research Program cost $833.6 million in 2011, or 16.5 % of its total budget [535]. However, NCI is currently in the process of implementing a comprehensive approach to transform its clinical trials system into a highly integrated, national clinical trials network [536].

10.3 NCI's Clinical Trials Program Network

At the urging of Sydney Farber, Mary Lasker, and other cancer advocates, Congress launched the Chemotherapy National Service Center in 1955 with an annual budget of $5 million. This initiative evolved into today's Cancer Therapy Evaluation Program (CTEP) within NCI's Division of Cancer Treatment and Diagnosis (DCTD). With its nine branches and offices, over 900 active trials enrolling 30,000 patients annually, nearly 400 grants and cooperative agreements, and about 100 investigational new drugs (INDs), including targeted agents, CTEP coordinates the world's largest publicly-funded oncology clinical trials network. Its international research sites are spread throughout the United States, Canada, and Europe to conduct cancer treatment trials through the Clinical Trials Cooperative Group Program (CTCGP). They include [537]:

- American College of Surgeons Oncology Group (ACOSOG)
- Cancer and Leukemia Group B (CALGB)
- Children's Oncology Group (COG)
- Eastern Cooperative Oncology Group (ECOG)
- European Organization for Research and Treatment of Cancer (EORTC)
- Gynecologic Oncology Group (GOG)
- National Cancer Institute of Canada Clinical Trials Group (NCIC CTG)
- National Surgical Adjuvant Breast and Bowel Project (NSABP)
- North Central Cancer Treatment Group (NCCTG)
- Radiation Therapy Oncology Group (RTOG)
- Southwest Oncology Group (SWOG).

Together these organizations engage nearly 15,000 investigators at over 3,100 institutions to accrue approximately 25,000 patients annually to either group-designed or NCI-sponsored clinical trials. Other NCI-sponsored clinical trials programs include the Community Clinical Oncology Program (CCOP), the CCR, the Office for Cancer Centers, and the Cancer Imaging Program, among others. Launched in 1983 to engage community physicians in NCI clinical trials, CCOP engages approximately 3,000 community-based physicians at nearly 400 hospitals in 37 states and

Puerto Rico to participate in NCI-sponsored cancer-control studies. In 1990, the program was extended to include a minority-based CCOP (MB-CCOP) to facilitate access to clinical trials at institutions that serve large minority and underserved communities [538]. However, while most clinical cancer trials in the US have been sponsored and funded by public funds, the pharmaceutical industry has more recently taken an increasingly prominent role in sponsoring and funding clinical trials, enticed by the implied riches from mining data from the Human Genome Project and its preeminent role in drug marketing, accounting for most new anti-cancer drugs being developed today.

The value of clinical trials extends beyond cancer. Indeed, reliance on clinical trials to assess the therapeutic value and toxicity of new drugs for any disease or condition is so widespread that applications for any drug approval by the FDA requires submission of scientific data gathered via clinical trials. Consequently, incorporation of clinical trials in experimental therapeutics as a prelude to official sanction and widespread drug use can be viewed as one of the major advances in modern medicine, especially as it pertains to the promotion and safeguard of public health. This approach of using the scientific method to assess the potential benefit of new drugs via human trials that we now take for granted was first proposed in 1834 by French physician Pierre Charles Alexandre Louis (1787–1872). In a treatise entitled *Essays in Clinical Instruction*, Louis advocated the numerical method for assessing the benefit of therapies when he wrote, "It is necessary to account for different circumstances of age, sex, temperament, physical condition, natural history of the disease, and errors in giving therapy" [539]. Anticipating resistance to his scientific approach to medicine, he wrote, "The only reproach which can be made to the numerical method is that it offers real difficulties in its execution…it requires much more labor and time than the most distinguished members of our profession can dedicate to it." His demonstration that resorting to bleeding for treating pneumonia was an illusion sanctioned by theory, tradition, and personal perception rather than by scientific proof [540] was hailed as "one of the most important medical works of the present century, marking the start of a new era in science" by the editor of the American Journal of Medical Sciences, where his article was published [541]. It was, he added with remarkable foresight, "the first formal exposition of the results of the only true method of investigation in regard to the therapeutic value of remedial agents." At first, Louis' approach to medical practice encountered fierce resistance, for physicians were unwilling to have their therapeutic decisions held in limbo until sanctioned by the numerical method, nor were they prepared to discard treatments sanctioned by tradition and by their own personal preference. Skeptics were unwilling to hold "their decisions in abeyance till their decisions received numerical approbation… [and were not prepared to discard therapies] validated by both traditional and their own experience on account of somebody else's numbers" [542]. Some of the raging arguments surrounding Louis's work launching "evidence-based medicine" were recently published [543]. Eventually, when practitioners recognized that Louis' numerical method enhanced rather than hindered their clinical skills and brought objectivity to their therapeutic choices, his method gained acceptance, eventually becoming the norm for assessing and validating the usefulness of new and old therapies. Louis attracted many notable foreign disciples, including Austin Bradford Hill, whose studies on streptomycin for pulmonary tuberculosis reinforced the notion of clinical trials [544], and William Osler, who applied Louis' and other principles of medical practice to medical education at Johns Hopkins University in 1893. Today, Louis is considered the direct or indirect mentor of most American and English scientists in public health, epidemiology, medicine, and biostatistics. As of this writing (June 2013), NIH lists 147,963 clinical trials in 50 states and 185 countries [545].

10.4 Clinical Trials: Types, Phases, Design, and Interpretation

In order to understand how cancer research is translated into patient care, and how it impacts the War on Cancer, it is necessary to have an understanding of the nature of clinical cancer trials, especially how they are designed, conducted, and interpreted [546]. Clinical trials are the final stages in the long process of evaluating the positive and negative biological effects of an agent potentially useful in the prevention, diagnosis, or treatment of any disease, though the focus here is cancer. There are three types of clinical trials according to their purpose: Preventive, Diagnostic, and Therapeutic. While they differ somewhat in design, this section will focus on the treatment trial model, and more specifically, drug trials.

The review process of potential anti-cancer drugs follows successive steps that include:

- Preclinical (animal) testing.
- An IND outlines the sponsor's proposed new drug for human testing in clinical trials.
- Phase-1 studies (typically involves 20–80 people).
- Phase-2 studies (typically involves a few dozen to about 300 people).
- Phase-3 studies (typically involves several hundred to about 3,000 people).
- The pre-NDA period to allow time for the FDA and drug sponsors to meet.
- Submission of an NDA formally asking the FDA to consider a drug approval.
- Within 60 days FDA must review the file, file an NDA if approved, assess the sponsor's drug safety and effectiveness data, review the content of the drug's professional labeling, inspect the manufacturing facilities, and either approve the application or issue a letter to the drug sponsor [547].

This process ensures that new drug sponsors, whether research institutions or drug manufacturers, take responsibility for developing a drug, and gives the FDA oversight of an orderly and sequential process ranging from preclinical animal testing to evaluating the safety (phase I) and activity of a drug administered alone (phase II) or in combination with other drugs (phase III). For the clinical phases of a study to proceed, an IND must be reviewed and approved by FDA and by the institutional review board (IRB) that oversees clinical research at the sponsor's institution, as well as an informed consent form to ensure that risks of the study are minimized and fully disclosed to participants, respectively. Although participants must sign an informed consent form before entering a study acknowledging understanding the potential risks and benefits to themselves and other details of the study, they can withdraw their participation at any time without prejudice.

The main purpose of phase I trials, which take an average of 1.5 years to complete and enroll between 20 and 80 usually healthy volunteers, is to determine the drug's most frequent side effects and how it's metabolized and excreted. The type and severity of side effects are assessed relative to the new drug's clinical purpose. That is, a relatively high level of toxicity that might be acceptable for treating a resistant cancer will be unacceptable for treating a type of responsive cancer for which other efficacious therapies exist. If a drug successfully completes phase I trials, it will proceed to phase II, a process that enrolls between 100 and 500 patients and averages 2 years to complete. The goals of phase II trials are primarily to establish anti-cancer activity using doses, schedules, and routes of administration associated with acceptable toxicity, and secondarily, to further assess toxicity. Participants of phase II trials are usually of two categories: patients with refractory cancers and, to a lesser extent, newly diagnosed patients with advanced cancers usually unresponsive to established therapies. Occasionally, phase II studies are controlled trials where a group of patients receiving the new drug (the experimental group) are compared with matched patients receiving either a placebo or a standard drug (the control group). Once a phase II is successfully completed, the new drug is eligible to proceed to the next phase. In phase III trials, which are always comparative trials involving 1,000–5,000 participants and take on the average 3.5 years to complete, more information about safety and effectiveness is gathered on different experimental groups, each compared to a control group receiving the standard regimen for the particular type of cancer under study.

The value of a clinical trial rests on its design, conduct, and analysis of results, its clinical relevance, and the quality of reporting. A well-designed trial must ensure that differences observed between groups with respect to anti-cancer activity and toxicity are drug-related and not due to dissimilarities in demographic or biological variables, as discovered by Louis nearly two centuries ago. This is because, contrary to the physical sciences where experiments can be reproduced with little variation, clinical research is adversely impacted by the complexity and heterogeneity of human biology, leading to a wide range of responses often amenable to biased interpretation. In general, factors that negatively impact the trustworthiness of clinical trials include selection bias (e.g., non-random treatment allocation), performance bias (e.g., knowledge of treatment allocation influencing outcome assessment), detection bias (e.g., biased assessment of outcome), and attrition bias (e.g., exclusion of patients or those lost to follow-up impacting group composition) [548]. Given the law of probabilities, two very large groups composed of thousands of individuals should be nearly homogeneous with respect to distribution by age, sex, and other major variables, rendering them comparable. However, despite efforts to match experimental and control groups for such variables, most clinical trials remain dissimilar because the total number of patients enrolled seldom exceeds a few hundred individuals. Moreover, given their high cost and labor-intense execution, and the need for swift enrollment and long follow-up of substantial numbers of patients, most phase III clinical trials are conducted in a multi-institutional setting, increasing the probability of selection and attrition bias. For example, some physicians might be less inclined to treat debilitated patients with a new drug perceived to be more toxic than the standard regimen and fail to recognize that patients dropped off study might alter homogeneity within groups. On the other hand, some patients might refuse a new drug on the basis of perceived toxicity, personal bias, or other reasons, while others might insist on participating in the study of a drug touted in the mass media to be a "miracle drug", an evocative label often associated with targeted therapeutics. Finally, performance and detection bias can tarnish interpretation and reporting of study results.

Several study designs have been developed in attempts to reduce selection biases. Of these, "randomized controlled trials" that aim to create groups comparable for any known or unknown potential confounding factors have become the gold standard [549]. In randomized trials, treatment is allocated by chance alone, without the knowledge of either caregiver or patient, before entering the trial. In practice, each patient eligible for accrual is assigned a given treatment randomly selected by a central computer. The randomization process, also known as allocation concealment, ensures that each patient has an equal chance of being assigned any of the therapies in the trial and that random assignment of participants to treatment groups will minimize uneven distribution of factors that might affect the endpoints of the trial, other than the treatment received. Randomization also ensures that, regardless of treatment assigned, all patients are handled uniformly with respect to their management, supportive care, and follow-up evaluation while on study. In certain (double blind) trials, neither patients nor researchers are aware of the treatment assignment until completion or termination of the study. However, some physicians feel that enrolling patients in such studies compromises the patient–physician relationship. After randomized to a treatment group, patients can further be "stratified" to subgroups according to well-defined criteria, such as age, disease stage, etc. Benefits of stratification include early detection of side effects or unusual response to treatment by particular patient subsets but not by the group as a whole. Other important considerations when designing clinical trials include study objectives, choice of end points, eligibility criteria, and sample size, to name but the most important. Many of these are intertwined, thus compounding the degree of difficulty in clinical trial design. For example, a phase III trial in lung cancer will be quickly completed given the modest objectives dictated by the known unresponsiveness of this disease, and a speedy accrual made possible by its high incidence in the population. Alternatively, a trial designed to assess a drug for the treatment of advanced Hodgkin's disease would have to be very large and lengthy given the success of doxorubicin-containing regimens that yield up to 90 % complete remission rates, with 75 % 5-year relative survival [550]. When survival is the main endpoint of a trial, treatment off-study of patients who fail to respond or relapse after an initial response to the experimental drug might have an impact on outcome and must be taken into consideration when analyzing trial results. This is accomplished by assessing disease-free interval, time to relapse, or time to progression as endpoints rather than survival at a designated time-point.

A most important feature of the modern clinical trial is the use of statistics to determine whether the outcome of a trial, either positive or negative, is likely to be drug-related or a chance occurrence. It is based on the frequency theory of probability that a given outcome of an experiment will be confirmed if sufficient repetitions of the experiment are undertaken. When comparing the potential effect of two drugs or events on a chosen study endpoint, two outcomes are possible: the effect of both drugs is equivalent or it differs, also called the *null* and *alternate* hypothesis, respectively. Statistical tests enable assessing the level of probability that apparent differences in outcome or lack thereof are erroneous (α or type I, and β or type II errors, respectively). In practice, a calculated probability above 5 % (p value >0.05) is accepted as evidence that differences in outcome could well be due to chance or experimental variations, whereas a p value <0.05 infers that the differences, whether positive or negative, are real. Additionally, the level of significance and the magnitude of the expected differences between experimental and control groups will determine the number of patients required in the trial in order to avoid type I or II errors. For example, a drug toxic to 10 % of individuals will have a 65 % chance of inducing toxicity in at least 1 of 10 patients, but an 89 % chance if toxicity affects 20 % of individuals. Conversely, in the same example, the chances of eliciting at least one toxic episode will rise with sample size, from 65 % if 10 individuals are studied to 96 % if 30 subjects are exposed. Thus, the impact of expected differences and sample size on study outcome are pivotal to the design of clinical trials. For example, to confirm with a 90 % confidence level the superiority of a drug with an expected 60 % response rate over an alternate drug with a known 55 % response rate would require accruing 4,100 individuals to the trial, whereas only 112 patients need be enrolled if the response rate of the alternate drug is only 30 % [551]. The likelihood that a positive outcome is truly positive is strengthened by the "prior probability of success" (or "θ" factor) for that drug in prior studies. It is tantamount to saying that positive outcomes are more likely than not to be true-positive if the drug under study has yielded positive results in prior studies. In addition to these basic statistical tests, there are far more sophisticated tools for assessing the discriminant value of multiple variables to a specific endpoint of a study, such as multivariate or logistic regression analysis [552]. However, they are beyond the scope of this coverage.

Finally, because today's cancer drugs are largely inefficacious, phase III clinical trials often yield no differences between the experimental and standard treatment arms or small differences that are statistically significant but clinically irrelevant [553, 554]. Attempts to magnify such inconclusive results revolve around two strategies. The first is to enroll large numbers of patients in a single trial to increase the discriminant power of the statistical analysis. The second is to use a statistical technique called *meta-analysis* that analyzes the combined results of several small trials in hopes of uncovering even small differences not revealed in individual small trials. However, the latter strategy is invalid when applied to trials that differ in design, therapies, types of patients, quality, or goals. The rationale and relevance of large trials and meta-analysis of small ones is that uncovering small differences in survival, especially in cancers with high incidence rates, might benefit thousands of patients each year. Meta-analysis can also lead to unexpected findings counter to the prevailing perceptions. For example, a meta-analysis of all phase III clinical trials conducted in North America between 1973 and 1994 in non-small cell lung cancer revealed that these patients' survival remained unchanged after two decades of clinical trials [555]. It is noteworthy that, instead of emphasizing this point, the authors concluded: "Future phase III trials should be sized appropriately, with at least 200 patients per treatment arm, in order to detect an expected 2-month prolongation of survival between therapeutic regimens". The prevailing tendency towards large studies, necessitated by the inefficacy of cytotoxic drugs, is illustrated by the fact that 26 of 33 active phase III trials sponsored by the EORTC in 2013 were designed to enroll between 532 and 3,806 patients [556].

Because available drugs to treat cancer yield modest survival outcomes at best, an extensive search for cancer chemoprevention agents has been underway and, given expected low yields, very large clinical trials were deemed necessary to provide useful clinical data. Yet, these attempts have been no more conclusive than small ones, as illustrated by the Breast Cancer Prevention Trial (BCPT), a clinical trial sponsored by the NSABP and funded by NCI. This study, which by 1998 had enrolled 13,388 women at a cost of $68 million, reported that, compared to placebo, Tamoxifen, a selective estrogen receptor modulators (SERMs), reduced the risk of breast cancer by 49 % after 4 years follow-up, but increased the risk of endometrial cancer by 150 %, not to mention increased risks of deep-vein thrombosis and pulmonary embolism [557]. Understandably, it has been suggested that unless a woman has a Gail index of 5 % or greater (that is, a >5 % 5-year risk for breast cancer, compared to a risk >1.66 % for women entered in the trial), chemoprevention with Tamoxifen should not be considered [558, 559]. On the other hand, two smaller studies, one British, the other Italian, did not yield a reduction in breast cancer incidence after a median follow-up of nearly 6 years, but confirmed the increased risk of endometrial cancer and of vascular events associated with Tamoxifen [560, 561]. The International Breast Cancer Intervention Study (IBIS-I) randomized 7,152 women with an increased risk of breast cancer to Tamoxifen or placebo. After a median follow-up of 50 months, an absolute reduction from 6.7 to 4.6 breast cancers per 1,000 woman-years was observed. Interestingly, the prophylactic effect of Tamoxifen persisted after completion of treatment, ER–negative cancers were not affected, and mortality from all causes was increased in the Tamoxifen group [562]. Another breast cancer prevention trial used Raloxifen, another SERM. In a first trial, called Multiple Outcomes of Raloxifene Evaluation (MORE), 7,705 post-menopausal women with osteoporosis with breast cancer as a secondary end-point were randomized to take Raloxifen or placebo between 1994 and 1998, with the participation of 180 centers in the US. After a median follow-up of 47 months, 79 cases of invasive cancer occurred in 39 women on placebo compared to 22 treated with Raloxifen. Interestingly, DCIS occurred in 11 women treated with Raloxifene vs. 5 women on placebo. Lastly, a very large randomized double-blind trial, called the *Study of Tamoxifen and Raloxifene* (STAR), was launched by the NCI in early 1999 to compare the relative effectiveness of Raloxifene and Tamoxifen in preventing breast cancer in post-menopausal women with a >1.66 % breast cancer risk. Five hundred centers across the United States, Puerto Rico, and Canada enrolled 19,747 women through 2004. After 81 months median follow-up, Raloxifene proved somewhat less effective than Tamoxifen in reducing invasive breast cancer, twice as effective in reducing uterine cancer, but was associated with 1.5-times the rate of pulmonary embolism and deep-vein thrombosis [563]. The cost of the STAR project that exceeded Tamoxifen's by a nearly 2:1 margin was apportioned as follows:

> To date, the National Cancer Institute has spent $88 million through peer-reviewed grants to the NSABP to support STAR. In addition, Eli Lilly and Company, Inc. provided NSABP with $30 million to defray recruitment costs at the participating centers and to help local investigators conduct the study. The maker of Tamoxifen, AstraZeneca Pharmaceuticals, Inc., Wilmington, Del., and the maker of Raloxifene, Eli Lilly and Company, Indianapolis, Ind., provided their drugs and matching placebos for the trial without charge to participants [564].

Hence, despite their very large size, long duration, and high cost, these breast cancer chemoprevention trials failed to provide definitive answers applicable to individual patients in the clinical setting, suggesting that, "perhaps the main conclusion is that there are no clear conclusions at this stage" [565].

Chapter 11
Factors that Impact Oncology Research and Practice

> We look for medicine to be an orderly field of knowledge and procedure. But it is not. It is an imperfect science, an enterprise of constantly changing knowledge, uncertain information, fallible individuals, and at the same time lives on the line. There is science in what we do, yes, but also habit, intuition, and sometimes plain old guessing. The gap between what we know and what we aim for persists. And this gap complicates everything we do.
>
> –Atul Gawande, M.D.

Given the fact that approximately 98 % of all cancer patients are treated outside of clinical trials, community oncologists find themselves as the final arbiters of cancer care. Hence, we must examine the various factors that might impact their practice.

11.1 Oncologists Qualifications

11.1.1 Training and Board Certification

Hematologists and Oncologists are highly trained subspecialists of Internal Medicine with special expertise in the diagnosis and treatment of malignant diseases. In the US, Hematology emerged as a separate medical discipline from an organizational meeting convened on April 7, 1957 at Boston's Harvard Club with 150 physicians in attendance. The first American Society of Hematology (ASH) meeting took place in April 1958, and the American Board of Internal Medicine (ABIM) held its first certifying examination in 1972 when 374 physicians became Diplomates in Hematology [566]. Medical Oncology became a subspecialty of Internal Medicine in 1972, and the first certifying examination was offered in 1973, with the first 351 Oncology diplomas being issued that year.

> Board Certified doctors voluntarily meet additional standards beyond basic licensing. They demonstrate their expertise by earning Board Certification through one of the 24 Member Boards that are part of the not-for-profit American Board of Medical Specialties (ABMS). Before a doctor can become Board Certified, each must complete: four years of premedical

education in a college or university, a course of study leading to an MD or DO degree from a qualified medical school, and three to five years of full-time experience in an accredited residency training program [567].

The ABIM, one of 24 member Boards of the ABMS, administers Board certification in all Medical specialties in the US (20 in 2012) and sets detailed "Policies and Procedures for Certification", including rules for disciplinary actions, revocation of certification, and other issues [568]. Only physicians certified in Internal Medicine can apply for certification in a Medical subspecialty such as Medical Oncology or Hematology, which require an additional 24–36 months of training in an approved post-graduate program. As of February 5, 2013, the ABIM had issued 254,929 certificates in Internal Medicine, 8,967 in Hematology, and 14,158 in Medical Oncology. The passing rate in 2012 was 85 %, 86 %, and 90 %, respectively. A number of these individuals obtain certification in both Hematology and Medical Oncology. Both subspecialties have evolved considerably since their inception. At present, Medical Oncology is strongly entrenched in the diagnosis and treatment of cancer, particularly the delivery of cancer chemotherapy. Oncologists have become the focal point for the management of cancer patients, often coordinating the input of Radiation and Surgical Oncologists, and of other members of the interdisciplinary cancer treatment team. Likewise, Hematology has evolved from a discipline initially dedicated to benign blood diseases and coagulation disorders to one that increasingly focuses on transplantation, genetics, and cellular transduction medicine at one end, and merges with Medical Oncology at the other. In the practice setting, Hematologists, Oncologists, and Hematology-Oncologists manage the vast majority of advanced cancers in the US, and derive most of their income from administering chemotherapy rather than from cognitive services. Given the overlap in training requirements, and the convergence of Oncology and Hematology with regards to cancer diagnosis and treatment, the term Oncologists will hereafter refer to all physicians whose primary clinical focus is cancer, whether their original training was primarily Oncology, Hematology, or both. Because of their well-organized and strictly supervised training in all aspects of cancer, American Oncologists are, at the outset, highly competent physicians superbly qualified to diagnose and treat all cancer types. Most update their knowledge database and clinical skills on a regular basis through Continuing Medical Education and periodic re-certification.

11.1.2 Continuing Medical Education

Cancer specialists update their knowledge database, as part of an ongoing and even compulsory continuing medical education process, through formal and informal channels. These include: oncology journals and books addressing the broadest range of subjects; national meetings organized annually by cancer societies offering diverse professional activities ranging from carefully prepared educational sessions to reports of bench and clinical research; and national or regional seminars focused on specific cancer issues. Of the numerous journals addressing cancer that make at least part of their content available on-line, the highly respected biweekly *Journal of Clinical Oncology* alone contributed 4,589 pages to its subscriber's bookshelves in 2,012, mostly of clinical trial reports with many appearing online before print. Likewise, *Blood*, the official ASH journal, published 5,252 pages of hematology and oncology articles in 2012, ranging from single case reports, to clinical trials, to immunobiology, to gene therapy. Additionally, a substantial number of single- and multi-authored books addressing a wide variety of cancer subjects are published with regularity. The former are usually theme-driven and are usually neither tutorial nor updated, whereas the latter are didactic with periodic updates. Some multi-authored books are part of multi-volume series with a broad range of subjects that are published over many years. Perhaps the best known and respected book, titled *Cancer: Principles and Practice of Oncology*, by DeVita and associates, now in its 9th edition, compiles 2,800 pages organized in 181 didactic chapters, written by numerous authoritative contributors [569]. Additionally, Oncologists have the opportunity to attend a variety of scientific meetings, seminars, and conferences that range from the highly informative and updated organized by cancer societies, universities, or research centers, to conferences of variable content and quality held by local oncology groups, often assisted by one or more guest speakers sponsored by the pharmaceutical industry. ASCO is one of the cancer societies with the greatest impact on Medical Oncologists, mostly through its yearly spring meeting. ASCO's 2013 meeting was attended by 25,500 professionals, mostly physicians (46 %), eager to learn the results of a variety of ongoing clinical cancer trials directly from the very investigators conducting the trials, and to gage the direction of cancer research [570]. Forty seven percent of attendees were from the US, with the balance from 116 countries. Specialties most represented included Medical Oncology (24 %), Internal Medicine (16 %), and Hematology (9 %). At the 2013 ASCO meeting, 2,720 eclectic reports were chosen for presentation out of the more than 5,306 that competed for the spotlight, 61 % of which reported on clinical trials [571]. Another group with great influence on providers of cancer care is the ASH. As of 2010, the ASH had 14,212 members, of which 34 % are from overseas. The ASH's 2012 annual fall meeting was attended by 20,578 scientists, clinicians, and guests to participate in a well organized program that included oral and poster presentations, a substantial portion of which addressed clinical issues and reported results of clinical trials, an educational program, and corporate-sponsored symposia. Because of ASCO's and ASH's large constituencies and broad reach, most of the nation's basic science and clinical cancer research is reported at one or the other of these societies' meetings. Attendance at one or both of the meetings each year by the vast majority of American Oncologists suggests the enormous influence these societies exert on continuing medical education and on the practice and direction of cancer care. This bewildering array of broadly disseminated scientific information, addressing everything from the broadest of issues to the narrowest of subjects on cancer, constitutes a source of continuing medical education widely utilized by most cancer care providers.

Finally, the interplay among Oncologists sharing an academic or community practice is a frequent source of exchange of information. Depending on the level and location of practice, this interplay can be informal or take place in one of two more formal settings: case discussions and journal clubs. As the name suggests, case discussions involve selecting individual cases for presentation to the group based on their didactic value or to seek a consensus regarding an uncertain diagnosis or a difficult management problem. Typically, in an academic center, case discussions are held weekly at the institution, and involve Medical, Surgical, and Radiation Oncologists, as well as Pathologists, Cytogeneticists, Flow Cytometrists, and other members of the medical team involved in patient care. On the other hand, the purpose of journal clubs is to review recent medical literature, focusing on a single subject. More informal and with the dual purpose of learning and socializing, journal clubs are often held monthly, usually at the home of each group member on a rotational basis. Finally, a variant of the journal club format involves oral presentations, frequently held in a restaurant setting, by remunerated speakers selected and sponsored by pharmaceutical companies based on both their experience and familiarity with one or more of the company's drugs and their willingness to serve on its speaker's panel. Here, the level of speakers' expertise and the quality and objectivity of the information presented varies greatly. In fact, by exalting the benefits of the promoted drug and building goodwill towards the manufacturer hosting the meeting, such speakers serve the company's goals more than the audience's needs.

Hence, the evidence shows that, if the War on Cancer remains stagnant, it is due not to Oncologists' faulty training or lack of expertise but to multiple extrinsic factors that directly or indirectly impact their practice, as we explore below.

11.2 Factors that Influence Oncology Practice

As described previously, cures are possible in some patients with some hematologic malignancies and certain germinal cancers, and modest prolongation of survival can be achieved in subsets of patients with advanced-stage cancer. Yet, unless medically or psychologically contraindicated, the vast majority of patients with advanced-stage cancer receive chemotherapy alone or in combination with surgery or irradiation, often switching from one drug or drug combination to another through the end of life in futile attempts to influence the course of the disease. For instance, a retrospective analysis of the cost of end-of-life care for 28,530 cancer patients surveyed between 2002 and 2009 showed mean cancer-related costs of $74,212 in the last 6 months before death, comprising hospital costs of $40,702 (55 %), outpatient costs of $30,254 (41 %), and hospice costs of $3,256 (4 %). Remarkably, more than 50 % of hospital costs ($20,559) were incurred in the last month of life [572]. This obstinacy towards concentrated healthcare expenditures at the end of life is not unique to cancer caregivers. Indeed, in 2011, Medicare spent $179 billion on end of life care or 28 % of $550 billion spent that year [573]. Furthermore, the average Medicare payment for deceased beneficiaries was 6.5-fold that for survivors ($39,975 vs. $5,993) in 2006, a ratio little changed since 1988 [574]. Taken together, these figures suggest that physicians engage in overuse of services through the end of life, remaining undeterred by the vainness and cost of their efforts. In addition to the financial burden imposed on terminal patients and their families, such a practice is associated with human suffering resulting from the multiple and often severe side effects of drugs and from complications of mostly needless procedures. In order to comprehend this apparent incongruity, we must analyze the perceptions, expectations, and motives of the parties directly involved, and their origins focusing on cancer caregivers and their patients. It is customary for physicians to consider a diagnosis of cancer as a "carte-blanche" for instituting aggressive management to be pursued while tumor responses are possible. Such an attitude, cemented in the notion of "standard of care" and reinforced by the imperative of avoiding medical malpractice, is further encouraged by revenue-driven practices such as the "chemotherapy concession". Physicians' attitudes towards cancer are reinforced by patients' strong desire to overcome the dire consequences of cancer left unchecked, although that determination is often based on an incomplete and often cursory understanding of the potential benefits and risks of treatment, and an inherent self-preservation instinct that, given the circumstances, is likely to prejudice a rational choice of action.

11.2.1 Standard of Care

Standard of care is primarily a legal concept that refers to the level of practice that any average, prudent, and reasonable physician would provide under similar circumstances of disease, time, and place. It must reflect the art (consensus of opinion) and the science (peer-reviewed literature) of medicine. In essence, from a legal standpoint, standard of care is not necessarily the best, most expensive, or most technologically advanced care available, but one that is considered acceptable and adequate under similar circumstances. Thus, providing treatment that is inferior to the norm and under- or over-utilizes medical services is unacceptable, unethical, and renders the physician liable to malpractice suits. Under these circumstances, and notwithstanding physicians' assertions to the contrary, standard of care determines to a large extent medical practice in the United States. To the Oncologist, standard of care acquires the additional connotation of being the "best" treatment modality for a particular cancer. This conceptual evolution led to the current design of phase III clinical trials where an experimental drug is compared to the standard or "best" treatment regimen for the particular cancer under study. Based on clinical trials, an ever evolving standard of care for every cancer is promulgated or implied in medical publications, at cancer society meetings, and at national and local seminars and conferences, all reinforced by a legion of guest speakers sponsored by the pharmaceutical industry, coordinated and supported by their field representatives, who eagerly distribute copies of the pertinent articles praising the advantages of drug(s) in question. Because negative reports are seldom published, the vast majority of the information conveyed describes "progress", "improvements", and "advances" in cancer management, along with the subliminal message that cancer management is choosing between two or more drugs or drug combinations, rather than whether the potential benefits justify the risks. Under these circumstances, substantial departures from standard of care practice, including withholding either an inefficacious drug or a treatment of widespread use elsewhere, could be construed as negligence and malpractice.

When applied to malignancies amenable to cures or 5-year DFS in substantial patient subsets such as Hodgkin's disease, testicular cancer, and a few other cancers, standard of care has profound practical and ethical implications. Indeed, in such cases, the benefit to risk ratio is dramatically shifted towards benefit, thus justifying a relatively high degree of risk to achieve a distinctly favorable outcome. Ironically, risks associated with such treatments are generally no greater than those linked to inefficacious regimens, with the notorious exception of acute leukemia, for which a complete ablation of patients' bone marrow, a prerequisite to achieving complete remissions and some cures, contributes to serious complications, including deadly infections, more often than to cures. In contrast, when applied to non-curative regimens that do not prolong survival meaningfully, standard of care essentially means "the best" of a group of fundamentally inefficacious therapies, a highly dubious honor. Yet, many cancer drugs and treatment regimens shown to be inefficacious over the years remain in use today because, in the absence of better alternatives, they are considered standard of care. For instance, a 2000 review of two decades of chemotherapy experience in the treatment of advanced non-small cell lung cancer by the ECOG reported an average tumor response rate of 25 %, a median survival of 25 weeks with 20 % surviving 1 year, regardless of the drugs or drug combinations used [575]. Based on these rather meager results, the author concluded, "It is appropriate to offer chemotherapy to all NSCLC patients with advanced disease, a good performance status, and no medical or psychological contraindications to its use". Recommendations such as this, made by leading experts in their field, especially when published in high-profile medical journals, are uncritically embraced by community Oncologists as the standard of care for day-to-day patient management.

Standard of care is also shaped by an unending barrage of clinical trial reports, particularly Phase III trials, each describing the merits and advantages of a drug or drug combination over alternatives for treating a particular cancer, enticing practitioners to "follow the lead". However, given the marginal efficacy of cancer drugs, many phase III clinical trials yield statistically significant differences in outcome with no clinical relevance, a concept few clinicians understand [576]. Rather than definitive, results from such studies should be viewed as exploratory and a springboard towards definitive studies. Oncologists' tendency to apply results of the latest clinical trials to their day-to-day practice is exemplified by the saga of the chemotherapy regimen known by its acronym "CHOP" (Cyclophosphamide, Hydroxydoxorubicin, Oncovin, and Prednisone), a drug combination that, developed in the early 1970s, became the treatment of choice for diffuse large B-cell lymphoma. Despite CHOP's superior efficacy, many alternative regimens were proposed and studied, including those known by the acronyms COMLA, ESAP, MACOP-B, m-BACOP, PROMACE-CYTABOM, and VACOP-B. Over the years, many patients were treated with these drug combinations and, despite some claimed advantages, the average outcome was inferior to CHOP's. More recently, CHOP has been combined with other agents with varied results. For instance, CHOP plus

Rituximab for lymphoma was reported to "significantly increase the rate of complete responses, decrease the rates of treatment failure and relapse, and improve event-free and OS as compared with standard CHOP alone" [577]. Yet, a companion editorial cautioned, "the difference between the survival curves begins to shrink at 2.5 years.... it is of concern that more patients treated with CHOP plus rituximab died from infection, cachexia, or cardiac disease" [578]. Nevertheless, CHOP remains a useful regimen for the treatment of certain forms of non-Hodgkin's lymphomas. Reports of some clinical trials reveal a therapeutic advantage for a small subset of study participants discovered after much statistical data triage, rather than for the majority, as anticipated. In general, such trials should be considered negative and published only if the mined data establishes a new standard of care for the patient subset.

11.2.2 Overutilization of Services and the Chemotherapy Concession

With very few exceptions, the outcome of an office visit is a prescription for medications, for laboratory tests, an imaging procedure, or a referral. In most cases, physicians have no financial interest in the pharmacy filling the prescription or in the facilities performing the procedures, and kickbacks are virtually unheard of, thus averting major conflicts of interest. Yet, in the United States, most health care is based on fee-for-service, which impacts physicians' practices as underlined by the very existence of incentive programs implemented by drug companies and health maintenance organizations [579, 580], a phenomenon well-documented in reports of over-utilization of services, especially those owned by physicians [581]. Over-utilization of services by physician-owners of equipment adds another source of income generation for medical practices [582, 583]. This has been amply documented in a very large retrospective analysis of an insurance claims database conducted on 526,000,000 diagnostic medical imaging claims between 1999 and 2003 that included the specialty of provider and referring physicians. Analysis of 18,123,121 episodes of care revealed,

> Physicians who referred patients to themselves or to other same-specialty physicians for diagnostic imaging used imaging between 1.12 and 2.29 times as often, per episode of care, as physicians who referred patients to radiologists (P<.005 for all comparisons). Adjusting for patient age and comorbidity, the likelihood of imaging was 1.196–3.228 times greater for patients cared for by same-specialty–referring physicians…These findings were consistent across the eight combinations of conditions and imaging procedures evaluated and cannot be explained by differences in case mix, patient age, or comorbidity [584].

In cancer care, the profit motive of many diagnostic and therapeutic decisions is obvious, ubiquitous, and hard to escape. Profit-driven practices are typified by over-utilization of standard services, by offering non-essential though convenient services, but first and foremost by the chemotherapy concession. Oncologists' tendency to offer additional income-generating services within the office is well-documented. For instance, the National Practice Benchmark 2010 report, derived from 117 Oncology practice responders nationwide, reported,

Nearly all of the reporting practices provide medical oncology and hematology services; three quarters of the respondents offer laboratory services and clinical research; and a third of the practices provide imaging, a closed-door pharmacy, genetic counseling, and radiation oncology services [585].

However, the most lucrative source of revenue for most Oncologists is the Chemotherapy Concession, also called "The Buy-and-Bill" model, which refers to the sale of chemotherapy drugs from doctors' offices [586]. This unique practice has been an economic reality for more than 30 years and accounts for two thirds of the income of Oncologists in private practice [587]. As could be expected, there are sound rational justifications for such a *modus operandi*, even if it raises serious ethical issues and often results in practices ranging from questionable to borderline unethical. The origins of the Chemotherapy Concession was the decision by Oncologists in private practice to combine delivery of cognitive and drug delivery services at their offices. This decision was professionally sound, given its convenience to themselves and their patients, and its many advantages. The most obvious benefits include: stocking on site most chemotherapy drugs common to a practice; minimizing the risk of errors in administration (intravenous medications are mixed and delivered by trained nurses); presence on the premises of the prescribing Oncologist (or an experienced nurse) to respond to any drug reaction or unforeseen treatment complication; and providing cancer patients a convenient and soothing environment where they can share experiences and support one another. That decision was also very astute financially. Indeed, Oncologists purchase drugs in bulk, at discount prices, from wholesalers, and sell them to patients one by one and at retail prices. Drug price markups, which range between 10 or 20 % to as high as 200 %, have been justified to cover overhead costs and to amortize chemotherapy facilities. Although such a practice is not in itself unethical, the opportunity for financial rewards from choice of drugs and practice patterns create conflicts of interest.

Oncologist compensation can be ascertained from a 2012 survey of 24,216 US physicians across 25 specialties [588]. After excluding "expert witness services, speaking engagements, and product sales", responding Oncologists' mean compensation was $295,000, with 15 % earning less than $100,000 but 10 % earning $500,000 or more. Oncologists in multispecialty group practices earned the most ($347,000), while those in academic settings earned the least ($164,000). The majority of Oncologists (56 %) spent an average 13–20 min with each patient, whereas 10 % spent less than 12 min and 33 % spent more than 21 min. The impact of non-cognitive services on Oncologists' income can be enormous [589]. Indeed, 117 Hematology/Oncology practices responding to a recent survey, including approximately 30 % who offered imaging and closed-door pharmacy, provide a window on current Oncology practice and income. Approximately 3,500 patients per FTE[1] were seen annually, and 90 % of practices sold drugs through the traditional Buy-and-Bill system, using an average 11 chairs per practice to administer an average 1,000 infusions per FTE. Average total income per FTE (gross revenue minus operating expenses) from 37 practices was approximately $1 million,

---

[1] Full-Time Equivalent.

including approximately $250,000 from imaging services, $60,000 from laboratory services, and $30,000 from closed-door pharmacy. Medicare was the main payer (46 %) [590]. Surprisingly, despite being in the top 10 best-remunerated specialties, 49 % of private Oncologists feel undercompensated [591]. In contrast, academic Oncologists' incomes are based solely on collections from charges for the time-consuming but less lucrative cognitive services: i.e., office visits, consultations, and the like. In academia, profits from drug sales are credited to the hospital pharmacy and receipts from laboratory tests are credited to the hospital laboratory. In addition, the demographics of patients attracted by private and academic Oncology practices have a major financial impact: The former is patronized by patients who, through insurance or their own funds, pay their full share of their health care costs, whereas academic Oncology practices accept and therefore attract indigent and low-income patients seeking health care subsidized by the state or the institution. Thus, because a large portion of charges at academic centers are non-collectable and some of the rest are lost to unsound accounting practices, collection rates by academic Oncologists can be as low as 20 % (20 cents collected for each $1.00 charged), whereas they reach 95 % in tightly-run private Oncology practices. While income discrepancies between private and academic practices are unjustified from knowledge and workload standpoints, the profit motive is so ingrained into healthcare that some proponents of equalization yearn to "Make the practice profitable...[by] maximizing the clinical revenue from each patient" [592] and that "It is critical [for hematology and medical oncology divisions] to acquire access to infusion center profits" [593].

While abuses of the chemotherapy concession are not rampant, there are countless circumstances and opportunities for engaging in subtle practices that base treatment decisions on financial considerations. Examples include: using CSF and erythropoietin outside of recommended ASCO indication guidelines [594]; selecting intravenous rather than oral cancer drugs of comparable efficacy; newer and more profitable but not necessarily more efficacious drugs; drug regimens that require more frequent office visits; or embracing highly profitable though unproven cancer management approaches, as was the choice of high-dose chemotherapy with stem cell rescue as the preferred treatment for some cancers without evidence-based support of its benefits [595]. While pressures from patients, patient advocates, and policymakers played crucial roles in the premature adoption of bone marrow transplantation, private and academic transplanters were quick to oblige. Universities, cancer centers, and large private practices scrambled to offer transplanting services, less to improve or complement their existing programs than as an income-generating procedure that eventually proved no better than standard chemotherapy for breast cancer, its major indication at the time. However, notwithstanding the ethical implications of the chemotherapy concession and its potential abuse, perhaps the most questionable Medical Oncology practice, adhered to by most private and academic Oncologists, is the administration of chemotherapy to patients with advanced cancers historically proven not amenable to cures or survival prolongation and to do so through the end of life. The sequence begins with "first line" drugs or drug combinations that historically have elicited the best tumor responses. Unresponsive patients and those whose cancer relapses after an initial response are then treated with "second line" regimens that, as the name suggests, are generally less inefficacious but equally toxic. Ultimately, most patients are treated with "salvage" therapies, a euphemism with little practical meaning. Finally, from time to time, Oncologists witness unexpected long-term survivors among patients expected to succumb to progressive cancers regardless of treatment. Such cases tend to be more vividly remembered than those who died of their disease within the anticipated time frame, tempting the physician to treat comparable future patients similarly. Though well-intentioned, such treatment decisions allow emotions to prevail over good judgment and unnecessarily expose patients to additional chemotherapy-induced side effects in an attempt to recreate a few memorable, though unexplained, outcomes.

The outlined medicine-as-a-business adhered to by virtually all medical specialty practices have a major and growing impact on the cost of health care, leading to a number of cost-containment proposals, including the "Top Five List" proposal [596] and my own [597]. Unlike my comprehensive blueprint for a global healthcare reform that would curb healthcare costs by redesigning the system's structure, the care delivery, and the payment model, plus restraining malpractice litigation and political interference, the Top Five List consists of a limited cost-containment approach based on discouraging the use of,

> [the top] five diagnostic tests or treatments that are very commonly ordered by members of [every] specialty that are among the most expensive services provided, and that have been shown by the currently available evidence not to provide any meaningful benefit [598].

William Osler, a renowned Canadian physician and medical historian, reputed to have been the most brilliant and influential teacher of medicine of his day, preached that, "The practice of Medicine is an art, not a trade; a calling, not a business; a calling in which your heart will be exercised equally with your head". Little did he know that modern medical practice would bear little resemblance to that ideal.

11.2.3 Medical Malpractice

Notwithstanding other major factors that impact Oncology practice, malpractice litigation is an overriding concern that hangs over physicians' heads like Damocles' sword. In private, most physicians will admit that malpractice concerns lead to defensive medicine. In one study, 65.4 % of practicing physicians felt the threat on a day-to-day basis, ranging from 51.4 % for the least exposed specialists (e.g., psychiatrists) to 82 % for the most vulnerable (e.g., emergency room physicians). By age 65, 75 % and 99 % of physicians in low- and high-risk specialties have faced a malpractice claim, respectively [599]. Unsurprisingly, a survey designed to assess how often high-risk specialists alter their practice patterns to reduce the threat of malpractice liability reported, "nearly all (93 %) reported practicing defensive medicine. Assurance behavior such as ordering tests and diagnostic procedures, and referring patients for consultation, was very common (92 %)" [600]. A portrayal of defensive medical practice in the emergency room follows:

> Today, if you go to an emergency room with head trauma, you will get an MRI (or at least a CT scan). It does not matter that you were not unconscious, that your pupils are round, equal and reactive to light and accommodation, that you know your full name and the date and time of the week, that you are well oriented and that you will not even require sutures. If you have a bump on your head, you will get an MRI (sometimes even before a physician examines you). If you cough and have lost some weight you will get a chest CT scan. If your joints ache they will be x-rayed. If you have indigestion, you will get an exercise electrocardiogram (stress test) and maybe a multigated acquisition scan and cardiac ultrasound, just in case [601].

The role of malpractice litigation as a cause of service overutilization and spiraling health care costs, and trial lawyers' abuse of tort law, will be addressed briefly here, as summary of a broad coverage provided elsewhere [602]. Medical malpractice is defined as a significant deviation from accepted standards of practice that causes harm. Under tort law, malpractice lawsuits are designed to compensate, financially, plaintiff's economic and non-economic losses caused by the *willful, negligent, or unskilled* actions of a defendant physician. While the fear of malpractice litigation keeps physicians vigilant, prudent, and thorough in the care of patients, in practice, many medical malpractice lawsuits are frivolous, which are triggered not by malpractice but by the greed of trials attorneys and of their clients, and are eventually withdrawn or dismissed. Yet, of the approximately 20 % of medical malpractice lawsuits that that went forward as early as 1992, and after 3–5 years of litigation, 24.8 % of awards from all successful cases surpassed $1 million [603]. In order to maximize awards, trial attorneys commonly resort to a practice called *deep-pocket defendants* or to selecting a friendly jurisdiction instead of the plaintiff's own. The former consists of casting a wide net around the physician defendant to include the hospital and the drug or device manufacturer and anyone remotely connected to the case. The latter is illustrated by the case of the Bankston Drugstore in Lafayette, MS.

> Then, in 1999, Bankston Drugstore was named as a defendant in a national class-action lawsuit against the manufacturer of Fen-Phen, an FDA-approved drug for weight loss. At that point, the small pharmacy went from serving its community's needs to becoming prey to money-driven litigants and the attorneys representing them. Though the drug maker was based in New Jersey, the plaintiffs' attorneys named Bankston in the lawsuits so the case could be kept in Jefferson County – a known plaintiff-friendly jurisdiction that, between 1995 and 2000, had twice the number of plaintiffs as actual residents [604].

Other strategies range from focusing on tangential issues likely to sway juries in the defendant's favor to challenging accepted principles of standard of care when everything else fails. One humiliating experience of a young defendant physician trainee is both revealing and heartbreaking. He described his case as follows,

> During closing arguments the plaintiff's lawyer put evidence-based medicine [EBM[2]] on trial. He threw EBM around like a dirty word and named the residency and me as believers

---

[2] Conscientious and judicious use of current best evidence in making clinical decisions.

in EBM, and our experts as the founders of EBM. He defined EBM as a cost saving method and stated his belief that the few lives saved were not worth the money. He urged the jury to return a verdict to teach residencies not to send any more residents on the street believing in EBM. The plaintiff's lawyer was convincing. The jury sent a message to the residency program [found liable for $1 million], that they didn't believe in evidence-based-medicine. They also sent a message that they didn't believe in the national guidelines and they didn't trust the shared decision-making model. The plaintiff's lawyer won. As I see it, the only way to practice medicine is to keep up with the best available evidence and bring it to my patients. As I see it, the only way to see patients is by using the shared decision-making model. As I see it, the only way to step into an examination room is to look at a patient as a whole person, not as a potential plaintiff. As I see it, I'm not sure I'll ever want to practice medicine again [605].

Trial lawyer practices have been denounced by many. For instance, on its website, the Center for Legal Policy of the Manhattan Institute for Policy Research describes the *Litigation Industry* as follows,

Plaintiffs' lawyers aggressively pursue clients through advertisements on television and radio, in newspapers and on the Internet. Through tort litigation, the plaintiffs' bar in America, which the CLP has dubbed Trial Lawyers, Inc., grosses almost $50 billion per year—significantly more than the annual revenues of Microsoft or Intel, and more than twice the global sales of Coca-Cola. The litigation industry in turn spends its earnings to block legal reform through one of the most powerful public relations and government relations lobbies in America. Since 1990, trial lawyers have donated over a half-billion dollars to federal political campaigns alone—a figure far higher than any other industry group [606].

11.2.4 Clinical Researchers and Publications

The aim of all medical research is to accrue scientific knowledge to the medical database, and in so doing, provide the foundation for ultimately improving health care. In a perfect world, all parties involved in the process would adhere to entirely altruistic principles focused on a common goal, the scientific truth, and be able to pursue that goal resolutely and without interference. However, a variety of pressures brought to bear on clinical researchers by their employers, sponsors, and publishers often influence the tone and content of most study reports and of virtually all press releases. Articles submitted for publication to medical journals are screened by anonymous "*peer-reviewers*", or experts in the field who are expected to ensure that the study for review was designed, implemented, analyzed, and reported according to established standards, and that the conclusions reached are commensurate with the findings. This process, which takes at least 2 months to complete, has been challenged as a closed system with known deficiencies and biases but no proven benefits that stifles, for profit, the widest and timely dissemination of scientific knowledge [607]. A constellation of reasons, some obvious, some less so, drives medical researchers to publish, one of which is highlighted by the ominous "*publish or perish*" aphorism. Indeed, the world of medical researchers is subject to pressures and biases that take many forms, including career advancement, shifting priorities in research funding, and the increasing link between research productivity and job security. For example, at most universities and research centers, salary and career advancement, such as rank promotion and tenure, are formally linked to scientific productivity that is judged by the number of research publications within a certain time frame, and to revenue generation. However, neither addresses scientific merit or social impact. Indeed, a single publication in a high-profile journal is likely to have a greater impact, at least on other scientists if not on society at large, than several articles in second-rated journals. Yet, the same high-profile journal might reject an article addressing a seemingly mundane issue of substantial social impact while publishing another judged of greater scientific value by reviewers, despite lacking social impact [608]. On the other hand, some reports lacking a solid scientific basis are published in reputable journals because they involve thousands of individuals followed for extended periods of time and have high media appeal. For instance, a recent study examined the association between height and cancer risk in 144,701 women [609]. After a median follow-up of 12 years, a positive correlation was found for all 19 sites surveyed in the 20,928 women who developed cancer; for every 10-cm increase in height, the relative cancer risk rose by 13 %. The cancer-height correlation remained unchanged after "adjusting for known variables that influence the risk of these cancers (weight, age, hormone therapy, smoking, alcohol consumption, age at menarche, education, ethnicity, and weight/height ratio)" [610]. Within days, seizing the opportunity for increased visibility and sales, the mass media the world over cited the study. Such "fishing expeditions", the results of which will eventually prove fallacious, waste financial and human resources in the pursuit of a questionable hypothesis. However, far more damaging to the advancement of science is the unbecoming or even dishonest behavior of a minority of researchers, as exposed in a recent book by the Emeritus Chair at a prestigious U.S. School of Medicine [611].

Clinical researchers often must contend with outside pressures that impact their work. Scientific merit and productivity often take a back seat to institutional or programmatic priorities, making revenue generation the deciding factor [612]. This is because priorities, at both the national and local levels, change with time in response to political, societal, and economic pressures, not to mention the whims of administrators at many universities and research centers who value medical research solely as a source of revenue. In such an environment, clinical researchers must adapt their research interests and direction in order to secure funds for their laboratory and adequate salaries for themselves. These multiple pressures might lead some clinical researchers to a "*follow the crowd*" mind-set studying the "*drug-du-jour*", either as part of multi-institutional cancer groups mainly supported by NCI or as "*solo*" investigators funded by pharmaceutical companies in their quest to market a new drug or to expand the clinical indications for an old one. It is ironic that the lack of progress in the conquest of cancer guarantees the survival and continued prosperity of the current status quo. Indeed, as an implicit indication of success, the NSABP and SWOG, among the oldest cancer study groups, proudly include on their respective web sites 50-year and 57-year longevity statements and the large number of patients accrued to their studies since inception [613, 614].

11.2.5 Pharmaceutical Companies

NIH research spending ranged from approximately $7 billion in 1980 to $30 billion in 2003, subsequently decreasing to $28 billion by 2008 [615]. NCI's budget, NIH's largest, increased from $1 billion in 1980 to $5.7 billion in 2012. In addition, through R&D spending, pharmaceutical companies have positioned themselves to play a preeminent role in clinical research and drug development. The 36 members of the Pharmaceutical Research and Manufacturers of America (PhRMA) has invested more than $500 billion for R&D since 2000, including an estimated $48.5 billion in 2012 alone [616]. Yet, not only does the financial muscle allocated to R&D by the pharmaceutical industry surpass NIH's, but the latter's expenditure is skewed towards basic science research, while the former's focuses on drug development for financial gain. At this writing (July 2013),

> America's biopharmaceutical research companies are testing 981 medicines and vaccines to fight the many types of cancer affecting millions of patients worldwide, according to a report released today by the Pharmaceutical Research and Manufacturers of America (PhRMA). These potential medicines, which are either in clinical trials or under review by the Food and Drug Administration, include 121 for lung cancer, 117 for lymphoma and 111 for breast cancer [617].

According to "Fortune 500", the pharmaceutical industry ranks as the US' third most profitable industry (19.3 % ROI[3] in 2009). It justifies its profitability, pointing out that, in addition to saving lives, "the biopharmaceutical sector generates high-quality jobs, powers economic output for the U.S. economy…[and] employs more than 650,000 workers and supports a total of four million jobs across the country" [618]. Drug pricing is justified by drug development's extremely low yield. Indeed, out of approximately 1,000 agents considered, only 5 reach the clinical trial stage, only 1 receives FDA-approval for human use, and only 3 out of 10 marketed drugs generate sufficient revenues to recover the up to $1 billion R&D per drug investment [619]. Yet, the pharmaceutical industry is highly profitable, not least because of financially successful business strategies: concentrating on potential blockbuster drugs and, more recently, focusing on the extremely profitable targeted therapeutics, all promoted by direct-to-consumers marketing since 1997, when FDA dropped most restrictions on media advertising of medical products. Direct-to-consumers and provider-targeted drug promotion reached $36 billion or 13.4 % of sales in 2004.

Drug marketing to doctors is ensured by an army of nearly 100,000 highly paid, well-dressed, affable, and attractive men and women "drug reps" whose role is to persuade or cajole physicians into prescribing drugs they promote, often including free samples and free food for the office staff. Other perks to physicians include free books, free tickets to events of their choosing, all-expenses-paid trips to medical meetings held in upscale settings, and payments for acting as consultants or speakers. One high-profile example is a Harvard psychiatrist who earned over $1.6

---

[3] Return on Investment.

million in consulting fees between 2000 and 2007 [620]. The extent of such practices was revealed in a report exposing seven drug companies (Eli Lilly, GlaxoSmithKline, AstraZeneca, Pfizer, Merck, Johnson & Johnson, and Cephalon) for paying $282 million to thousands of physicians for participating in their speakers' bureau programs since 2009 [621]. On the other hand, direct-to-consumer TV advertising, the most successful and profitable advertising venue, follows a description of symptoms many viewers recognize as their own (e.g., the medical student syndrome), accompanied by the advice "ask your doctor" or a statement by the presumed actor-patient such as "after checking with my doctor, he and I chose…" In fact, in a survey of 3,500 randomly selected physicians, approximately 40 % admitted to acquiescing to patient demands for brand-name drugs when equally efficacious generic drugs were available [622]. These various strategies helped propel a number of drugs to blockbuster status, including Lipitor® for lowering cholesterol (peaked at $14.3 billion in 2006), Plavix® for inhibiting blood clots ($6 billion in 2006), Nexium® for ulcers ($5 billion in 2006), Procrit® ($3.3 billion in 2003), Vioxx® for arthritis ($2.5 billion in 2003), Claritin® for allergies (peaked at $2.5 billion in 2001), and Viagra® for erection disorders ($2 billion in 2011).

The pharmaceutical industry's pricing power also relies on the unbridled support of Congress. Numerous examples of active congressional intervention in support of the health industry's bottom line are described elsewhere [623]. Suffice it to cite two representative examples here. When Merck decided to expand the indications for its drug Fosamax® in order to capture millions of women with a dubious entity called "osteopenia", it lobbied Congress to change Medicare reimbursement guidelines to include bone scans, which led to the Bone Mass Measurement Act (1997). This legislation was instrumental in an explosion of bone scans that reached into the millions each year ($2.6 million Medicare claims in 2004 alone) and catapulted worldwide Fosamax sales to $3.2 billion in 2005. Another example is the Medicare Prescription Drug, Improvement, and Modernization Act (2003) that prohibits Medicare from negotiating drug prices, costing the agency an unjustifiable additional $21 billion in 2006 alone. Another example of interest groups' support of the health industry's profit strategy is the case of a new breed of expensive CT scanners that were imposed on Medicare by cardiologists, radiologists, medical societies, and patient advocacy groups, with the final push coming from Congress. According to a report,

> General Electric's latest $1.4 million 'LightSpeed' CT scanning machine, which records 64 high-resolution images or slices [was shown in] a study that appeared in December 2008 in the Journal of the American College of Cardiology that over 50 percent of all CT detected coronary obstructions were false positive. 'This high false-positive rate has potentially serious implications, leading to unnecessary and potentially risky procedures that threaten to accelerate already excessive health care costs,' said an accompanying editorial by Steven Nissen, chair of the Cleveland Clinic's cardiovascular medicine division… Despite those risks, when Medicare announced a plan in December 2007 to rein in spending on CT angiography by requiring clinical trials and limiting CT scan use to patients with symptoms of heart disease, it was bombarded with 649 protest letters from cardiologists and radiologists, their professional societies, patient advocacy groups and equipment manufacturers. Even

Congress got involved, with 79 members of the House sending a letter noting their opposition to Kerry Weems, the acting administrator of the Center for Medicare and Medicaid Services. The agency backed off. Three months after its December announcement, Medicare reversed course, saying it would cover the test without restrictions and offering only 'hope' for future studies of the scans' effectiveness [624].

On the other hand, the extremely high expectations that mining the human genome will in time lead to definitive means for controlling formerly uncontrollable diseases such as cancer is shared by virtually all physicians, including Oncologists. Such enthusiasm unhindered by mostly modest survival benefits associated with most new cancer drugs helps the drug industry's pricing power for cancer drugs, as demonstrated by the fact that 11 of 12 targeted drugs approved by FDA in 2012 cost over $100,000 annually [625], with the most expensive drug costing $410,000 per patient per year. Such abuses of pricing power are another indication that the American health system is in need of a major overhaul, as I recently proposed [626].

PhRMA's deep pockets enables its members to pay $1,000–$3,000 per patient enrolled in clinical trials, a lucrative source of revenue for clinical researchers and their employers or for the multi-institutional cancer group of their affiliation. Non-academic research organizations often are hired as alternatives to academic researchers at a lower cost and with greater control over the process [627]. That gives drug companies leverage when dealing with cash-poor clinical researchers, often dictating the trial design, sequestering the raw data generated, and allowing little outside input in data interpretation and conclusions. As a result, published trials supported by the pharmaceutical industry tend to favor the innovative rather than the standard treatment arm more often than NCI-funded trials, and trials with unfavorable outcome might never be published [628, 629]. A 2002 survey of the influence of private industry on clinical trials conducted at 108 participating US medical schools concluded,

> Academic institutions routinely engage in industry-sponsored research that fails to adhere to International Committee of Medical Journal Editors guidelines regarding trial design, access to data, and publication rights. Our findings suggest that a reevaluation of the process of contracting for clinical research is urgently needed [630].

Concerned about conflicts of interest issues regarding research funded or sponsored by the pharmaceutical industry and the potential harm to society of biased research reports published vicariously in the name of academic researchers, most scientific journals now require authors to report potential conflicts of interest, including payments from or financial interest in any company involved in the study. Ironically, clinical investigators' widespread acceptance of financial support from drug companies, of one type or another, will, in time, dampen the intended effect of tagging research reports. Indeed, not unlike health warnings on cigarette packs that leave smokers blasé, author disclosure statements of financial interest in drug company-funded research seem not to diminish the clinical value of such research in the eyes of prescribing physicians.

11.2.6 The Media

The popular press often reports medical "breakthroughs", especially in short pieces about cancer, or conducts short interviews with "leading scientists" to enquire about recent "discoveries" and their potential benefits. Not surprisingly, most reports of breakthroughs are based on preliminary *in vitro* or animal studies accompanied by unrealistic future health care projections, years ahead of any potential clinical applications. Understandably, when medical breakthroughs fail to materialize, follow-up stories are seldom if ever reported, for negative medical news attracts neither audiences nor advertisers, and the public's short memory can be trusted. On the other hand, many interviews are not the result of the inquisitiveness of journalists but the self-interest of researchers and pharmaceutical companies, who, eager to promote their own agenda, seek reporters willing to oblige. This modus operandi, justified by the "public's right to know" the fate of public funds for medical research, but driven by the profit motive (e.g., selling periodicals or advertising), has become standard reporting. Moreover, journalists' sketchy scientific background limits their ability to comprehend and communicate complex medical subjects shaping the content and tone of their reports. For example, an analysis of 306 representative newspaper articles on cancer chosen at random revealed major deficiencies, including: misleading titles in 47.5 %; no traceable citations (name of journal, researcher, or institution) in 40 %; and erroneous information or lack of clarifying data in 55 %. Only 13.6 % placed the information conveyed in the proper context [631]. In an effort to improve journalistic communication to the public of results of medical research and to place each report in the proper context, in 2002, NIH launched an annual symposium for journalists entitled *Medicine and the Media: The challenge of reporting on Medical research*. The symposium was designed to "prepare participants for the crucial task of evaluating research findings, selecting stories that hold meaningful messages for the public, and placing them in the appropriate context" [632]. Astonishingly, only 28 participants attended the first symposium. In order to lure public interest in medical issues, news media have resorted to hiring physicians, as illustrated by CNN's chief medical correspondent Sanjay Gupta, MD and NBC News' chief medical editor Dr. Nancy Snyderman. In addition to hosting the network's weekend health program *House Call*, Dr. Gupta makes frequent appearances on their programs *American Morning* and *Anderson Cooper 360°*. He also publishes a column in *Time* Magazine and participates in CBS's *Evening News* and *60 Minutes* as a special correspondent. Though an Emory University neurosurgeon, Dr. Gupta reports on a wide range of medical subjects, encompassing the dangers of sugar, heart attacks, cell phones, and cancer. As I reach this point in the narrative, *Time* Magazine has just published a cover story titled, "How to Cure Cancer" [633]. The 23-page story is an amalgam of "feel-good" bits of cancer news intertwined with the names and full-page images of prominent cancer researchers at prestigious cancer centers reminiscent of industry-sponsored TV programs. In it, the author speculates on a new approach to cancer research funded by Stand Up to Cancer (Su2C), an organization launched by the entertainment industry, presumably embraced or emulated by major cancer centers, that is expected to accelerate anti-cancer drug discovery, the success of which he backs by citing a few anecdotal tumor responses, as is always the case. Such a prominent display of journalistic presumptuousness suggests the unending relevance of a 13-year old Lancet editorial on breast cancer. It remarked, "If one is to believe all the media hype, the triumphalism of the profession in published research, and the almost weekly miracle breakthroughs trumpeted by cancer charities, one might be surprised that women are dying at all from this cancer" [634]. It must be acknowledged that, at the other end of the spectrum, there are some remarkably well-documented and superbly edited medical reports, especially in specialized print and electronic media. However, given their focus on topical health issues of human interest with a happy ending and their limited reach confined to a small segment of the population with a higher level of formal education, the impact of such reports on the public at large is negligible.

In conclusion, many factors impact the direction and trend of cancer research and Oncology practice. On the one hand, clinical cancer researchers and their sponsors, employers, and publishers are motivated by altruism, career advancement, notoriety, financial gain, and other incentives. In short, they are human. Additionally, the vast majority of cancer reports, whether published in the scientific literature or the popular press, and regardless of source, are carefully crafted to convey progress. This is because the parties involved in reporting clinical cancer research, notably medical editors, are not interested in negative reports and the mass media prefers news susceptible to a "breakthrough" label. This creates a spiral of collective optimism that reinforces the self-delusion within the medical community and the erroneous perception by the public that the *War on Cancer* is on track and the cure of cancer is at hand. Drug manufacturers contribute to that perception through direct-to-consumers and direct-to-physician advertising claiming advantages for each and every new drug, which, along with heavy lobbying on Capitol Hill, supports the industry's pricing power, especially for cancer drugs. Oncologists, on the other hand, find themselves at the "receiving end" of the ever-evolving cancer information chain that shapes standard of care to which they are ethically bound but also need to observe in order to avoid malpractice litigation. Beyond that, the rewarding fee-for-service payment model, the lucrative chemotherapy concession, and other revenue-generating practices also mold treatment selection, hopefully without affecting patient survival or QOL.

Chapter 12
The Complex Physician-Patient Interaction: Expectations *vs*. Reality

> *Some see a hopeless end, while others see an endless hope.*
> – Unknown

12.1 From the Patient's Perspective

12.1.1 First the Basics

Facing a diagnosis of cancer can be psychologically devastating. The state of mind of most patients facing a catastrophic life event evolves through five stages: denial, anger, bargaining, depression, and acceptance [635]. In the denial phase, patients' reaction often is "this can't be happening, not to me", which evolves to "why me? It's not fair" characteristic of the anger phase. Then comes the "I'll give anything for…" of the bargaining stage, followed by the "why bother" of the depression phase, shifting to "It's going to be OK" of the acceptance phase. In cancer patients, the latter phase is often translated into a resolute determination to "fight" and "beat" the disease, which culminates in inner peace and the acceptance of death when it becomes clear that treatment has failed. Thus, it is not surprising that most patients opt for treatment: any treatment that offers some hope. This forward-looking fighting spirit, anchored on the primeval human instinct of self-preservation, often is bolstered by a subjective understanding of information disclosed by the physician, retaining positive elements while misinterpreting or unconsciously dismissing negative ones. Hence, in the US and some Western societies where "breaking bad news" has become an accepted practice, the physician must provide hope and emotional healing throughout the disclosure process. This can be accomplished by ensuring that the patient is ready to assimilate bad news, that information provided meets the patient's wants, needs and preferences, and that the emotional impact of bad news is mitigated or retrieved by emphasizing whatever positive aspects of the case. Factors that can affect the patient's understanding benefits and risks of treatment should be taken into account. They include the disclosure venue and timing (hospital, office, and context settings); the content of the disclosure (thoroughness, clarity, and specificity); and the level of personal interest and empathy conveyed by the physician [636]. Only then should the Oncologist formulate a management plan, taking into account the biological, psychological, behavioral, and social aspects of the patient's disease and his/her input [637, 638]. The founder of the Schwartz Center movingly described his own experience with lung cancer only days before his death to illustrate the enormous power of caregivers' empathy on a patient's frame of mind [639].

In many regions of the World, physicians censor the information shared with cancer patients in misguided attempts to protect them from the potential emotional harm of bad news [640–642]. Sheltering patients from bad news has had unintended consequences. It increases fear and anxiety, prevents a trusting physician-patient relationship to develop, and deprives patients from the empowering feeling of actively participating in the decision-making process and ongoing care. In societies where disclosing bad news is accepted practice, patients often control the type and amount of medical information disclosed to them depending on their level of anxiety, ability to cope, and other personal factors. For example, while some patients demand full disclosure in order to actively participate in their own care, patients with the greatest fear of death and a perception of poor prognosis intuitively prefer minimal disclosure, relinquishing all decisions to the physician [643]. In the end, most cancer patients defer to their physicians the choice of therapy, especially when treatment recommendations are presented with empathy but self-assurance. The preceding general guidelines ensure appropriate physician-patient communications, safeguard patients rights, and enable treatment plans that respond to patients' needs and wishes. Special guidelines apply to clinical trials and are regulated by Federal laws requiring all human research to be conducted according to basic ethical principles that ensure respect for the individual, beneficence, and justice, and that patient participation be informed, voluntary, and not influenced or coerced in any way.

12.1.2 More Details

12.1.2.1 Disclosure in the Community Setting

It is stating the obvious to assert that the Oncologist planning treatment and the cancer patient being advised should both be aware of the risks and benefits of the recommended treatment and have a clear understanding of potential outcomes. Thus, it might be expected that a substantial number of patients afflicted by advanced cancer of the types proven over the years to follow a relentless course not substantially altered by treatment would not be offered treatment or decline it if offered. However, the vast majority of cancer patients are treated despite the fact that fewer than 2 % achieve a cure and a meager prolongation of survival is the best hope [644]. This is due not only to Oncologists' pro-treatment stance, but also to patients' attitudes regarding cancer treatment. Indeed, studies have shown that cancer patients are willing to assume greater risks when facing imminent death than would caregivers and the public. According to one survey, 53.1 % of cancer patients expressed a willingness to suffer *severe* treatment side effects in order to reach a 1 % cure rate, 42.1 % to survive an additional 3 months, and 42.6 % to achieve symptom relief, compared to 20, 10.2, and 6.8 % of Oncologists, 13.5, 6.0, and 5.9 % of Oncology nurses, and 19, 10, and 10 % of healthy controls [645]. Is this risk-taking attitude by cancer patients a rational, weighted decision? Is it the result of over-enthusiastic physicians emphasizing small benefits while minimizing risks? Or, is it the result of desperate decisions of individuals in despair when confronting imminent death? In most instances, patients' role in the decision-making process is limited to acquiescing to the physician's choice of action after asking but a few questions, despite surveys indicating that most patients in all age groups prefer to participate actively in decision-making [646, 647]. Indeed, not only do the psychological and emotional impacts of a cancer diagnosis diminish patients' analytical power and discerning capacity at a time it is most needed, but most patients make no attempts to research their disease or treatment options independently. Given the circumstances, the instinct of self-preservation usually prevails, leading most patients to hear what they wish to hear, particularly if the content and setting of the disclosure process and empathy of the caregiver are sub-optimal [648, 649].

Trust in the physician is an essential element of the patient-physician relationship. However, a physician becomes a perfect agent for the patient only when the latter would make the same decision if in possession of the same clinical information and expertise. Such a circumstance rarely exists in practice, for few patients will ever achieve a level of understanding comparable to that of their physicians, and the latter often fail to meet patients halfway [650]. In practice, multiple Oncologist-patient encounters will take place over the course of the disease, involving three stages each time: exchange of information, discussion, and decision-making. The type of interaction depends on the patient-physician relationship, which generally takes one of three forms [651]. The first is the traditional *paternalistic* model, where information flows in one direction: from physician to patient, all decisions regarding treatment and patient management are made by the physician, and the patient acquiesces to professional authority and expertise. At the other extreme lies the *informed* model where information flows from physician to patient but the patient makes all decisions. Between these extremes is the *shared* model where exchange of information proceeds both ways: the physician thoroughly informs the patient of treatment options along with their benefits and risks, and the patient voices preferences, and both contribute to the decision-making process. While by virtue of their training and expertise, and for expediency, most physicians tend to adopt the *paternalistic* approach, patients' preferences vary according to age, sex, educational level, and type and severity of the disease. For example, a study of 1,012 women with breast cancer revealed that 22 % wanted to select their own treatment, 44 % elected to share the task with their physician, and 34 % preferred to delegate the responsibility to their physician [652]. Additionally, many patients are receptive to substantial amounts of information, even if they do not wish to participate in making treatment decisions. Under the *shared* model, patients must be in possession of substantial clinical information in order to participate effectively in treatment decisions that will profoundly impact their lives and often determine their survival. Yet, because communication skills are not taught in medical schools and there are no standard guidelines, the physician disclosure process is often inadequate, not geared to patients' needs and preferences, and often overestimates benefits and underestimates risks. A good point of departure is to practice *patient-centered care*, defined as "respecting and responding to patients' wants, needs and preferences, so that they can make choices in their care that best fit their individual circumstances", as the cornerstone of quality care delivery [653].

It might surprise the reader to know that there are no specific guidelines for cancer care, though generalities have been addressed over the years. For instance, in 1999, the Institute of Medicine (IOM) concluded that cancer patients did not receive state-of-the-art care and its National Cancer Policy Board Cancer Care System made 10 recommendations for promoting optimal care delivery. While reasonable, the measures recommended are broad and designed to become pubic policy rather than apply to individual care. For instance,

> Recommendation 3: Measure and monitor the quality of care using a core set of quality measures. Cancer care quality measures should span the continuum of cancer care and be developed through a coordinated public-private effort: be used to hold providers, including health care systems, health plans, and physicians, accountable for demonstrating that they provide and improve quality of care; be applied to care provided through the Medicare and Medicaid programs as a requirement of participation in these programs; and be disseminated widely and communicated to purchasers, providers, consumer organizations, individuals with cancer, policy makers, and health services researchers, in a form that is relevant and useful for health care decision-making [654].

On the other hand, ASCO's "Measures of Quality of Care for Patients With Cancer" recommends "The selection and proper application by clinicians of clinical treatments that optimize the outcomes of care" as part of the "initial therapeutic management" [655]. Under its Quality Oncology Practice Initiative, ASCO lists 97 items with subdivisions, all of which are very general, such as "core 9: Documented plan for chemotherapy, including doses, route, and time intervals." Or "core 13a1: Chemotherapy administered to patients with metastatic solid tumor with performance status of 3, 4, or undocumented (Lower Score – Better)" [656]. Likewise, the National Comprehensive Cancer Network Clinical Practice Guidelines in Oncology lists the following specific guidelines:

- For treatment of cancer by site.
- For detection, prevention, & risk reduction.
- For supportive care.
- For age-related recommendations.
- For patients [657].

Yet, none address the initial physician-patient phase that sets the stage for a mutually satisfying relationship and in large measure determines a seamless course of action and peace of mind for the patient. There is consensus that this relationship should rest on a transparent disclosure of diagnosis, proposed intervention with reasonable alternatives, intended benefits, and associated risks. However, there are no specific guidelines addressing when to initiate treatment towards what outcome and whether to discontinue treatment when it becomes clear that the intended outcome cannot be reached or when the burden of treatment becomes unacceptable. What Oncologists must correct is the widespread practice of assessing treatment efficacy based on tumor response rather than on patient outcome, which explains in large measure why cancers historically shown to progress relentlessly regardless of treatment are routinely treated, often to the end of life. Indeed, potential benefits of cancer treatment in the clinical setting should be measured not by tumor responses but by patient outcome benchmarks, including OS, 5-year survival, and DFS. Such information is readily available from the medical literature for most cancers in all stages and should be used as the sole guide for deciding whether or not chemotherapy will be of benefit to a particular patient, and so inform the patient. Tumor outcomes, such as average response rates and partial or complete remissions gathered from the literature, should be discussed. However, physicians must inform patients that the latter represent not goals in themselves but interim measurements of tumor size that are useful for determining whether the therapy instituted is efficacious and worth pursuing or inefficacious and should be abandoned. Physicians should stress that tumor responses have little relevance to the ultimate course of the disease or to patient survival. Likewise, potential complications, especially life-threatening toxicity of the treatment contemplated, and their management, should also be disclosed at the outset. Alternative treatments, including withholding or delaying treatment, and the effect of each on survival and QOL, should be discussed. Likewise, because pain is one of the most feared complications of cancer, patients must be reassured that pain control is easy to achieve in most circumstances given today's potent analgesics, and physicians should not flinch from prescribing opioids when appropriate [658]. Finally, patients should be encouraged to ask questions, to discuss their options with loved-ones or seek second opinions, and be allowed time for reflection. Oncologists who adopt this advisory role are rewarded by enlightened patients who tend to become participants in their own care, and who have a greater appreciation of the highly complex issues involved in cancer management and, having understood and accepted the risks involved, are less likely to resort to unwarranted legal action.

All factual information described above should be recorded on a written informed consent form that could follow recommendations by the Office of Human Research Protections for clinical trials [659]. The form, to be written in easy to understand language, should prominently display the following information:

- Short text or tabular description of the patient's diagnosis (e.g., cancer type – stage), and special circumstances of the case likely to skew expected outcome.
- Best drug or drug combination recommended, plus one or two alternative options.
- Anticipated patient outcome (e.g., DFS – 5-year survival) and risks associated with each drug option, stratified by severity and probability of occurrence.
- Summary of pertinent medical literature data on benefits and risks of treatment options recommended, along with the actual references.
- Disclosure of patient rights, including well-being and privacy protection, and autonomy.

- Description of patient-triggered issues and other subjects that were discussed.
- Disclosure of the physician's financial interest in drugs and tests recommended.

In order to streamline and standardize the process, inform consent forms could be developed for the ten most frequent cancers (e.g., prostate, breast, lung, colorectal, melanoma, bladder, lymphoma, kidney, thyroid, and pancreas) that accounted for 74.8 % of all cancers in 2012. Alternatively, the ten most lethal cancers could be targeted initially (e.g., lung, colorectal, breast, pancreas, prostate, lymphoma. ovary, esophagus, bladder, and brain), which accounted for 66.2 % of all cancer deaths in 2012. The task of designing such specific consent forms could be assigned to panels of experts from NCI, ASCO, ASH, cancer cooperative groups, universities, or research centers and, after securing input by the Medical Oncology community, be made freely available on the Web to anyone. Some will argue, correctly, that such a document cannot apply to all situations. However, sufficient flexibility could be built into the document to allow timely modifications according to the individual's disease and psychosocial profiles, with the added advantage that each would be discussed with the patient and recorded as rationale for treatment adjustments. There is precedent for this in clinical trial protocols where initial and subsequent adjustments to the treatment proposed are allowed in order to individualize care and reduce risks. Moreover, the expanded information disclosure process and informed consent form would codify, organize, and bring uniformity, transparency, and objectivity to a process that many community Oncologists follow in principle, but in an inconsistent and poorly-documented manner. Additionally, a thorough, transparent, and objective initial disclosure would serve as a basis for future physician-patient communications and facilitate subsequent management decisions as they become necessary during the course of the disease. This approach is applicable to all cancer patients, including those who choose a "paternalistic" physician-patient relationship model and prefer to be in possession of rudimentary rather than detailed information about their disease and its treatment. In cases of extreme reluctance, detailed information can be conveyed primarily to the patient's surrogates. By providing written evidence that patient and physician reviewed the case management specifics together, a signed consent form of this nature would encourage and generalize the practice by allaying physicians' fears of litigation and ultimately be helpful in court cases.

12.1.2.2 Disclosure Within Clinical Trials

The first international codification of ethical principles to guide clinical researchers involved in human experimentation is known as *The Declaration of Helsinki*. This document entitled *Ethical Principles for Medical Research Involving Human Subjects* was adopted by the 18th World Medical Association (WMA) general assembly meeting in Helsinki, in June 1964. The 9th of its 12 *Basic Principles* reads,

> In any research on human beings, each potential subject must be adequately informed of the aims, methods, anticipated benefits and potential hazards of the study, and the discomfort it may entail. He or she should be informed that he or she is at liberty to abstain from participation

12.1 From the Patient's Perspective

in the study, and that he or she is free to withdraw his or her consent to participation at any time. The physician should then obtain the subject's freely-given informed consent, preferably in writing [660].

The declaration was first revised in 1975 at the Tokyo 29th WMA meeting where the concept of *Independent Review Boards* was introduced, with the seventh and last revision being in 2008 at the 59th meeting in Seoul, which codified registration of clinical trials and reporting of results. The final document is universally regarded as the ethical cornerstone of human clinical research.

In the US, codification of human research began with the *National Commission for the Protection of Human Subjects of Biomedical and Behavioral Research* issued by the National Research Act signed into law on July 12, 1974. Among other tasks, the commission was charged with identifying the basic ethical principles that should underlie the conduct of biomedical and behavioral research involving human subjects, and to develop guidelines which should be followed to assure that such research is conducted in accordance with those principles. The commission first met on February 1976 at the Smithsonian Institution's Belmont Conference Center, followed by monthly deliberations over a period of nearly 4 years, which resulted in a Department of Health and Human Services' publication entitled: *The Belmont Report: Ethical principles and guidelines for the protection of human subjects of research,* best known as the *Belmont Report* [661].

The *Belmont Report* expanded the *Nuremberg Code* [662], drafted in 1947 as a set of standards for judging researchers who conducted unethical biomedical experiments on concentration camp prisoners during WWII, and was designed to prevent repetition of medical research abuses revealed in 1972 regarding the natural history of untreated syphilis [663]. This referred to a study conducted in the 1940s on 399 poor black males from Tuskegee, Alabama who were not informed of their disease (syphilis) and denied penicillin when it became available in 1947, leading to a full enquiry and an apology by President Clinton in 1997. Other infamous unethical experiments, highly implausible today thanks to legislation enacted since, came to light in a 1993 exposé by *The Albuquerque Tribune*. It revealed both the injection of radioactive tracers to thousands of unsuspecting human subjects and the radiation exposure of thousands of unaware individuals to several hundred secret and intentional releases of radiation over a 30-year period. Half a century later, on January 15, 1994, President Clinton created the Advisory Committee on Human Radiation Experiments to investigate reports of unethical conduct by the US government and by government-funded institutions, in the use of, or exposure to, ionizing radiation in human beings during the period of 1944–1974. In its final report, the panel described the following illustrative case:

> The subject, as it turned out, was already in the Oak Ridge Army hospital, a victim of an auto accident that had occurred on March 24, 1945. He was a fifty-three-year-old "colored male" named Ebb Cade, who was employed by an Oak Ridge construction company as a cement mixer. The subject had serious fractures in his arm and leg, but was otherwise "well developed [and] well nourished." The patient was able to tell his doctors that he had always been in good health. Mr. Cade had been hospitalized since his accident, but the plutonium injection did not take place until April 10. On this date, "HP-12"

(the code name HP – "human product")…was reportedly injected with 4.7 micrograms of plutonium… Measurements were to be taken from samples of Mr. Cade's blood after four hours, his bone tissue after ninety-six hours, and his bodily excretions for forty to sixty days thereafter. His broken bones were not set until April 15-five days after the injection-when bone samples were taken in a biopsy…One document records that Mr. Cade had "marked" tooth decay and gum inflammation, and fifteen of his teeth were extracted and sampled for plutonium. The Committee has not been able to determine whether the teeth were extracted primarily for medical reasons or for the purpose of sampling for plutonium…According to one account, Mr. Cade departed suddenly from the hospital on his own initiative… [664].

From the *Belmont Report* and subsequent legislative efforts was born the modern *informed consent*, a document that establishes three fundamental ethical principles that must be observed in any human research:

- Respect to persons by acknowledging participants' autonomy and protection for those with diminished autonomy.
- Beneficence that ensures that no harm will be done and to maximize possible benefits and minimize possible harms.
- Justice, the principle of shared burdens and benefits, to ensure that potential benefits of the research benefits study participants as well as non-participants.

Several reviews of the content and scope of the informed consent have been published over the years, including some quite recently [665]. The oversight and responsibility for implementing guidelines for experimentation in humans rests with the IRB at centers that conduct human research [666]. On the other hand, uniformity of the disclosure process is ensured by the informed consent, which informs and engages patients, and sets the stage for open and transparent communications between patient and physician for the duration of the study. However, the *Belmont Report* and a structured *informed consent* protect the approximately 2 % of the total US cancer population participating in clinical trials at any given time, but do not apply to the remaining 98 %, who receive non-investigational cancer treatment in the community setting [667–669]. In addition, critics contend that social or mind control experimentation are not covered. Another loophole is the use of cancer drugs *off-label*. This practice consists of using drugs for indications other than those approved by the FDA or in combinations not sanctioned by prior clinical research, especially for treating patients who have failed standard treatment. Yet, this is permitted by the *Belmont Report* in which "practice" is defined as "interventions that are designed solely to enhance the well-being of an individual patient or client and that have a reasonable expectation of success." In contrast, research is defined as "an activity designed to test an hypothesis… described in a formal protocol that sets forth an objective and a set of procedures designed to reach that objective." Although the use of cancer drugs off-label might be justified occasionally by seasoned Oncologists' breadth and depth of knowledge, the practice is widespread and often based on anecdotal personal experience rather than on clinical trial data. As a result, unsuspecting patients so treated are exposed to additional and often unforeseen side effects and complications without commensurate benefits. While most Oncologists are judicious in the use of drugs off-label, the unrestricted practice could theoretically extend to any drug and any cancer.

The quality of the disclosure, or lack thereof, can also be at issue, both in clinical trials and in the clinical setting. Audio- or video-taped surveys of Oncologists' interviews with prospective clinical trial participants demonstrated multiple deficiencies in the disclosure process that, in some cases, calls into question the validity of the informed consent [670, 671]. Indeed, while most Oncologists are conscientious and dedicated to their patients' welfare, the desire to communicate in simple language, poor communication skills, and time constraints often lead to insufficient or faulty disclosure. Alternatively, the zeal for thoroughness might result in disclosure of superfluous and confusing details, or the use of an overly complicated or technical language not readily comprehensible by some patients. Recent advances in research technologies often generate incidental findings, raising the issue of whether researchers and caregivers should disclose such information to patients when non-essential to the clinical study or to the treatment contemplated [672]. However, more troubling, though less common, is the conduct of some unscrupulous researchers who disregard ethical principles and violate Federal rules designed to protect research subjects for expediency or self-serving motives, putting patients at risk and exposing themselves to FDA censure, as in the case of an editor of the NEJM [673], loss of Federal research funding and academic standing [674, 675], humiliating retraction of published data [676], dismissal [677], or lawsuits [678]. More ominously, each new revelation of unethical conduct by medical researchers contributes to public distrust in clinical research and raises questions as to whether they represent isolated cases or the tip of an iceberg of research misconduct.

12.2 From the Caregiver's Perspective

12.2.1 Facing Difficult Decisions

Approximately 2 % of patients with disseminated or metastatic cancer treated with chemotherapy can be cured of their disease, and marginal to modest prolongation of survival, usually measured in weeks, is feasible in some types of cancer [679]. Hence, treating the vast majority of patients with advanced cancer unless contraindicated, as is the practice today, would seem to be an unwise if not futile exercise. Indeed, when the most desirable "quantitative" patient outcomes such as cure, 5-year survival, or meaningful prolongation of survival are not achievable, seeking "qualitative" outcomes such as palliation and improved QOL become the Oncologist's ultimate goal. While the above statement is intuitively obvious and unassailable, it embodies concepts and issues that, given their ethical, social, and legal context, are difficult to sort out in the clinical arena. For example,

- When is a cancer refractory and its treatment futile, leading to palliation?
- What is palliation?
- Is palliative chemotherapy justified when efficacious alternatives are available?
- How much chemotherapy toxicity is acceptable for what type and level of palliation?

- Does the placebo effect of chemotherapy justify its use in palliation?
- What is the preferred setting for providing optimal palliation?

The above questions and many others raise issues Oncologists are confronted with on a daily basis that encompass religious, moral, ethical, and socioeconomic factors, in addition to medical considerations. The sequence of the above list rests on the fact that the concept of palliation, its modality, and delivery setting are most pertinent and crucial in the context of terminal patients when treatment of the disease has failed and the physician must focus on ensuring the best possible QOL during the patient's final stages. Hence, the pivotal decision to initiate the palliative phase is triggered by the determination that further disease-specific treatment would be futile. Yet, the absence of guidelines as to timing and the controversy regarding rights of autonomy from the caregiver's and patient's perspectives and the definition of medical futility raise new questions. On the one hand, modern medical science enables physicians to maintain and prolong vegetative states through mechanical ventilation, feeding tubes, and other life-supporting means, and patients and patient surrogates increasingly assert their autonomy in life and death decisions, often with a limited understanding of the consequences. On the other hand, the concept of medical futility is misunderstood by the various stakeholders in its scope and timing. For instance, a survey of surrogates of 50 critically ill hospitalized patients revealed that most doubted the ability of physicians to predict medical futility [680]. Likewise, a Medline database search of studies on medical futility between 1980 and 2008 revealed that 47 studies supporting and 45 refuting the concept of medical futility provided insufficient clinical guidance for making such a decision [681]. Moreover, while the concept of QOL is intuitively obvious, it is neither definable nor quantifiable with any degree of consensus. More ominously, the closely related notion of palliation has two incompatible and widely divergent interpretations in the practice setting: one that properly views palliation in the context of alleviating suffering through symptom relief; the other that equates palliation with the administration of non-curative treatment, presumably aimed at controlling disease-related symptoms or, more unrealistically, at preventing future complications of progressive cancer. While the former addresses patients' immediate QOL concerns, the latter justifies inflicting additional pain and suffering now in exchange for a usually unfulfilled promise of a better future QOL. This attitude towards palliation suggests that cancer caregivers, for a variety of personal and extraneous reasons, are unable or unwilling to acknowledge in a timely manner that their efforts to change the course of their patients' cancer has come to an end. To do so should not be construed as abandonment but rather as a humane approach to prevent further suffering at the end of life by providing appropriate palliative care and an opportunity for patients and relatives to come to terms with the dying process and achieve peace and dignity. In contrast, terminal patients often receive more intensive care in the last few weeks of life than in the preceding months. This is documented yet again in a recent study of end-of-life health care costs incurred by 28,530 privately insured oncology patients between July 2002 and December 2009 [682]. In that study, the mean total cancer-related costs in the last 6 months before death was $74,212, of which 79 % was incurred for three types of acute services: Inpatient care, $40,702 or 55 %; Hospital outpatient procedures (Hosp. OPP), $10,123 or 13.6 %; and Chemotherapy, $7,595 or 10.2 %, with Hospice care accounting for only $3,256 or 4.4 % of the total. While on the sixth month before death, outpatient procedures, inpatient care, chemotherapy, and hospice cost $1,992, $1,785, $1630, and $28, respectively, hospice care cost rose to $2,464 in the last month of life, whereas inpatient care cost soared to $20,559 or nearly 85 % of total cost (Fig. 12.1).

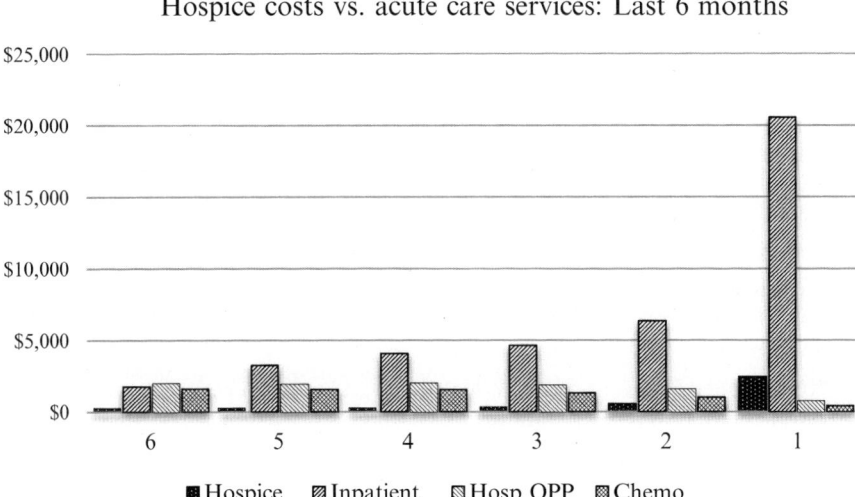

Fig. 12.1 Cost of leading cancer care services in last 6 months before death (Adapted from [602])

Likewise, a survey on handling end of life cancer care for 215,311 Medicare decedents between 2003 and 2007 showed that 64.9 % were hospitalized during the last month of life, including 24.7 % to ICU facilities, and 30.2 % died in the hospital. Although 53.8 % were enrolled in hospice care during the last month of life, the average stay was only 8.4 days. Revealingly, 48.1 % of Medicare beneficiaries were seen by 10 or more different physicians during the last 6 months of life [683]. Hence, data on the type and setting of medical services rendered to nearly a quarter of a million terminal cancer patients from both the private and public sectors between 2002 and 2009 demonstrate that, towards the end of life, physicians redouble their efforts to "save" or prolong their patients' lives by overutilizing acute inpatient services and by calling on consultants while making only a token and late use of hospice support as a venue for providing palliative care. In retrospect, acute care services patients received in the last few weeks before death were not only futile with respect to altering the course of the disease but often prolonged suffering. However, given the lack of consensus about the concept of QOL and the flexible interpretation of what constitutes palliation and how to achieve it in the clinical setting context, the following discussion addresses the concept of *futile* chemotherapy and its subservience to the notion of cancer *refractoriness*, and the relevance of both to cancer management, especially at the end of life.

A Google Scholar search for "medical futility" literature between 2002 and 2012 yielded 18,200 entries. This high level of interest was stimulated mainly by reports in the late 1980s of patients and their surrogates demanding life-sustaining measures judged by their physicians to be pointless [684, 685], and by the patients' autonomy movement. The latter emerged from a number of factors, including sophisticated therapies capable of artificially prolonging life, the commercialization of medicine that eroded the patient-physician relationship, and the *Patient Self-Determination Act* of 1991 that encouraged patients' self-assertiveness in decision-making, especially at the end of life. Such patient demands, based on a misinterpretation or misuse of the principle of patients' rights of autonomy, are neither ethically or legally defensible. This is because, well-established in law and ethics, the rights of autonomy are negative rather than positive rights. That is, patients have the right to choose among treatment options offered by physicians, including refusing treatment altogether despite negative consequences to themselves. However, patients have no legal or ethical right to demand a treatment of their choice, mainly because,

> Given the array of treatments now available for advanced and chronic illness, it has become nearly impossible for a patient or a patient's surrogate decision maker to fully anticipate or comprehend the intricacies, burdens, and benefits of all available options [686].

From the physician's standpoint, the debate and controversy centers on whether caregivers can withhold or withdraw a treatment they judge futile, and when they can ethically and legally do so. Resolution of these questions is directly linked to the definition of medical futility. The term futile derives from the Latin *futilis* or leaky, an idea rooted in Greek mythology that, through compelling imagery, illustrates the two main inherent attributes of a futile endeavor: pointlessness and endlessness. According to this mythical version, King Danaus of Egypt had 50 daughters and his brother Aegyptus had 50 sons. The latter demanded that his sons marry their cousins, an idea vehemently opposed by Danaus. On the wedding day, Danaus instructed his daughters to kill their husbands in the wedding bed. All complied but Hypermnestra, who defended her disobedience, claiming she remained a virgin after the wedding night. According to legend, the 49 daughters guilty of murder were punished in the underworld by having continually to fetch water carried in sieves [687].

As a complex concept that incorporates medical, social, ethical, and legal components, medical futility has escaped precise definition. The American Medical Association has opted to relegate its definition and implementation to health care institutions, stating,

> To assist in fair and satisfactory decision-making about what constitutes futile intervention: (1) All health care institutions, whether large or small, should adopt a policy on medical futility; and (2) Policies on medical futility should follow a due process approach [688].

Quantitative and qualitative elements known as *odds* and *ends* are crucial factors in decision-making regarding potentially futile medical interventions, though in the practice setting, there is no consensus on what thresholds should apply [689]. The most permissive definition of medical futility puts the quantitative threshold for *odds* at less than 0.01 (<1 %) [690]. That is, any treatment with less than 1 in 100 chance of benefiting the patient would be considered futile, a definition that gives licence to treat anyone any time. The *ends* can have a physiological component and a normative one. The former refers to the clinical objective of treatment (e.g., tumor response or patient survival) and the latter to the patient's perception of benefit, whether or not the physiological component was achieved. The latter falls in the subjective realm of QOL. In the abstract, a futile treatment is one that has low probability (e.g., the *odds*) of achieving a desired goal (the *ends*), but setting an arbitrary limit of 1 % is unrealistic. Indeed, such a degree of precision does not belong to clinical medicine where decision-making remains an art rather than an exact science. Arguments offered by pro-futility advocates include: professional integrity that asserts that physicians should not be required to offer useless or harmful treatments; physicians are the sole arbiters of how and when to treat; and stewardship of scarce resources to be used for beneficial purposes. Critics contend mainly that physicians have no grounds to impose their personal values regarding what *ends* to be pursued and at what *odds* [691, 692], especially because no consensus has been reached on the definition of medical futility or its application in the clinical setting; empirical evidence from clinical trials is not necessarily applicable to individual patients; it amounts to a usurpation of patients' autonomy; and evidence-based outcome standards are lacking in most medical fields. However, while conceptually defensible, critics' arguments become somewhat tenuous in the context of Oncology practice where average *odds* and *ends* are known for most cancers in most circumstances and the ethical principles of beneficence and non-maleficence are relatively easy to aim at based on the *ends* expected. Indeed, in Oncology, *odds* are well defined and generally quantifiable with respect to the desired *ends*, whether tumor response or survival prolongation, which, for "first line" treatment, signifies tumor size reduction or a few extra weeks of life in most cases (*physiological ends*), respectively. Positive *ends* benefit patients in other ways, including symptom relief and a sense of well-being (*psychological ends*). Because relief of suffering is the ultimate goal of medical care, the latter is especially important. On the other hand, the *odds* for "second line treatment" of unresponsive or recurrent cancer are limited to an occasional unexplained outlier (the *ends*) that should not be the rationale for subjecting most other patients so treated to drug toxicity and other treatment complications (e.g., burden). The *odds* of continuing treatment of patients with unresponsive or progressive cancer expecting to mitigate future symptoms is nil, and hence, futile. In addition to *odds* and *ends*, treatment burden is an important element in the decision-making equation. That is, the physical, emotional, financial, or social costs associated with treatment: the concept of proportionality. However, futility and burden, terms grounded in the ethical principles of beneficence and non-maleficence, are not to be confused. A treatment is futile when its prospects for achieving the intended *ends* are essentially nil (e.g., negative beneficence), and burdensome when it is likely to cause harmful *ends* (e.g., positive maleficence).

In the clinical practice setting, assessment of treatment efficacy is tumor-centered rather than patient-oriented where beneficence is generally judged as a function of tumor-size reduction and maleficence, to many, is implicitly justified by prolonged survival of a few. Is it ethical to risk harming many individuals in order to benefit a few? This issue is particularly pertinent to Oncology where drug toxicity and treatment complications can reach life-threatening severity, including bone marrow, heart, kidney, and lung failure, and fatal infections or bleeding, while objective benefits are modest at best for most patients with most types of advanced or metastatic cancer, as shown by average national survival statistics. Perhaps the best illustration of lack of proportionality between intended *ends* and *burden* to patients and society has been the relentless dose escalation of a variety of drug combinations for metastatic breast cancer, leading to high-dose chemotherapy with stem cell transplantation. An analysis of several metastatic breast cancer studies representing 30-years of clinical trials demonstrated little difference in OS (median of 2 years), whether patients were given standard-dose chemotherapy, high-dose chemotherapy, or high-dose chemotherapy with bone marrow rescue [693]. The latter group included some long-term survivors and, not surprisingly, some early deaths as well. These studies demonstrate that, compared to standard-dose treatment, high-dose chemotherapy of breast cancer with stem cells rescue is medically futile, for it increases the burden to patients (physical, emotional, and financial) and society (misallocation of resources), without clear benefits to most patients, notwithstanding an occasional outlying long-term survivor. While sobering in themselves, these results are the more humbling when considered in light of the current (2013) indications for bone marrow transplantation no longer includes breast cancer. Indeed, out of 17,938 transplants performed in the US between 2008 and 2011, only 1 case was for breast cancer [694]. Interestingly, a 1980 study reported a comparable 2-year OS in women with metastatic breast cancer before the chemotherapy era that remained unchanged during the early years of standard chemotherapy [695]. Moreover, after multiple clinical trials over four decades searching for efficacious drugs against advanced breast cancer, the average 5-year survival increased by a modest 15 % between 1975–1977 and 2001–2007, as shown in Fig. 9.1, and much of the improvement can be traced back to advances in general medical support rather than anti-cancer therapies. These data are cited not to suggest that all cytotoxic chemotherapy for advanced breast or other cancers is futile but to emphasize the need for the medical community to assess critically the consequences of the current practice of escalating and relentlessly treating most types of cancer that often becomes heroic at the end of life, prolonging not life but suffering, and the need to abide by ethical and humane standards of care. Such reassessment should lead to a medically and legally acceptable definition of futile treatment and an unambiguous description of procedures that, while protecting vulnerable patients, enable individual physicians to discharge their duties compassionately and legally through the end of life.

12.2.2 Managing Cancer Patients at the End of Life

Notwithstanding moralists' and bio-ethicists' views on end of life management, physicians who frequently face life and death situations throughout their careers have the experience necessary to steer the debate towards a realistic and practical definition of medical futility, and to guide the development of sensible guidelines for its application in the clinical setting. Yet, Oncologists view cancer as an enemy that must be defeated, accounting perhaps for their obstinate determination in pursuing treatment while hope persists, and for considering cures, survival prolongation, and even tumor responses as personal victories. This, despite decades of experience showing that most advanced cancers progress relentlessly regardless of treatment, and that patients inevitably reach a point of no return when it becomes obvious that the end is near and further cancer treatment would be of no benefit. In the clinical setting, recognition of this fact most often occurs when treatment modalities have been exhausted or chemotherapy tolerance has been reached or breached or the burden of treatment has become unacceptable. It is usually at this late juncture that further cancer treatment is judged futile and the focus becomes symptom relief and preservation of QOL. The psychological and emotional impact on patients of reaching that juncture can be reduced by a pre-existing, transparent, and proactive physician-patient relationship that will have prepared the patient and surrogates to anticipate, face, and accept the inevitable outcome and do so in a timely manner in order to ensure death with dignity. However, if such an outcome is inevitable for most non-hematologic and non-embryonal malignancies, the question is whether further treatment of cancers known to progress during "first-line" chemotherapy or recur soon thereafter should also be considered futile, particularly given the potential harm associated with the relentless administration of inefficacious but toxic drugs. This question is particularly relevant in view of the trend over the last 40 years to escalate from standard to high-dose chemotherapy to combination chemotherapy and other strategies attempting to enhance the efficacy of mostly inefficacious, non-specific cancer drugs. Regrettably, facing reality is often postponed, especially when reality contradicts preconceptions and entrenched practice patterns. Perhaps this explains why reports of near-stagnating survival rates in patients with advanced lung cancer between 1973 and 1994 and metastatic breast cancer between 1980 and 2002 have been all but ignored [696, 697]. Indeed, patients afflicted by these and other chemotherapy-unresponsive cancers continue to be treated with cytotoxic drugs, albeit in new combinations and permutations, including the recent use of drugs targeting molecular biomarkers, also with little likelihood of survival prolongation [698, 699].

The debate over medical futility in the US has had the salutary effect of highlighting the notion that a peaceful and dignified death, defined as the natural outcome of aging or the inevitable sequel of a terminal illness, is both desirable and achievable by instituting end-of-life palliative care. When the physiological objective of treatment (e.g., tumor response or patient survival) is no longer feasible, the emphasis shifts from disease treatment to palliative care. The social and family foundation of the palliative care concept was forcefully articulated by the former secretary of the US Department of Health, Education, and Welfare, Joseph Califano (1977–1979):

> It is time we recognize, in the dependency of the terminally ill, the dignity and beauty of dependency that we long celebrated in the early days of newborn babies. Those with irreversible illness deserve the same loving care as they leave this world that we provide the helpless infants as they enter it [700].

This age-old concept, ingrained in most cultures but forsaken in modern societies, has evolved into the *Hospice* movement. The term Hospice derives from the Latin *Hospis*, which means both host and guest, and *hospitium*, which refers to the dwelling where guests are greeted with hospitality. While hospitality to pilgrims and traveling strangers was offered from pagan antiquity to the Islamic world, it flourished during the times of the Christian crusades and pilgrimages when *hospitiums* were one of the responsibilities assumed by many monasteries where monks extended care to the sick and dying, but also to the hungry and weary on their way to the Holy Land, Rome, or other holy places, as well as to the woman in labor, the needy poor, the orphan, and the leper on their journey through life. The *Hospice du Grand-Saint-Bernard*, located at the Great St. Bernard Pass (2,500 m. altitude) in the Canton de Valais, Switzerland, founded around 1050 by St. Bernard of Menthon to protect pilgrims from local bandits and famous for its breed of giant St. Bernard rescue dogs, still shelters gratuitously thousands of mountain climbers and hikers every year. Travel shelters became widespread during the Middle Ages. For example, the four main pilgrimage routes through France (from Paris, Vézelay, Le Puy, and Arles) leading to Santiago de Compostela in Spain, each fed by numerous subsidiary routes, spanned over 3,000 miles of roads, dotted by over 800 *hospitiums* or hostels along the way that provided shelter and lodging to millions of pilgrims between the early twelfth century and the end of the eighteenth [701]. Many still offer rest, refuge from the elements, and bed-and-breakfast to modern-day pilgrims and backpackers. Likewise, the Knights of St. John of Jerusalem founded the first hospice on the Greek island of Rhodes to provide refuge to crusaders and care for the ill and dying. The concept of shelter, food, and comfort for the needy traveler was expanded to local populations in 1633 when a French priest, St. Vincent de Paul, founded the *Company of the Daughters of Charity* in Châtillon-sur-Chalaronne, France. The Daughters' vows were to shelter and care for orphans, the poor, the sick, and the dying. By 1789, the Daughters of Charity operated 426 shelters in France and hundreds more throughout Western Europe. Today, their organization operates hospitals, orphanages, homes for the poor, and schools worldwide. Their success inspired Baron von Stein of Prussia, a century later, to open Kaiserswerth, the first Protestant hospice, also staffed by nuns. However, historians and commentators generally credit Jeanne Garnier of France, Mary Aikenhead of Ireland, and Dame Cicely Mary Saunders of Britain for evolving the concept of hospice and promoting its worldwide adoption: Jeanne Garnier as founder of the *Association des Dames du Calvaire* and of the first hospice for dying cancer patients in Lyons, France, in 1842; Mary Aikenhead, founder of the *Religious Sisters of Charity,* for associating the concept of Hospice to end-of-life care at their Our Lady's Hospice, opened in 1879; and Dame Cicely Mary Saunders, co-founder of the *Cicely Saunders International*, for emphasizing the psychosocial dimensions to death and dying at St. Christopher's Hospice she founded in 1967, and for inspiring followers throughout the world [702].

While the Connecticut Hospice opened in 1974 launched the hospice era in the US, the palliative care movement failed to gain momentum, mainly due to physicians' over-reliance on scientific advances to address purely medical issues while neglecting patients' psychosocial needs and to the public's death-denying attitude that seeks "all that can be done" to the very end of life. However, two developments led to the recognition of the merits of the hospice concept and its adoption by the government, medical organizations, and society at large. They include the failure of physicians to provide adequate pain control to terminally ill patients, to acquiesce to their patients' end-of-life care preferences, or to ignore them altogether [703], and the convergence of critics of the right to physician-assisted suicide onto the opposing notion of "physician-assisted living" [704]. In 1990, the WHO defined palliative care as,

> The active total care of patients whose disease is not responsive to curative treatment. Control of pain, of other symptoms, and of psychological, social, and spiritual support is paramount. The goal of palliative care is the achievement of the best quality of life for patients and their families [705].

On the other hand, the American Academy of Hospice and Palliative Medicine view the issue differently, stating,

> The goal of palliative care is to prevent and relieve suffering, and to support the best possible quality of life for patients and their families, regardless of their stage of disease or the need for other therapies, in accordance with their values and preferences [706].

Certainly, palliation of physical symptoms and mental anguish caused by illness and the prospects of immediate death should be part of the overall patient care management throughout the entire course of the disease, but becomes critical towards the end of life, and must involve immediate relatives and be delivered at home preferentially, rather than in the hospice setting. This is because hospices are brick-and-mortar facilities specifically intended and organized to deliver palliative care to the terminally ill in an impersonal setting that isolates patients from their familiar environments and supporting relatives when most needed. Indeed, the evolution of the hospice movement in the US has led to a system that failed to capitalize on the enlightened recommendations of Dr. Elisabeth Kubler-Ross, one of the pioneers of the concept. Based on 500 interviews with dying patients she recounted in her 1969 book titled "On death and Dying", she pleaded for home rather than institutional care at her 1972 testimony before a Senate Special Committee on Aging, where she stated,

> We live in a very particular death-denying society...We isolate both the dying and the old... The majority of our [500] patients want[ed] to die very badly at home. Yet, close to 80 percent of all patients interviewed died in an institution...We should not institutionalize people...The biggest need [of a dying patient] is always [to] allow for hope. Hope is not the same as hope for cure treatment or prolongation of life. When a patient is dying, this hope will change to something that is not associated with cur[ative] treatment or prolongation of life...Besides the need for hope, patients need a reassurance that they will not be deserted, yet most of our patients who become beyond medical help felt deserted...We can give families more help with home care and visiting nurses, giving the families and the patients the spiritual, emotional, and financial help in order to facilitate the final care at home...It is a question of reeducating the whole public. Nursing schools, social work schools, and medical schools have now started to include the care of the dying patient in their curriculum [707].

Yet, hospice care in the US today is an outcome of a dehumanized, medicine-as-a-business enterprise that abandons terminal patients to confront their last anguishing days surrounded by unfamiliar faces and unsoothing if not outright hostile intensive care environments. In her 1972 Senate testimony, Dr. Kubler-Ross cites a typical case that populates our hospitals' intensive care units today,

> She was a 21-year-old girl with acute leukemia. She was young and full of life. When we interviewed her in our hospital, she said very loud and clear that although her chances were one in a million that her big dream was still that she could graduate in June from college, that she could get married in July. Her bargain was that she would not have any children for 5 years, and if she would still be alive, she would then have lots of children and live happily ever after. But, she also said she knew that her chances were one in a million. She came back into the hospital 5 weeks later, again because the family could not get enough home care for her. Her biggest dream was to live at home, and possibly to die at home. She was put into an intensive care unit. When I visited her in the intensive care unit on New Year's Eve, she was a picture of utter isolation, loneliness, and anguish. She was lying with tubes hanging out of her mouth, her lips cut, the infusion bottles going, a tracheostomy, [was on] the respirator, and she was desperately holding my hand. I covered her with a bed sheet (she was not even covered). A nurse came and says, 'Don't bother. She is going to push it off anyway.' I walked toward her and she grabbed my hands pointing her fingers to the ceiling. I looked up and said, 'Susie, I think this light bothers you. You're lying on your back and must stare into this light.' She grabbed my hands and kissed them obviously conveying 'You are understanding me.' I went to ask if these lights could be turned down, only to get a nice lecture about the rules and regulations of the intensive care unit. I also asked for two chairs for the mother and father to sit down when they visit, because I cannot comprehend why patients have to die alone in an intensive care unit and their families sit alone outside in a waiting room. I was told the mother cannot get a chair because she stayed more than 5 minutes last time [708].

Sadly, Dr. Kubler-Ross patient's agony will provoke a sense of déjà-vu in most cancer caregivers and in many relatives or acquaintances of terminally ill patients' final days. An avoidable agony, caused by the misguided belief that each patient is a potential treatment outcome outlier that can be salvaged by aggressive management to the bitter end, only to be proven wrong time and time again. Professionals who care for the terminally ill have only one chance to achieve the desirable goal of death with dignity forcefully advocated by Dr. Kubler-Ross and avoid painful memories from loved ones, as cautioned in Dame Saunders' tenet, "How people die remains in the memory of those who live on" [709]. Success in accomplishing both requires major changes in the public's attitude towards death and for physicians' to better understand their holistic role as healers, as outlined in the next chapter.

Part VI
A Paradigm Shift in Cancer Management

In my 2005 book titled *The War on Cancer: An Anatomy of Failure: A Blueprint for the Future*, I wrote,

> Predicting the next revolution in cancer care is admittedly an uncertain undertaking but cumulative evidence of a system gone astray and nascent trends for correction are unmistakable. Until recently, researchers and their sponsors focused their efforts, and clinicians and their patients centered their hope, more on the eradication of advanced cancer than on its prevention or detection in surgically curable early stages. Additionally, the notion that cancer represents a deadly tissue growth that is distinct from the host and therefore must be eradicated at all cost is a flawed hypothesis. Indeed, not only have the types of cancer drugs fostered by this notion proven inefficacious and treatment outcomes disappointing, but recent advances in cancer genetics have overturned the conceptual foundations upon which this notion rests. Moreover, it is increasingly clear that translational application of cancer genetics data is the foundation for the emerging pharmacogenomics of the future rather than the trial-and-error approach of the past. Thus, the time has come to develop a new approach to cancer control based not on eradication at any cost but on comprehensive, stepwise, and evidence-based measures. They include prevention, early stage diagnosis, and – when these fail – on controlling the aberrant molecular genetic pathways underlying the development, growth, and dissemination of cancer [710].

Uncertain undertaking indeed. Ten years later, efforts at developing cancer-specific prevention tools remain marginal, little progress has been made in generating methods to detect early stage cancer, and the implied promise of exploiting the human genome for diagnostic and therapeutic purposes remains unfulfiled. The most likely explanations include the difficulties involved, the inertia of entrenched practices geared towards the inefficacious treatment of advanced cancer neglecting prevention or early stage detection bolstered by financial interests of all stakeholders in preserving the status quo, and a state of nonchalance born from a widespread belief that unraveling of the human genome will eventually launch a new era in cancer control through pharmacogenomics, an expectation that remains unfulfiled.

As a result, and as detailed in previous chapters, cancer incidence rates, measured as cases per 100,000 population, rose 28 % between 1975 and 1992, after which they slowly declined 9 % through 2009. In the meantime, cancer mortality rates rose, albeit more slowly (8 %), between 1975 and 1991, after which they declined 19.5 % in 2009 (Fig. 5.2), 60–80 % of which is attributable to smoking cessation and to expanded screening for surgically resectable breast, colorectal, and prostate cancer [711]. On the other hand, 5-year survival, an accepted indicator of treatment success, reveals a very uneven but instructive picture. For instance, average 5-year survival gains between 1975 and 2008 for the ten most common cancers in all stages that together accounted for 71 % of new cases and 65.5 % of cancer deaths (Fig. 9.1) ranged from 4 % (pancreas) to 32 % (prostate), but declined in two (e.g., larynx, −3 % and uterus, −4 %). Moreover, ten advanced-stage cancers that accounted for approximately 45 % of total cases exhibited a dismal average 2–16 % 5-year survival between 2002 and 2008 (Fig. 9.2). Finally, the trend in incidence rates for approximately 40 % of all cancers continues to rise. For instance, between 1999 and 2008, increased incidence rates were recorded for cancers of the oropharynx, esophagus, skin melanoma, pancreas, thyroid, liver and intrahepatic bile duct, and kidney and renal pelvis [712]. The rise was caused by changes in cancer risk behaviors and, to a lesser extent, to improved early-stage detection practices. Together, these data lead to the inescapable conclusion that cancer control measures in place since President Nixon signed the National Cancer Act on December 23, 1971 have been inefficacious and a new paradigm must be developed if we are to avoid another four decades of near-stagnation, as outlined in the following two chapters.

Chapter 13
Prevention and Early Detection

> *My cancer scare changed my life. I'm grateful for every new, healthy day I have. It has helped me prioritize my life.*
>
> – Olivia Newton-John

In its 2012 annual plan titled "Cancer: changing the conversation", NCI seems to advocate continuation of the status quo that justifies its ongoing broad-based initiatives, rather than to re-directing its activities. For instance, under "Prevention and Screening", it states,

> Cancer prevention includes efforts to forestall the process that leads to cancer, along with the detection and treatment of precancerous conditions at their earliest, most treatable stages, and the prevention of new, or second primary, cancers in survivors [713].

Perhaps NCI's future direction in cancer prevention and screening will be better focused than outlined in the report. Indeed, while an in-depth knowledge of the specific molecular events that promote the development and progression of each type of cancer is lacking, we do know that approximately 53 % of all new cases of cancer are attributable to smoking, obesity [714], and alcoholism (Table 4.1). Another 10 % can be traced back to exposure to carcinogenic viruses, 1.5 % to alcoholism, and 1.0 % to exposure to ultraviolet radiation [715]. These five, mostly behavior-associated cancers account for more than one third of all cancer deaths in the US [716]. Their control calls for behavioral changes supported by appropriate motivational and even compulsory legislation when needed. Although human behavior cannot be legislated successfully, the usefulness of anti-smoking campaigns has been validated by a 54 % decline in the smoking US population since 1965 (Table 3.6), saving hundreds of thousands of lives each year. Altering other cancer-associated behaviors would generate similar results.

Except for immunization against cancer-causing viruses, any efficacious cancer prevention policy entails a long-term commitment to lifestyle changes of difficult implementation, reluctant participation by all parties involved, and deferred benefits. The success of such a policy hinges on being goal-oriented, realistic, and participatory, involving all stakeholders at the national, community, and caregiver levels. Hence, it must meet the following basic criteria:

- Focus on the root causes of most cancers.
- Target cancers with high incidence and death rates.

- Set progressively achievable goals.
- Adopt strategies to rally support from policy-makers, caregivers, and the public.

In the US, targeting smoking, obesity, alcoholism, and over-exposure to ultraviolet light and carcinogenic viruses would meet the first criteria. Focusing on lung cancer within this category would, in part, meet the second. For instance, re-invigorating anti-smoking campaigns would further encourage smoking cessation and reduce the incidence rate of all types of cancers linked to cigarette smoking, including lung, oral cavity, esophagus, stomach, bladder, kidney, pancreas, larynx, cervix, and acute myelogenous leukemia. A concomitant early detection program focused on lung cancer would have a greater impact on overall cancer deaths than all other smoking-related cancers combined. Indeed, with its 7,000-plus chemical components, including at least 70 carcinogens, a cancer risk well-known by the tobacco industry as early as 1961 [717], tobacco is the most lethal of human carcinogens, a distinction underlined in the 1982 Surgeon General report that branded tobacco "the major single cause of cancer mortality in the United States." However, despite successful national and local efforts to curb smoking, it retains its dominant position as the most hazardous cancer-promoting behavior, being responsible for approximately 28 % of cancer deaths in the United States [718]. Successful smoking cessation reduces disability and premature deaths by 50 % within 10 years of cessation. This is due to a 50 % reduction of coronary heart disease within 1 year, and a 50 % decreased incidence of strokes and of cancers of the lung, the oral cavity, and the esophagus after 10–15 years of abstinence [719]. After 15 years of tobacco abstinence, death rates fall to levels recorded in persons who never smoked.

Although obesity in itself does not cause cancer, unlike smoking, the strong correlation between obesity and several types of cancer is an indication that the obese individual has been exposed for many years to yet unknown cancer promoters contained in or mediated by certain types of diets. Diets deficient in cancer-protecting agents also have been postulated, leading to exploratory clinical trials designed to assess the potential cancer-preventive effect of selenium, retinoids,[1] vitamins, lycopenes,[2] and green tea, among others, with mixed results, at best. For instance, the Selenium and Vitamin E Cancer Prevention Trial (SELECT), launched to assess the long-term effect of vitamin E and/or selenium on risk of prostate cancer, enrolled 35,533 men. After 7–12 years follow-up, vitamin E was shown significantly to increase the risk of prostate cancer [720]. Instead, obesity prevention should rely primarily on national state, local, and caregiver-based educational campaigns modeled after smoking-cessation, aimed primarily at the general population but also at those who, for reasons of their own (e.g., ideological or financial), subscribe to the misguided and counterproductive hypothesis that obesity is a disease.

Likewise, vaccination against carcinogenic viruses such as HPV and HBV should be pursued aggressively, as should the development of new vaccines funded by the public purse, for the pharmaceutical industry is more interested in developing

---

[1] Chemicals related to Vitamin A.
[2] Red phytochemicals found in tomato and other red fruits and vegetables.

blockbuster drugs than revenue-poor vaccines. In fact, vaccination against HPV-16 and HPV-18 infections that cause 70 % of all cervical cancers [721], coupled with the safe and reliable Pap smear for detecting surgically curable early stage cervical cancer, provide the tools and the opportunity sharply to reduce the onset of the disease and progression to advanced stages and deaths, respectively. Regrettably, opposition to teenage vaccination and other factors have limited vaccine penetration to only 70 % of the eligible population and is responsible for a stagnant 5-year survival from cervical cancer between 1975 and 2008. In this context, it is ironic that recent research in cancer vaccines has focused not on developing vaccines against known carcinogenic viruses, but on vaccines designed to enhance the ability of the immune system to recognize alleged tumor antigens (e.g., MAGE, MART, CEA, HER-2, MUC-1, PSA) in attempts to mediate tumor rejection. Yet, after 20 years of attempts to coax the immune system into rejecting cancers using various forms of immunotherapy, only anecdotal successes have been reported. How then to explain researchers' enduring fascination with the concept of immunotherapy? The answer is multifaceted but includes three major factors. First, the intellectual attractiveness of extending the concept of immune rejection of non-self (e.g., bacteria, viruses, transplanted organs) to cancer cells, even after the latter have been shown to be part of the self, albeit harboring genetic alterations. Second, the complexity of the immune system is challenging to immunologists, molecular biologists, and geneticists interested in probing its multifaceted dimensions. Third, the anticipation of academic and financial rewards and media acclaim that are sure to accompany any breakthrough in this domain, especially when compared to what is perceived as the lackluster endeavor of prophylactic anti-viral vaccine development.

Given the unassailing logic and safety of adopting the outlined cancer prevention approach as a national policy, the current practice of cancer chemoprevention is a misguided and often harmful concept emanating from our drug culture. There are several reasons for this. First, chemoprevention consists of administering agents expected to reduce the incidence or recurrence of cancer, especially in high-risk individuals, rather than to curbing the five unhealthy behaviors responsible for over 50 % of all cancers in the entire population. Second, the mechanism of action of chemoprevention is ill-defined and long-term side effects often offset cancer-preventing benefits. Moreover, because benefits are expected to accrue to a subpopulation of participants and long-term harmful effects and the size of the affected participants are unpredictable, very large studies and years of follow-up are necessary to establish their safety, efficacy, and risk-benefit ratio, at a very high cost, as demonstrated by the SELECT study and the Tamoxifen for Prevention of Breast Cancer trial [722]. Chemoprevention is another facet of the hit-and-miss approach that is the foundation of the search for anti-cancer drugs and has met the same fate: decades of stagnation. On the other hand, the outlined evidence-based prevention initiative focused on curbing smoking, obesity, and alcoholism that together account for more than 50 % of all cancers, year after year, constitutes the first step of a highly focused, evidence-based, three-prong approach to cancer control that offers the best prospects of achieving incremental reductions in national cancer incidence and mortality rates that should validate its well-grounded foundation, promote stakeholders' cooperation and support, and ensure its long term success.

At present, most cancers are diagnosed in relatively advanced stages or reach that level when treatment fails or as disease progresses after partially successful therapy. Because not all cancers can be prevented and the outcome of patients with advanced cancer is largely unaffected by current therapies, a change in direction also must include a greater emphasis on detection of cancer in surgically excisable stages. In order to achieve the latter goal and ensure stakeholders' continued support, cancer screening must target cancers responsible for most cancer deaths. Cancers concerned include lung and bronchus in men and women, female breast, prostate, and colorectal in men and women. Together, these cancers are expected to cause 472,370 deaths or 81.4 % of the total (580,350) expected in 2013 (Table 4.2). Ideally, cancer-screening tests should be low-tech, dependable, reproducible, noninvasive, inexpensive, harmless, and simple to perform in the physician's office or at the local laboratory. Yet, except for the reliable Pap smear, there is a tendency towards high-tech tools, such as CT scans, MRIs, flow cytometry, and molecular techniques, that are more useful for assessing the tissue of origin, stage, presence of metastases, and growth potential of cancer and predicting treatment responses or relapses, than for screening purposes. Because of their non-specificity, current screening tools, sophisticated or not, often lead to false positive and false negative results that negatively impact patients' subsequent management, QOL, and survival. This has led to controversial changes in screening guidelines, as illustrated by PSA and mammography for prostate and breast cancer, respectively.

PSA is a protein produced by prostate cells that can be measured in blood. Easy performance, harmlessness, and low cost helped its widespread acceptance by patients and physicians alike, becoming a routine yearly test for men age 50 and beyond. Patients with blood PSA concentrations above a certain level (controversial and ever-changing) were usually submitted to a prostate biopsy to further assess for presence of cancer and a prostatectomy if the biopsy proved positive. As experience accumulated, it became clear that such an approach was as harmful as it was beneficial. First, prostate biopsies are not without risk, as revealed by a study showing a 6.9 % rate of hospitalization following an outpatient procedure [723]. Second, whereas "active surveillance" of patients with low-grade prostate cancer is the recommended course of action, approximately 80 % opt for treatment, most often radiation therapy or radical prostatectomy [724, 725]. Choosing either for asymptomatic, slow growing prostate cancer can lead to an increased morbidity and mortality. Indeed, radical prostatectomy is associated with 0.5 % mortality and 4.5 % re-hospitalization rates within 30 days of the operation, and lead to complications in 28 % of patients, mainly urinary incontinence (7–21 %) and impotence (35–60 %). External beam radiation can lead to short-term acute cystitis, proctitis, and enteritis. Today, PSA as a screening test for prostate cancer has lost support, and the U.S. Preventive Services Task Force recently recommended against PSA-based screening for prostate cancer, stating,

> Prostate cancer is a serious health problem that affects thousands of men and their families. But before getting a PSA test, all men deserve to know what the science tells us about PSA screening: there is a very small potential benefit and significant potential harms. We encourage clinicians to consider this evidence and not screen their patients with a PSA test unless the

individual being screened understands what is known about PSA screening and makes the personal decision that even a small possibility of benefit outweighs the known risk of harms [726].

In contrast to professional or self breast examination, the benefit of which is uncertain, mammography currently is the most widely used and useful screening test for breast cancer in women over age 40. It has been shown to reduce mortality due to breast cancer by 15–20 % [727]. However, it also can result in harm associated with the consequences of over- and under-diagnosis. A false-positive mammogram in women screened annually for 10 years occurs on average in 7.4 % of first mammograms, 26.0 % by the fifth, and 43.1 % by the ninth mammogram [728], and 7–17 % of them are biopsied [729]. Likewise, invasive breast cancer will be missed in 6–46 % of women, depending on age and certain characteristics of their breasts [730]. In addition, a percentage of biopsy-proven cancers, estimated to range between 0 and 54 %, are indolent types that remain asymptomatic and do not impact survival if left untreated. Although repeat mammography, ultrasound, and MRIs can reduce the percentage of false-negative and false-positive cases, a significant number of these women will require or choose mastectomy to allay any remaining doubt. While most patients experience an uneventful recovery post-mastectomy, some will develop lymphedema,[3] an early or late chronic complication often associated with axillary lymph node dissection frequently performed during the operation. The preceding short survey of the shortcomings of two of the most widely used cancer screening tools clearly demonstrates the need to develop better cancer screening tests, preferably through a robust national program sponsored and generously funded by NCI. As benefits of the outlined prevention policy become noticeable and new screening tools are developed, prevention and screening initiatives can be incrementally extended to other cancers chosen according to their rank by incidence and mortality rates. Such an approach, designed as a national policy to have the maximum impact on cancer control nationwide, does not exclude adding cancers based on cogent and justifiable criteria other than incidence and mortality rates.

Designing and implementing cancer prevention and screening policies such as the ones outlined are complex undertakings beyond the scope of this book that must be legislated by Congress and implemented by NCI [731, 732], with input from public and private organizations such as IOM [733] and ACS [734] and interested advocate groups. Success in formulating and enacting any evidence-based cancer control policy requires enlightened policymakers serving the general good rather than the interests of a few, including their own [735]. The Federal policy of subsidies and payments for tobacco growers is one of many examples of the latter. The Federal government maintains a deceitful policy of providing payments to tobacco growers (via the US Department of Agriculture) while it promotes anti-smoking activities (coordinated by the CDC), funds for research in smoking-related illnesses (sponsored by the NIH), and regulates tobacco products (through the Federal Trade Commission, the Substance Abuse and Mental Health Services Administration, and the FDA).

---

[3] Swelling of the arm caused by blockage of lymph circulation.

In its latest incarnation, the Fair and Equitable Tobacco Reform Act of 2004 replaced the Depression-era tobacco quota program. The new program provides annual "transitional" payments to eligible tobacco farmers that amounted to $189 million in 2012 [736]. State legislators also are mendacious in protecting the general good. For instance, on November 23, 1998, 46 Attorneys General signed the landmark Master Settlement Agreement (MSA) with the five largest US tobacco manufacturers that ended years of litigation. The MSA provides $206 billion, including $12.7 billion up-front payment and the balance paid in annual installments through 2025. The award was intended primarily to compensate involved states for tobacco-related health-care costs and dissuade youth from taking up smoking, Unsurprisingly, the lion's share of the proceeds is being used for purposes other than health issues [737]. At the supra-national level, the WHO issued cancer prevention and early detection guidelines [738, 739]. After identifying smoking as the cause of most cancer deaths worldwide, WHO chose tobacco as its main cancer prevention target, issuing the Framework Convention on Tobacco Control treaty in 2005. It confers its 170 signatories responsibilities and legal obligations to educate their populations about the ravages of tobacco, to adopt measures to reduce its demand, and to regulate its distribution [740].

Chapter 14
The Holistic Management of Advanced Cancer: A Three-Stage Blueprint

> *Constant kindness can accomplish much. As the sun makes ice melt, kindness causes misunderstanding, mistrust, and hostility to evaporate.*
>
> – Albert Schweitzer

In previous Chapters, I documented the failure of a five decades-old reliance on the cell-kill approach and more recently of molecularly targeted agents to control advanced cancer. I also identified multiple factors that perpetuate the status quo, documented the commercialization of Oncology practice, and the dehumanization of end-of-life care. Based on that evidence, I advocate a paradigm shift in the treatment of advanced cancer [741]. The shift must be radical but implemented gradually until successful alternatives are developed and in place. The task ahead is momentous but its formulation is beyond the scope of the book. However, some basic practical principles can be envisioned to reach our goal. I refer to the patient-centered principles of beneficence, non-maleficence, respect for patients' autonomy, and justice that are the ethical foundations of medical care [742, 743].

Simply stated, beneficence is the practice of doing good to others, such as rescuing someone from danger, whereas non-maleficence refers to the ethical principle of "do no harm", a medical standard inscribed in the Hippocratic Oath. In medical practice, beneficence almost always involves some degree of harm. Hence, caregivers are obligated to balance expected benefits against possible risks of any action, including ordering a test, a procedure, a medication, an operation or a treatment regimen, and ensure that the benefit-harm ratio be favorable. Although physicians are expected to possess the necessary knowledge to make that determination, patients' autonomy must be respected and any choice of action requires the patient's acquiescence after full disclosure and a signed informed consent, when appropriate. The policy of obtaining consent is linked to the principle of patient autonomy, even when the benefit-risk ratio of a proposed intervention is most favorable. Justice is perhaps the most controversial ethical principle and the most difficult to apply to individual cases. It refers to the fair adjudication of care between competing claims, which, in modern health care, has become almost synonymous with the fair apportionment of scarce financial resources. While few will challenge these principles' altruistic goals, their full application in medical practice is offset by the multiple pressures on caregivers and by the needs and beliefs of each individual patient.

As a result, ignoring one or more principles of ethical care is a widespread practice that is justified by doubtful arguments in the treatment of advanced cancer and is especially inappropriate at the end-of-life.

In preceding Chapters, I have shown that, once a diagnosis of advanced or metastatic cancer is confirmed, patients are treated with chemotherapy or more recently molecularly targeted drugs. The issue here is not to question the "raison d'être" of these mostly inefficacious agents, but their often-indiscriminate use that negatively impact patients' QOL and interfere with a dignified end-of-life without demonstrable benefits. The sequence begins with "first line" drugs or drug combinations chosen among the most efficacious against the targeted tumor. Unresponsive patients and those whose cancer relapses after an initial response are then treated with "second line" regimens that, as the name implies, are even less efficacious but equally toxic. Ultimately, most patients are treated with "salvage" regimens, an approach that rarely salvages anyone. Such a consensus approach to advanced cancer management, fostered by the belief within the medical community that, with powerful tools at our disposal, everything must be done regardless of cost, is a view bolstered by the multiple factors that shape Oncology practice, the emotionally-charged but misleading motto "when there is life there is hope", and by patients' attitudes when facing death. Yet, this caregivers' aggressive stance, clearly justified for the approximately 2 % of curable types, notably trophoblastic cancers (~90 % cure rate), germ cell cancers (~65 %), certain adult and childhood leukemias (~25–75 %), Hodgkin's disease (~65 %), and certain NHLs (~30 %) [744], induces only marginal survival benefits in most of the remaining 98 %. This is confirmed by the fact that, between 1975 and 2008, cumulative gains in 5-year survival for the 10 most frequent cancer sites that together accounted for 71 % of new cases and 65.5 % of cancer deaths in 2008 exceeded 15 % in only four cancers. Meager as they are, these gains must be credited to new and more efficacious antibiotics for treating chemotherapy-induced infections, easier access to blood product transfusions, and other life-sustaining measures, as much as to treatment of the underlying cancer. Most recent statistics show that patients with ten types of cancer accounting for nearly 50 % of new cases between 2002 and 2008 exhibited a dismal 2–16 % 5-year survival. These grim statistics call into question the value of aggressive practices that violate one or more ethical standards seeking goals seldom attained despite five decades of trying. One recently proposed solution to this predicament, called "personalized medicine", is based on the notion that clinical trial results are averages of the studied population, which, coupled with the enormous complexity of the disease process, preclude selecting the most appropriate agent for a particular individual. As a result, some patients are under-treated and others are over-treated, and the type and severity of adverse effects vary from patient to patient. However, this seemingly inarguable logic lacks clinical validation, an endeavor that promises to be arduous, long, and costly. Indeed,

> In the current climate of increasing molecular testing capabilities, clinicians are urged to approach commercially available biomarker tests with a healthy level of scrutiny of their clinical application and validation. At this juncture, various commercially available assays may be of little added value, and accelerated biomarker development with clinical validation is desperately needed [745].

Moreover, personalized medicine assumes the efficacy of available drugs for the treatment of cancer, which is not supported by the evidence. Yet, what is even more difficult to explain is the relentless pursuit of aggressive, acute care with renewed vigor at the end of life that, in addition to worsening a gradually deteriorating QOL, ultimately proves futile time and time again. Faced with these realities, it appears clear that a new cancer management paradigm guided by the ethical principles of beneficence, non-maleficence, and justice while respecting patients' autonomy must be developed. In order to be executed successfully, such a paradigm shift must be strongly endorsed and promoted at the national level by leading public and private health care organizations such as NCI and ACS & ASCO, and supported and implemented by caregivers who hold the key to its success.

14.1 Redesigning the Search for New Cancer Agents

While critics will point out that this is already underway through translational applications of newly acquired genome-based knowledge, the current search is conducted largely by individual and secretive pharmaceutical companies more interested in generating high-revenue products quickly than in contributing to the overall control of cancer. The extremely high price of most molecularly targeted anti-cancer agents and the emergence of biopharmaceutical companies dedicated to manufacturing unaffordable orphan agents for treating rare diseases, such as the $410,000 per patient per year price tag of Soliris®, are illustrative. Another example is the accelerated drug approval programs (e.g., Fast Track, Breakthrough Therapy, Accelerated Approval, and Priority Review) launched by the FDA in response to manufacturers' pressure that benefit, more drug sponsors' bottom line, than patients' health. Some will argue that free competition is the best road to better and cheaper products. Although this is certainly true for consumer products, health care is a supply-driven industry where physicians are arbiters of patient needs, making it impervious to market forces that operate in other industries where consumer demand drives supply and keeps costs in check [746]. Nevertheless, drug manufacturers should not be discouraged from participating in the search for better drugs. Yet, theirs are piecemeal efforts targeting specific diseases that are unsuitable as a cancer control strategy. Such a goal can be achieved only through a focused and centrally coordinated national program that, like the Manhattan project (1939–1946), involved 130,000 people to produce the first atomic bomb that ended WWII, and the Apollo Program that within a decade fulfilled President Kennedy's vision of "landing a man on the Moon and returning him safely to the Earth" when astronauts Neil Armstrong and Buzz Aldrin landed their Lunar Module on the moon on July 20, 1969. While the latter prowess was invoked by Mary Lasker and associates as a key argument for spearheading the movement that led to the National Cancer Act of 1971, I envision a joint national effort towards a single goal and a break with the past at all levels of the cancer research "enterprise". Such an approach was proposed by Benno C. Schmidt Sr., chairmanship of the President's Cancer Panel, in his 1971 statement before the Senate Committee on Labor and Public Welfare, "However, there is no comprehensive overall program plan today, and such a plan is a sine qua non of effective assault on cancer" [747]. For instance, the practice of awarding research funds to individual researchers to support their pet projects promotes, by design, a fragmented rather than cooperative approach to the War on Cancer. On the one hand, while the motto "one brick at a time" is frequently invoked in cancer research circles to support such an uncoordinated approach, it is more a catchy expression than a means to an end, as the War on Cancer demonstrates. On the other hand, "study section" members at granting agencies who review and recommend individual projects for funding are themselves researchers with expertise in the subjects assigned to them whose decisions are often questionable. This is illustrated by my own experience. Two interrelated applications for research funds were rejected by NCI; one to develop CLL and/or HCL cell lines ("not doable" I was told); the other to study our own anti-cCLLa[1] MoAbs [748] aimed at future human trials ("MoAbs are too dangerous for human use"). These projects, subsequently funded by the Department of Veterans Administration, led to the development of two HCL cell lines [749], their in vitro and in vivo characterization [750], and that of four MoAb-derived immunotoxins [751, 752]. If not biased, my reviewers' decision revealed a spectacular lack of vision. Indeed, a myriad of MoAbs, in one form or another, are currently part of our armamentarium for treating numerous diseases ranging from rheumatoid arthritis to cancer. To replace this disjointed and multidirectional approach, I propose enrolling tens of thousands of scientists in the medical, biological, biochemical, and other complementary fields of science, concentrated in a few campus-like environments to join forces and focus their interdisciplinary expertise towards a common goal of unraveling the secrets of cancer development and progression and developing tools for their mastery. Participants within each field would bring to the table expertise known or potentially relevant to cancer. Data generated within each field would be analyzed at pre-determined intervals and interpreted in the context of data generated in other fields to serve as a new point of departure for further collaborative study. Such an approach is more likely to uncover common underlying processes that lead to cancer development and progression and the means to block or reverse them than the current fragmented and uncoordinated hit-and-miss approach of developing and screening individual drugs aimed at individual types of cancers; an old technique pioneered by Paul Ehrlich in his 7-year quest for antimicrobials one century ago.

14.2 Restructuring the Treatment of Advanced-Stage Cancer

While the first proposed cancer control phase is being planned and implemented, and until efficacious means for controlling cancer have been developed, I propose treating all patients according to the four ethical principles of patient care. Given the

---

[1]A cell surface antigen common to CLL cells.

enormous complexity involved, the transition time is likely to be considerable, during which patient care must continue using drugs and means at our disposal but administered judiciously rather than heroically, as is current practice. Hence, patients with advanced-stage cancer types known to be curable should be aggressively treated with one or more highly efficacious regimens (e.g., chemotherapy with or without adjuvant surgery, radiation, or molecularly-targeted therapy) for that particular tumor. While this approach is known to be associated with substantial morbidity and mortality, most caregivers and patients agree that, when the ultimate goal is a cure, the risks are worth taking. On the other hand, patients with advanced-stage cancer of the types known to be incurable should be offered the best available treatment in hopes of prolonging survival guided by national statistics. In most cases, such regimens exhibit an acceptable risk-benefit ratio with acceptable negative impact on QOL, unless injudiciously pursued beyond the duration recommended for each treatment and appropriate for each case. Finally, patients with tumors that fail to respond to or progress during appropriate first-line treatment, or relapse after an initial response, should be advised of the unlikely usefulness and the increased risks associated with further treatment. At this stage, the emphasis should shift to palliative care as the main goal, instituted and supervised by the same caregiver, whether in a hospice or home setting. However, in order to respect patients' autonomy, caregivers should be prepared to continue treatment with second-line regimens for patients who demand it after a detailed disclosure of potential complications and adverse effects that might negatively impact QOL or worse without meaningful survival benefits. Disclosed information must be easy to grasp and skillfully delivered. Yet, information available from the medical literature is often insufficiently clear to serve as the basis for caregivers to reach the most appropriate decision. Indeed, reports of clinical trials and other studies include an array of statistical information (e.g., means, standard deviations (SD), Student's t-test, chi-square, p values, confidence intervals, hazard ratio, and others) that, while useful for scientifically buttressing the conclusions reached, are often barely glanced at without much comprehension by the majority of clinical Oncologists who lack statistical training or time to interpret such details. The following example chosen at random illustrates the point:

> During the median follow-up of 10.0 years, 171 of 364 men (47.0 %) assigned to radical prostatectomy died, as compared with 183 of 367 (49.9 %) assigned to observation (hazard ratio, 0.88; 95 % confidence interval [CI], 0.71 to 1.08; P=0.22; absolute risk reduction, 2.9 percentage points). Among men assigned to radical prostatectomy, 21 (5.8 %) died from prostate cancer or treatment, as compared with 31 men (8.4 %) assigned to observation (hazard ratio, 0.63; 95 % CI, 0.36 to 1.09; P=0.09; absolute risk reduction, 2.6 percentage points). The effect of treatment on all-cause and prostate-cancer mortality did not differ according to age, race, coexisting conditions, self-reported performance status, or histologic features of the tumor. Radical prostatectomy was associated with reduced all-cause mortality among men with a PSA value greater than 10 ng per milliliter (P=0.04 for interaction) and possibly among those with intermediate-risk or high-risk tumors (P=0.07 for interaction). Adverse events within 30 days after surgery occurred in 21.4 % of men, including one death [753].

Drug study reports, which serve as bases for treating future cancer patients, focus on mean tumor response and patient survival outcomes, usually including standard deviations (σ) that indicate dispersion from the mean, and "*p*" values that establish whether or not the difference observed between the experimental (drug) and control arms of a study is the result of random chance alone (e.g., $p \geq 0.05$ or $p \leq 0.05$, respectively). While such statistics are necessary for correctly assessing the relative efficacy of a drug, they are of limited value to a caregiver who must extrapolate such data to an individual patient, who in turn wants to know the odds of surviving X number of months or years. For instance, mean survival might be neither representative of any patient within a study nor applicable outside of it, especially when outcomes are distributed over a wide range or include outliers. On the other hand, median survival is more representative of most study participants' outcome distribution than mean survival, and survival probabilities are more valuable to patients, and both should be included in all drug study reports. Such information would facilitate caregivers' tasks of presenting to patients information easy to assimilate and decide upon, as illustrated in Table 14.1. The top of the table displays relevant survival statistics of a hypothetical study of drug "X" involving eight patients with a relatively narrow survival range (2–7 months) plus one outlier at 76 months.

Table 14.1 Participant survival of two studies of drug "X" with survival probability at various endpoints

Patients (n = 9)	Survival[a]	2	3	4	4	5	5	6	7	76	Mean 12.4	Median 5.0
	Probability	100 %								11 %	11 %	56 %
Patients (n = 104)[b]	Survival[a]	2	3	4	4	5	5	6	7	50–70	Mean 6.5	Median 5.0
	Probability	100 %								3.6 %	16 %	52 %

[a]Months
[b]See text

As shown, the median survival is more representative of most patients' survival within the group than the mean that is significantly skewed by the single outlier's, and therefore more likely to apply to future patients. Indeed, a future patient offered drug "X" following the same protocol used in the study will have a 100 % chance of surviving at least 2 months and 56 % chance of matching the group's median survival (5 months), but only 11 % of surviving as long as the mean or the longest survivor (12.4 and 76 months, respectively). In order to mimick drug studies that usually involve 100 participants or more, let us expand our hypothetical study to involve 104 patients with similar survival distribution (e.g., 13 patients surviving 2 months, 13 surviving 3 months, etc.) plus three outliers surviving 50, 60, and 70 months each. As shown at the bottom of Table 14.1, while the probabilities of surviving at least 2 months or reaching the group's median survival are equal or comparable to the first group (100 % and 52 %, respectively), the probabilities of matching the group's mean and surviving 50 months or longer are 16 % and 3.6 %, respectively. The large differences between mean and median survival probabilities are due to the fact that over 50 % of patients matched or exceeded the median survival in either group, whereas only 11 % and 16 % matched or exceeded the mean survival in the first and second group, respectively. Given most caregivers' lack of training and time to dissect the meaning of standard statistics, and in the interest of full and transparent disclosure, probability data for several points, especially the shortest, mean, median and longest survival, should be an integral part of every clinical trial report. Yet, even assuming an optimal patient-friendly disclosure, including survival probabilities, the process requires special skills on the part of caregivers that, while acquired with experience, should be taught in medical schools as part of an ethics curriculum, a necessary training neglected by most US medical schools. Ideally, the disclosing caregiver should be knowledgeable about the potential benefits and risks of the intervention proposed and of alternatives and be a "good listener". That is, allow sufficient time for each patient to express his/her doubts, concerns, fears, and other emotions triggered by the circumstances that should be incorporated in the decision-making process. In addition, the venue (e.g., hospital, office, and context settings), content of the disclosure (e.g., thoroughness, clarity, and specificity), and the level of personal empathy conveyed by the physician are paramount for terminal patients and their relatives to achieve peace of mind when most needed. A careful adherence to these guidelines from the outset and at each management stage will both prepare patients and relatives to face increasingly difficult physiological, emotional, spiritual, religious, financial, and legal decisions and facilitate each inevitable transition.

14.3 Reviving the Art of End of Life Care

There is no empirical evidence to support a precise definition of the interval referred to as end of life or its transition point. For our purposes, end of life is defined as the period of time patients with terminal cancer enter after exhausting first- or second-line disease treatments. This period, which covers the last few months of life, represents the phase when the primary goal of treatment must shift from disease treatment to palliative care. Its duration can range from as short as 2 weeks to 6 months or longer. Such a wide range has several advantages. First, it recognizes that the art of medicine does not enable caregivers to predict with any degree of certainty the remaining life of a terminal patient. Second, it provides flexibility for each caregiver and each patient to decide on the most appropriate time to switch from disease treatment to palliation as the primary focus, based on individual circumstances. Third, a late transition point (e.g., 2-weeks) respects the autonomy of patients who unwisely demand continuation of disease treatment not warranted by an expected unfavorable benefit-risk ratio. In such cases, the switch can be progressive in order to comply with a patient's wishes while reducing the negative impact of such a decision on QOL. Fourth, a 6-month transition point matches the maximum life expectancy to qualify for Medicare hospice benefits and precludes a premature switch under average circumstances. However, a subset of patients with unresponsive but slowly progressive cancer will survive beyond 6 months even without treatment extending the period of palliation. Today, most terminal patients are unnecessarily subjected to acute inpatient care and procedures often delivered in ICU facilities through the last month of life, often without eliciting patients' input, a practice that has increased in the last decade. In a recent editorial on a study comparing sites of death and types of care delivered to nearly 850,000 Medicare beneficiaries who died in 2000, 2003, and 2009, the author commented,

> The frequency of hospitalizations and intensive care (ICU) stays during the last months of life increased [between 2000 and 2009]...The increased availability of palliative and hospice care services does not appear to have changed the focus on aggressive, curative care [in the last months of life]...Palliative and hospice care [must be] offered earlier in the process than is the current norm [754].

The author attributed recurrent hospitalizations of terminally ill patients not congruent with patients' health goals to "Providing curative care in the acute hospital regardless of likelihood of benefit or preferences of patients," which should determine what services are offered [755].

The proposed three-tier approach to the management of advanced and terminal cancer patients ensures a favorable beneficence-maleficence ratio during each phase of cancer management. It also respects the principles of patient autonomy that enables patients to remain in control of their own destiny and of justice by biasing use of resources towards patients with the best chances for a meaningful survival while reducing unwise and counterproductive expenditures beyond a point of no return. The proposed guidelines for end of life care do not constitute a disguised form of "active euthanasia", defined as "causing the death of a person through a direct action", which I strongly oppose, or "passive euthanasia" if defined as "hastening the death of a person by altering some form of support", which I do not condone, but allowing a natural process to take place following strict ethical principles focused on finding a timely balance between disease treatment and palliation agreed to by both the caregiver and the patient after full disclosure and discussion of the pros and cons of each course of action. Adoption of such an approach would restore patient care to its traditional intent and allow terminal patients to die with dignity and help their families achieve closure. Yet, it is such a departure from entrenched views and practices within and outside the medical community today that resistance to its adoption is likely to arise from stakeholders interested in maintaining the status quo, as described in Chap. 11, but also from those who cling to the idyllic misconception that "where there is life there is hope", a slogan that leads to harm more often than not when used as a guide to the management of terminal cancer patients. Adoption of the proposed three-tier approach to advanced and terminal cancer management also will necessitate that western societies come to grips with the notion that death is an inevitable part of life that cannot be put on hold in spite of caregivers' good intentions and heroic efforts, even when using the best tools modern medicine has to offer.

Conclusions

Despite a constant barrage of reports of breakthroughs in cancer management, the balance sheet of the War on Cancer since President Nixon signed into law the National Cancer Act on December 23, 1971 is disappointing, whether one looks at interim incidence or death rates, 5-year survival, or cure rates. Indeed, cancer incidence rates rose 16 % overall between 1975 and 2009 while death rates declined 15 % and 5-year survival improved by a mere 19 % between 1975 and 2008. Meager as they are, most of the gains in death rates and 5-year survival are attributable to smoking cessation (e.g., lung cancer), early stage diagnosis (e.g., breast, prostate, and colorectal cancers), and improvements in surgical techniques, anesthesia, antibiotics, and general medical support. Moreover, these averages conceal an even gloomier picture. Indeed, only 2 % of patients with advanced cancers are curable (e.g., trophoblastic ~90 % cure rate, germ cell ~65 %, certain adult and childhood leukemias ~25–75 %, Hodgkin's disease ~65 %, and certain NHLs ~30 %) while the remaining 98 % derive only marginal to modest survival benefits from treatment, often vigorously pursued to the end of life. For instance, in the decade of 2000–2009, cancers with decreasing cancer mortality trends (e.g., ovary, non-Hodgkin's lymphoma, bladder, brain, stomach, and AML) accounted for 30.7 deaths per 100,000 population, but cancers with increasing mortality trends (e.g., pancreas, liver, and uterus) were not far behind at 20.5/100,000. Likewise, out of the ten most prevalent cancer sites that together accounted for 71 % of new cases and 65.5 % of all cancer deaths in the 2002–2008 period, the 5-year benchmark was reached by only 15 % of four cancers (e.g., breast, kidney, non-Hodgkin's lymphoma, and prostate), by 10 % in another four (e.g., pancreas, lung, thyroid, and bladder), and declined in two (e.g., larynx −3 % and uterus −4 %). And, let us not forget that 597,689 Americans died of cancer in 2010 or 1,637 each day, the most ever. Yet, the nation's response to this killer is tame, for the enemy is from within.

Certainly, the complexity of the processes underlying the development and progression of cancer and the sheer number of types of cancer are at the core of the slow progress in cancer management. However, other critical factors are at play, including a series of flawed hypotheses regarding the nature of cancer that consumed vast human and financial resources but generated little progress and the uncoordinated search for answers that followed the implementation of the National Cancer Act. For instance, implicit in the term neoplasm (new growth) was the notion that, like invading bacteria, these processes were inherently different from the host and had to be thoroughly eradicated in order to prevent metastases and death. The application of the infectious disease model to cancer steered cancer research, diagnosis, and treatment. From this, two major practical corollaries followed. The first is that cancer research was oriented towards the search for therapeutically exploitable differences between cancer and normal cells, guided by successive hypotheses ranging from excessive cancer cell proliferation, a misconceived generalization that drove drug development and use for decades, to targetable tumor-specific antigens, an illusion not yet abandoned. The second corollary was the concept of "cytotoxicity" (e.g., cell-kill), introduced to describe the quintessential property drugs must exhibit in order to eradicate disseminated cancer. The notion of cell-kill as the cornerstone of cancer treatment became untenable when the carcinogenic process was shown to involve oncogenes that promote cell growth, mutated tumor suppressor genes that fail to counteract oncogenes, defective DNA repair genes that enable replication of unstable genomes, microRNA that control the expression of most human genes, or defective cell death pathways that confer a survival advantage to cancer cells. Yet, cancer non-specific cytotoxic drugs remain at the core of cancer treatment today, though new agents are being developed to target cancer biomarkers albeit, with limited therapeutic success. Other hypotheses include the purported role of the immune system in rejecting cancer cells presumed to be non-self, a misconception that, vigorously pursued since the 1980s, has yet to show positive results, and the virus link that, bolstered by the discovery of HTLV-1 in 1981, eventually led to identifying eight cancer-causing viruses and to two FDA-approved prophylactic vaccines against the HPV types 16 & 18 and one therapeutic vaccine intended to strengthen the body's natural defenses against prostate cancer, again with limited success. It is unfortunate that ideological objections have limited vaccination of the most HPV-susceptible population in the US.

Although Mary Lasker and associates invoked the conquest of the moon within a decade as a key argument that spearheaded the movement leading to the National Cancer Act, what followed was an uncoordinated effort that did not achieve the intended goal of controlling cancer. In contrast, I envision a coordinated national effort towards a single common goal and a break with the past at all levels of the cancer "enterprise", both research and patient care. For instance, the practice of awarding research funds to individual researchers to support their pet projects promotes, by design, a fragmented rather than cooperative approach to the conquest of cancer. Indeed, while the motto "one brick at a time" is frequently invoked in cancer research circles to support such an uncoordinated approach, it is more a catchy expression than a means to an end, as the stagnant War on Cancer attests. On the other hand, "study section" members at grant funding agencies assigned to review and recommend individual projects for funding are experts whose mandate is to fund viable individual projects of narrow goals unrelated to each other. Instead,

I propose to replace this disjointed and uncoordinated approach by enrolling tens of thousands of scientists in the medical, biological, biochemical, and other fields of science to join forces and focus their efforts towards a common goal of unraveling the secrets of cancer development and progression and develop tools for their mastery. Participants within each field would bring to the table expertise known or potentially relevant to cancer. Data generated within each field would be analyzed at intervals, interpreted in the context of data generated in other fields to serve as a new point of departure for further collaborative study. Likewise, I propose to launch sustained cancer prevention campaigns coordinated at the national, state, regional, and caregiver levels initially aimed at altering cancer-associated behaviors including smoking, obesity, and alcoholism that together account for approximately 53 % of all new cases of cancer and more than one third of all cancer deaths in the US. Another 10 % of cancers, traceable to exposure to carcinogenic viruses and 1.0 % to ultraviolet radiation exposure, also could be targeted initially. Prophylactic vaccination against carcinogenic viruses such as HPV and HBV should be pursued aggressively as should the development of new vaccines funded by the pubic purse, for the pharmaceutical industry is more interested in developing blockbuster drugs than revenue-poor prophylactic vaccines. Major efforts should be devoted concomitantly to develop tools to detect early-stage, surgically curable cancer focusing initially on those with the highest mortality. To succeed in generating substantial and early results, the proposed cancer prevention and screening policy must be goal oriented, realistic, and participatory involving all stakeholders at the national, state, community, and caregiver levels. As benefits accrue and new screening tools are developed, prevention and screening initiatives could be incrementally extended to cancers based on cogent and justifiable criteria beyond incidence and mortality rates.

In the clinical arena, I propose a holistic approach to the management of advanced cancer based on the patient-centered principles of beneficence, non-maleficence, respect for patient autonomy and justice that are the foundations of ethical patient care. This approach represents a radical shift to be implemented gradually until efficacious anti-cancer agents have emerged from the nationally coordinated efforts aimed in that direction. Hence, patients with advanced-stage cancer types known to be curable should be treated aggressively with the most appropriate available regimens (e.g. chemotherapy with or without adjuvant surgery, radiation, or molecularly targeted therapy) for that particular tumor. While this approach is known to be associated with substantial morbidity and mortality, when the ultimate goal is a cure the risks are worth taking. On the other hand, patients with advanced-stage cancer of the types known to be incurable should be offered the best treatment available in hopes of prolonging survival while preserving QOL. Patients with tumors that fail to respond to or progress during appropriate first line treatment, or relapse after an initial response should be advised of the unlikely usefulness and the increased risks associated with further treatment. At this stage, the emphasis should shift to palliative care instituted in a hospice or home setting. However, in order to respect patients' autonomy caregivers should be prepared to acquiesce to a patient's demand to continue treatment with second-line regimens unless otherwise contraindicated and after a detailed disclosure of potential complications and the adverse impact on

QOL of such a course of action without compensatory survival benefits. The disclosed information must be easy to grasp and skillfully delivered from the outset and at each subsequent stage in order to prepare patients and relatives to face increasingly difficult decisions and facilitate each inevitable transition. Finally, I propose to revive the lost art of end of life care. This period, that covers the last few weeks or months of life represents the phase when the primary goal of treatment must shift from disease treatment to palliative care rather than unnecessarily subjecting these physically and emotionally fragile patients to acute inpatient and ICU care despite the unlikelihood of benefits and often without eliciting patients' preferences at a great cost to themselves and to society. This approach does not constitute a disguised form of "active euthanasia" defined as "causing the death of a person through a direct action", which I strongly oppose, or "passive euthanasia" if defined as "hastening the death of a person by altering some form of support", which I do not condone, but allowing a natural process to take place following strict ethical principles focused on finding a timely balance between disease treatment and palliation agreed to by both the caregiver and the patient after full disclosure and discussion of the pros and cons of each course of action. Only then will end of life care become humane and ethical once again, allowing terminal patients to die with dignity and their families to achieve closure. The proposed strategy to advanced and terminal cancer management ensures a favorable beneficence-maleficence ratio during each management phase. It also respects the principles of patient autonomy, enabling patients to remain in control of their own destiny, and of justice by biasing use of resources towards patients with the best chances of extending life meaningfully while reducing unwise and frequently counterproductive expenditures beyond the point of no return. Adoption of such an approach would necessitate that western societies come to grips with the notion that death is an inevitable part of life that cannot be put on hold in spite of caregivers' best intentions and heroic efforts, even when using the most sophisticated tools modern medicine has to offer.

References

1. Faguet, GB. *The War on Cancer: An Anatomy of failure: A Blueprint for the Future*. Dordrecht, The Netherlands, Springer, 2005.
2. Ibidem.
3. Faguet GB. *The Affordable Care Act: A missed opportunity; a better way forward*. New York, NY. Algora Publishing, 2013.
4. Fromer MJ. How, After a Decade of Public & Private Wrangling, FDR Signed NCI into Law in 1937, *Oncol Times* 2006;**28**:65–67. 10.1097/01.COT.0000295147.30150.9e
5. Rettig A. *Cancer Crusade: The Story of the National Cancer Act Of 1971*. Bloomington, IN, Authors Choice Press, 2005.
6. Patterson JT. *The Dread Disease: Cancer and Modern American Culture*. Cambridge, MA, Harvard University Press, 1987
7. Henderson B, Maverick M. A political Biography. Austin, University of Texas Press, TX, 1970. pg. 144.
8. Jakobi PL, Jackson, D, Sr. *Handbook of Texas Online* Web 20 Jun. 2012. http://www.tshaonline.org/handbook/online/articles/fja44
9. Epstein SS. *The Politics of Cancer Revisited*. Hankins, NY, East Ridge Press, 1998.
10. Ibidem.
11. Office of Government and Congressional Relations: Legislative History; National Cancer act of 1937. Web 10 Jun. 2012. http://legislative.cancer.gov/history/1937
12. National Cancer Institute: Fact book 1974. DHEW Publication number (NIH) 74–512, January 1974. Web 19 Jun. 2012. http://obf.cancer.gov/financial/attachments/NCI-Fact-Book-1973-Actuals.pdf
13. Cox M. *Ralph W. Yarborough, the People's Senator* (Focus on American History). Austin TX, University of Texas Press, 2002.
14. Ibidem.
15. The Mary Lasker Papers: Biographical information. The National Library of Medicine: Profiles in Science. Web. 26 Jun. 2012. http://profiles.nlm.nih.gov/ps/retrieve/Narrative/TL/p-nid/199
16. The Mary Lasker Papers. Letter from Ralph W. Yarborough to Mary Lasker. The National Library of Medicine: Profiles in Science. Web 26 Jun. 2012. http://profiles.nlm.nih.gov/ps/retrieve/ResourceMetadata/TLBBJZ
17. The Mary Lasker Papers: Biographical information. Op. cit.
18. Farber S, Diamond LK, Mercer RD, et al. Temporary remissions in acute leukemia in children produced by the folic acid antagonist, 4-aminopteroylglutamic acid (Aminopterin). *N Engl J Med* 1948;**238**:787.
19. Garb S. Cure for Cancer: *A National Goal*. N.Y. New York, Springer, 1968.

20. Cited in Groopman J. The thirty year war: Have we being fighting cancer the wrong way? *The New Yorker*, June 4th, 2001, p 53.
21. Mr. Nixon: You can cure cancer. The Mary Lasker Papers. Profiles in Science. National Library of Medicine. Web. 26 Jun. 2012. http://profiles.nlm.nih.gov/ps/retrieve/ResourceMetadata/TLBBBY
22. The Richard Nixon Library and Birthplace, Web. 20 Jul. 2010. http://nixonfoundation.org/Research_Center/1971_pdf_files/1971_0026.pdf
23. Ibidem.
24. National Cancer Institute: Mission. Web. 16 Jul. 2012. http://www.nih.gov/about/almanac/organization/NCI.htm#programs
25. NCI Budget Requests: Quick facts. National Cancer Institute. Web. 20 Jul. 2012. http://www.cancer.gov/aboutnci/servingpeople/nci-budget-information/requests
26. NCI mission statement. National Cancer Institute. Web. 20 Jul. 2012. http://www.cancer.gov/aboutnci/overview/mission
27. Rothschild BM, Tanke DH, Helbling M. Epidemiologic study of tumors in dinosaurs. *Naturwissenschaften* 2003;**90**:495–500. doi:10.1007/s00114-003-0473-9
28. An ancient Medical Treasure at your fingertips. U.S. National Library of Medicine. The Edwin Smith Surgical Papyrus. Web 29 Sept. 2012. http://archive.nlm.nih.gov/proj/ttp/flash/smith/smith.html
29. Gods of Ancient Egypt: Sekhmet. Ancient Egypt Online. Web Nov 15, 2012. Web 04 Nov. 2012. http://ancientegyptonline.co.uk/Sekhmet.html
30. Shultz M, Parzinger H, Posdnjakov DV, et al. Oldest known case of metastasizing prostate carcinoma diagnosed in the skeleton of a 2,700-year-old Scythian king from Arzhan (Siberia, Russia). *Int J Cancer* 2007;**121**:2591–5.
31. Prates C, Sousa S, Oliveira C, et al. Prostate metastatic bone cancer in an Egyptian Ptolemaic mummy, a proposed radiological diagnosis. *Int J Paleontology* 2011;**1**:98–103.
32. Gourevitch D. Reinventing Hippocrates (book review of David Cantor, ed. *Reinventing Hippocrates. The History of Medicine in Context*). *Bull History of Med* 2003;**77**:1418–1419.
33. Aphorisms by Hippocrates, Translated by Francis Adams. Web Nov 12, 2012. http://classics.mit.edu/Hippocrates/aphorisms.html
34. The Hippocratic Oath. Translated by Michael North, National Library of Medicine, 2002. Web 04 Nov. 2012. http://www.nlm.nih.gov/hmd/greek/greek_oath.html
35. Hippocrates. On forecasting diseases. MedLibrary.org: Hippocrates. Web 04 Nov. 2012. http://medlibrary.org/medwiki/Hippocrates
36. Hippocrates Aphorism 165–6. Aphorisms of Hippocrates from the Latin version of Verhoofd with literal translation. Web Nov 12, 2012. http://archive.org/stream/AphorismsOfHippocratesFromTheLatinVersionOfVerhoofd/Aphorisms_of_Hippocrates_from_the_Latin_version_of_Verhoofd_djvu.txt
37. Hippocrates Aphorism 131–38. Aphorisms of Hippocrates from the Latin version of Verhoofd with literal translation. Web 12 Nov. 2012. http://archive.org/stream/AphorismsOfHippocratesFromTheLatinVersionOfVerhoofd/Aphorisms_of_Hippocrates_from_the_Latin_version_of_Verhoofd_djvu.txt
38. Celsus AC, *De Medicina*, (with English translation by W.G. Spencer), Book V. 28, 2C-F William Heinemann Ltd, Cambridge, MA: Harvard University Press, 1938. Web 12 Nov. 2012. http://wwww.archive.org/stream/demedicina02celsuoft/demedicina02celsuoft_djvu.txt
39. Zeis E. *Die Literatur und Geschichte der plastischen Chirurgie*. Leipzig: W Engelmann; 1863, p 187.
40. Celsus AC, De Medicina. Op. cit.
41. Celsus AC, De Medicina. Op. cit.
42. Celsus AC, De Medicina. Op. cit.
43. Kühn C.G., *Claudii Galeni Opera Omnia*. Leipzig: C. Cnobloch, 1821–1833. Reprinted in facsimile by rpt. Hildesheim: Georg Olms, 1964–5. (Greek, Latin trans.) Editio Kuchniana Lipsiae.

44. Hankinson, R. J. ed. *The Cambridge Companion to Galen*. Cambridge Collections Online. Cambridge University Press, 2008. Web 14 Dec 2012. http://universitypublishingonline.org/cambridge/companions/ebook.jsf?bid=CBO9781139001908
45. Nutton V. *Heirs of Hippocrates*. The UCL centre for the history of medicine. Web 08 Nov. 2012. http://www.ucl.ac.uk/histmed/people/academics/nutton
46. *Galeni Opera Omnia*, Op. Cit.
47. Nutton V. *Galen, On my own opinions. Text, translation and commentary*, CMG V.3.2, Berlin, Akademie Verlag, 1999.
48. Aëtius of Amidenus. Sixteen books by Aëtius Amidenus, whom some call the most distinguished physician of Antioch, in three volumes; Book 14, chapter 4. Edited by Janus Cornarius, Venice, 1534.
49. Adams F. *The Seven Books of Paulus Ægineta*. Translated from the Greek with Commentary (Digitized version). Vol. II London: Printed for the Sydenham Society, 1844–47. Vol. 1, p xviii. Web 23 Nov. 2012. https://archive.org/stream/sevenbooksofpaul02pauluoft#page/n7/mode/2up
50. Ibidem, v.6, p 332.
51. Ibidem, v.6, p xvii.
52. O'Leary, De Lacy. *How Greek Science Passed to the Arabs; chapter IV*. Routledge & Kegan Paul, London, 1949.
53. Ibidem, Chapter III.
54. Hunt J. *The Pursuit of Learning in the Islamic World: 610–2003*. Web 08 Dec. 2012. http://books.google.co.uk/books?id=KTWDxDEY-Q0C&pg=PA99#v=onepage&q&f=false
55. Hamid Naseem Rafiabadi. Saints and Saviours of Islam. Web 08 Dec. 2012. http://books.google.co.uk/books?id=ysB4DTRgh5sC&pg=PA295#v=onepage&q&f=false
56. Hunt J., Op. cit.
57. Tschanz DW. *Saudi Aramco World* 2011;**62**:34–39. Web 8 Mar 2014. https://archive.org/details/avenzoarsavieets00coliuoft
58. Faguet GB. *The War on Cancer*. Op. cit.
59. Andreae Vesalii Bruxellensis, scholae medicorum Patavinae professoris, *De humani corporis fabrica libri septem*. Basilae: Joannis Oporini (printer), Mense Junio, 1543.
60. Copernicus Nicolaus. *De Revolutionibus Orbium Coelestium*. [On the Revolutions of the Heavenly Spheres]. Norimbergae: apud Ioh. Petreium, 1543.
61. Paré A. *La Méthod de traicter les playes faites par les arquebuses et aultres bastons à feu*, 1545 Reprinted 2008, Paris, Presses Universitaire de France.
62. Paré A. In: Hamby WB. *The Case Reports and Autopsy Records of Ambroise Paré*. 1960 Springfield, IL: C.C. Thomas [cited in Shimkin MB, *Contrary to Nature:* Cancer. 57p.
63. Cited by Wolff J, in: *The Science of cancerous disease from earliest times to the present*. Science History Publications, 1989, p 42.
64. Descartes R. *Discours de la méhode pour bien conduire sa raison et chercher la vérité dansles sciences, 4e partie, 2e Méditation*. 1824, Paris. Antoine Augustin Bossourd. Web 6 Mar. 2013 (digitized original version) https://archive.org/details/discoursdela00desc
65. Aselli G. *De lactibus sive Lacteis venis*, 1627. (facsimile reprint of the Latin original), Whitefish, MT: Kessinger Publishing, LLC, 2009.
66. Bett WR: *Historical aspects of cancer*, in: Raven RR (ed) Cancer, vol I. London: Butterworth, 1957. 1–5pp.
67. Petit J-L. Oeuvres completes, Limoges, 1837, pg 438 (cited in Wolf J. The Science of cancerous diseases from earliest times to the present). 1989, Sagamore Beach, MA, *Science History Publications/USA*, pg 50.
68. Petit J-L. Essai sur le cancer des mammelles, cited by Darmon P, in Les céllules folles, *Plon*, Paris 1993.
69. Peyrilhe B. Dissertatio academica de cancro, Lyon, 1773 (cited in Wolf J. The Science of cancerous diseases from earliest times to the present. 1989, Sagamore Beach, MA, *Science History Publications/USA*, pp 54–55).
70. Halsted WS. The results of operations for the cure of cancer of the breast performed at the Johns Hopkins Hospital from June, 1889, to January, 1894. *Ann Surg*. 1894;**20**:497–555.

71. Pinell P. Naissance d'un fléau: Histoire de la lute contre le cancer en France (1890–1940), Editions Métailié, 1992. 21p.
72. Ramazzini B. De Moribus Artificum Diatriba. 1713. [Translation by Wright WC Birmingham, AL: *Classics of Medicine Library*; 1983].
73. Franco G, Franco F. Bernardino Ramazzini: The Father of Occupational Medicine. *Am J Public Health* 2001;**91**:1382.
74. Collegium Ramazzini: Mission. Web Apr 2, 2014. http://www.collegiumramazzini.org/about.asp
75. Griffiths, M. Nuns, virgins, and spinsters: Rigoni-Stern and cervical cancer revisited. *Brit J Obstet Gynaec* 1991;**98**:797–802.
76. Bosch X, Manos M, Muñoz N, et al. Prevalence of Human Papillomavirus in Cervical Cancer: A Worldwide Perspective. *J Natl Cancer Inst* 1995;**87**:796–802.
77. Hill J. Cautions against the immoderate use of snuff and the effects it must produce when this way taken into the body. London, R. Baldwin & J. Jackson. 1761. [In: Redmond DE. Tobacco and Cancer: The first clinical report, 1761. *N Engl J Med* 1970;**252**:21.
78. Brown JR, Thornton JL. Percivall Pott (1714–1788) and Chimney Sweepers' Cancer of the Scrotum. *Br J Ind Med*. 1957;**14**:68–70. Web 30 Nov. 2012. http://www.ncbi.nlm.nih.gov/pmc/articles/PMC1037746/?page=2
79. Ibidem.
80. Ibidem.
81. Cook JW, Hewett CL, Hieger I. The isolation of a cancer-producing hydrocarbon from coal tar. Parts I, II, and III. *J Chem Soc* 1933, 395–405. DOI: 10.1039/JR9330000395
82. Brown JR, Thornton JL, Op. Cit.
83. Brown JR, Thornton JL, Op. Cit.
84. Bayle GL et Cayole JB. Cancer, in: *Dictionnaire des sciences médicales*, Paris, Pankouke, 1812, vol III, 671p.
85. König, F. Die Bedeutung der Durchleuchtung (Röntgen) für die Diagnose der Knochenkrankheiten. *Dtsch Med. Wochensch* 1896;**22**:113–114.
86. Broca PP. *Mémoire sur l'anatomie pathologique du cancer*. Bulletin de la Société anatomique de Paris, 1850, 25: 45 et seq.
87. Who invented the microscope? A complete microscope history. Web 06 Dec. 2012. http://www.history-of-the-microscope.org/history-of-the-microscope-who-invented-the-microscope.php
88. Meeusen J. The junkyard Chevalier and the 11 year old girl'1 Simple and compound microscope by Charles Chevalier, 1832–1849. Web 06 Dec. 2012. http://www.meeusen.com/chevalier/
89. Virchow R. 1858 *Die Cellularpathologie, 4th ed.* Berlin: Hirschwald, 1871.
90. Velpeau AALM. *Traité des maladies du sein et de la régoin mammaire*, Paris: Masson, 1853.
91. Harris H. *The Birth of the cell*. New Haven, Yale University Press. 1999.
92. Otis, L. *Müller's Lab: The story of Jacob Henle, Theodor Schwann, Emil Du Bois-Reymond, Hermann von Helmoltz, Rudolf Virchow, Robert Remak, Ernst Haekel, and their brilliant, tormented advisor*. Oxford, Oxford University Press, 2007.
93. Rutherford, A. The Cell: Episode 1; The hidden kingdom. BBC4 (August 2009).
94. Bard L. *Anatomie et Classification des tumeurs*, Paris: Masson, 1895.
95. Calkins GN. Boveri T, Zur Frage der Entstehung maligner tumoren. *Science* 1914;**40**;857–859.
96. Holmes OW. Currents and countercurrents in medical science, with other addresses and essays (Boston: Ticknor and Fields, 1861), p. 39. cited in Parascandola J. From germs to Genes: Trends in drug therapy, 1852–2002. *Pharm Hist* 2002;**44**:3–11.
97. Peller, S. *Cancer research since 1900. An evaluation*. New York: Philosophical Library, 1979. 158p.
98. The Nobel Prize in Physiology or Medicine 1926. Nobelprize.org. 6 Dec 2012. Web 20 Apr. 2004. http://www.nobelprize.org/nobel_prizes/medicine/laureates/1926/index.html
99. Weiss RB. The anthracyclines: will we ever find a better doxorubicin? *Sem Onc* 1992;**19**:670–86.

100. Asghar RJ, Parsonnet J. Helicobacter pylori and risk for gastric adenocarcinoma. *Semin Gastrointest Dis* 2001;**12**:203–8.
101. Isaacson PG. Extranodal lymphomas: the MALT concept. *Verh Dtsch Ges Pathol* 1992;**76**:14–23.
102. Seto M. Genetic and epigenetic factors involved in B-cell lymphomas. *Cancer Sci* 2004;**95**:704–710.
103. Blaser MJ. Helicobacter pylori and gastric diseases. *BMJ* 1998;**316**:1507–1510.
104. Herrera V, Parsonne J. Helicobacter pylori and gastric adenocarcinoma. *Clinical Microbiology and Infection*, 2009;**15**:971–976.
105. Coley WB. The treatment of malignant tumors by repeated inoculations of erysipelas: with a report of ten original cases. *Am J Med Sci* 1893;**105**:487–511.
106. McCarthy EF. The Toxins of William B. Coley and the Treatment of Bone and Soft-Tissue Sarcomas. *Iowa Orthop J* 2006;**26**:154–158.
107. Herr HW, Schwalb DM, Zhang ZF, et al.: Intravesical bacillus Calmette-Guérin therapy prevents tumor progression and death from superficial bladder cancer: ten-year follow-up of a prospective randomized trial. *J Clin Oncol* 1995;**13**:1404–8.
108. Long CW. An account of the first use of sulphuric ether. *Southern Med & Surg J* 1849;**5**:705–713.
109. Lister J. On the antiseptic principle in the practice of surgery. *Lancet* 1867;**90**:353–356.
110. Asimov I. *Asimov's biographical encyclopedia od science and technology.: The living stores of more than 1,000 great scientists from the Age of Greece to the Space Age, chronologically arranged.* Garden City, NJ. Doubleday.
111. Paschoff N. *Marie Curie and the science of radioactivity.* Oxford: Oxford University Press, 1996.
112. Curie E. *Madame Curie: A biography.* New York, Da Capo Press, 2001.
113. Fröman N, Marie and Pierre Curie and the Discovery of Polonium and Radium. NobelPrize.org. Web 8 Dec 2012. http://www.nobelprize.org/nobel_prizes/physics/articles/curie/
114. Ibidem.
115. Paschoff N. Op. cit.
116. Rous P. A transmissible avian neoplasm. (sarcoma of the common fowl) *J Exp Med* 1910;**12**:696–705.
117. Goodman LS, Wintrobe MM, Dameshek W, et al. Use of methyl-*bis*-(β-*chloroethyl*) amine hydrochloride and tris-(β-*chloroethyl*) amine hydrochloride for Hodgkin's disease, lymphosarcoma, leukemia, and certain allied and miscellaneous disorders. *JAMA* 1946;**132**:126–132.
118. Jacobson LO, Spurr CL, Barron ES, et al. Studies of the effect of methyl methyl-*bis*-(β-*chloroethyl*) amine hydrochloride on neoplastic diseases and allied disorders of the hemopoietic system. *JAMA* 1946;**132**:263.
119. Encyclopedia of the First World War: Deaths from gas attacks. Web 10 Dec. 2012. http://www.spartacus.schoolnet.co.uk/FWWgasdeaths.htm
120. Cook T. *No Place to Run: The Canadian Corps and Gas Warfare in the First World War*. UBC Press, 1999.
121. Swerdlow SH, Campo E, Harris NL, et al. WHO Classification of Tumours of Haematopoietic and Lymphoid Tissues. Lyon, France: *International Agency for Research on Cancer*; 2008.
122. *Chronic lymphocytic leukemia: Advances in Molecular biology, Cytogenetics, Diagnosis, and Management.* Ed Guy B. Faguet, Totowa, NJ, The Humana Press, 2003.
123. Surveillance Epidemiology and End Results, SEER Stat Fact Sheets: Pancreas Cancer. Web 11 Dec. 2012. http://seer.cancer.gov/statfacts/html/pancreas.html
124. DOE Genomics Timeline Program Developments: 1990. Web 12 Dec. 2012. http://genomicscience.energy.gov/program/timeline.shtml
125. Venter JC, Adams MD, Meyers EW, et al. The sequence of the human genome. *Science* 2001;**291**:1304–1351.
126. International Human Genome Sequencing Consortium. Initial sequencing and analysis of the human genome. *Nature* 2001;**409**:860–921.
127. Roberts L. Controversial from the start. *Science* 2001;**291**:1182–1188. DOI: 10.1126/science.291.5507.1182a
128. Ibidem.

129. Kerem B, Rommens JM, Buchanan JA, et al. Identification of the cystic fibrosis gene: genetic analysis. *Science* 1989;**245**:1073–80.
130. Polymeropoulos MH, Lavedan C, Leroy, SE et al. Mutation in the α-Synuclein Gene Identified in Families with Parkinson's Disease. *Science* 1997;**276**:2045–2047.
131. Greenman C, Stephens P, Smith R, et al. Patterns of somatic mutation in human cancer genomes, *Nature* 2007;**446**, 153–158 | doi:10.1038/nature05610
132. Watson J. *The double Helix: A personal account of the discovery of the structure of DNA.* New York, Atheneum. 1968
133. Ibidem.
134. Parshall G, Licking EF. James D. el al. Double-Teaming the Double Helix. US News & World Report, August 17, 1998, Web 14 Dec. 2012. http://www.usnews.com/usnews/issue/980817/17dna.htm
135. Watson J., Op. cit.
136. Watson J, Crick F. A structure for deoxyribose nucleic acid. *Nature* 1953;**171**:737.
137. Sayre A. *Rosalind Franklin and DNA*. New York, W.W. Norton & Company, (2000).
138. The Nobel Prize in Physiology or Medicine 1962. Nobelprize.org. Web 14 Dec. 2012. http://www.nobelprize.org/nobel_prizes/medicine/laureates/1962/
139. US National Library of Medicine. Web 20 Apr. 2004. http://ghr.nlm.nih.gov/handbook/illustrations/dnastructure
140. Mendel, J.G. (1866). *Versuche über Pflanzenhybriden* Verhandlungen des naturforschenden Vereines in Brünn, Bd. IV für das Jahr, 1865 Abhandlungen:3–47.
141. The Ascent Of Man: Complete BBC Series. Web 12 Dec. 2012. http://www.amazon.co.uk/The-Ascent-Of-Man-Complete/dp/B000772842
142. Griffiths AJF, Miller JH, Suzuki DT, et al., An Introduction to Genetic Analysis, 7th edition. New York: *W.H. Freeman*, 2000.
143. Ibidem.
144. Bateson W. Mendel's Principles of Heredity: A Defence. Cambridge, *Cambridge University Press*, 1902.
145. Chromosome 1: DOE Human Genome Project. Genomics.energy.gov. Web 12 Dec. 2012. https://public.ornl.gov/site/gallery/originals/Chrom01.jpg
146. Ibidem.
147. Sandberg A, Chen Z. *Cytogenetic Analysis*, In: Hematologic Malignancies: Methods and Techniques, Ed Guy B Faguet, Totowa, New Jersey, The Human Press Inc., 2001.
148. Sandberg A, Chen Z. *FISH Analysis. in* Hematologic Malignancies: Methods and Techniques, Ed Guy B Faguet, Totowa, New Jersey, The Human Press Inc., 2001.
149. Baudis M, Bentz M. *Comparative genomic hybridization, in* Hematologic Malignancies: Methods and Techniques, Ed Guy B Faguet, Totowa, New Jersey, The Human Press Inc., 2001.
150. Higenfeld E, Padilla-Nash H, Haas OA, et al. *Spectral karyotyping (SKY) of hematologic malignancies, in* Hematologic Malignancies: Methods and Techniques, Ed Guy B Faguet, Totowa, New Jersey, The Human Press Inc., 2001.
151. Mohr S, Leikauf GD, Keith G, et al. Microarrays as cancer keys: An array of possibilities. *J Clin Oncol* 2002;**20**:3165–3175.
152. Polymerase Chain Reaction. In: Hematologic Malignancies: Methods and Techniques, Ed Guy B Faguet, Totowa, New Jersey, The Human Press Inc., 2001. 83–176p.
153. Cooper GM. The Cell: A Molecular Approach. 2nd edition. Sunderland (MA): *Sinauer Associates*; 2000. The Eukaryotic Cell Cycle. Web 18 Dec. 2012. http://www.ncbi.nlm.nih.gov/books/NBK9876/
154. Ibidem.
155. Ibidem.
156. Donehower LA, Levine AJ. 2008. p53, cancer and longevity, In *Molecular Biology of Aging*, (eds) Guarente Leonard, Partridge Linda and Wallace Douglas, Cold Spring Harbor Laboratory Press, 6, 127–152.
157. Cooper GM. Op. Cit.

158. HGNC Database, HUGO Gene Nomenclature Committee. Symbol Report: CDN2A. Web 21 Dec. 2012. http://www.genenames.org/cgi-bin/gene_symbol_report?hgnc_id=1787
159. Elmore S. Apoptosis: A Review of Programmed Cell Death. *Toxicol Pathol* 207;**35**:495–516. doi: 10.1080/01926230701320337
160. Ibidem.
161. Ibidem.
162. Ibidem.
163. Ibidem.
164. Ibidem
165. Tsujimoto, Y., Gorham, J., Cossman, J., et al. The t(14;18) chromosome translocations involved in B-cell neoplasms result from mistakes in VDJ joining. *Science* 1985;**229**:1390–1393.
166. Moyzis RK, Buckingham JM, Cram LS, et al. A highly conserved repetitive DNA sequence (TTAGGG) present at the telomeres oh human chromosomes. *Proc Natl Acad Sci USA* 1988;**85**:6622–6626.
167. Shay JW, Wright WE, Werbin H. Defining the molecular mechanism of human cell immortalization. *Biochim. Biophys. Acta*, 1991;**1072**:1–7.
168. Shay JW, Bachetti S. A survey of telomerase activity in human cancer. *Eur J Cancer* 1997;**33**:787–791.
169. Bodnar AG, Ouellette M, Frolkis M, Holt SE, et al. Extension of life-span by introduction of telomerase into normal human cells. *Science* 1998;**279**:349–352.
170. Jiang H, Schiffer E, Song Z, et al. Proteins induced by telomere dysfunction and DNA damage represent biomarkers of human aging and disease. *Proc Natl Acad Sci USA* 2008;**105**:11299–11304.
171. Valdes AM, Andrew T, Gardner JP, et al. Obesity, cigarette smoking, and telomere length in women. *Lancet* 2005;**366**:662–664.
172. Lavarino C, Cheung N, de Torres C, et al. Specific gene expression profiles and unique chromosomal abnormalities are associated with regressing tumors among infants with disseminated neuroblastoma. *J Clin Oncol*, 2007 ASCO Annual Meeting Proceedings Part I. Vol 25, No. 18S (June 20 Supplement), 2007: 9501.
173. D'Angio GJ, Evans AE, Koop CE: Special pattern of widespread neuroblastoma with a favourable prognosis. *Lancet* 1971;**1**:1046–1049.
174. Hiyama E, Hiyama K, Yokoyama T, et al.: Correlating telomerase activity levels with human neuroblastoma outcomes. *Nat Med* 1995;**1**:249–55.
175. Clarke MF, Dick JE, Dirks PB, et al. Cancer Stem Cells – Perspectives on Current Status and Future Directions: AACR Workshop on Cancer Stem Cells. *Cancer Res* 2006;**66**:9339–9344.
176. Powell AA, Talasaz AH, Zhang H, Coram MA, Reddy A, et al. (2012) Single Cell Profiling of Circulating Tumor Cells: Transcriptional Heterogeneity and Diversity from Breast Cancer Cell Lines. PLoS ONE 7(5): e33788. doi:10.1371/journal.pone.0033788
177. Knudson, AG. Mutation and cancer: Statistical study of retinoblastoma. *Proc Natl Acad Sci USA* 1971;**68**, 820–823.
178. Faguet GB, Webb HH, Agee JF, et al. Immunologically diagnosed malignancy in Sjogren's pseudo-lymphoma. *Am. J. Med.* 1978;**65**:424–429.
179. Nowell PC, Hungerford DA. A minute chromosome in human chronic granulocytic leukemia. *Science* 1960;**142**:1497.
180. Futreal PA, Kspryk A, Birney E, et al. Cancer and Genomics. *Nature* 2001;**409**:850–855.
181. Hamblin TJ. Heterogeneous origin of the B-CLL cell, In: Chronic Lymphocytic Leukemia: Advances in Molecular genetics, Biology, Diagnosis, and Management. Ed Guy B Faguet. Totowa, NJ, The Humana Press, 2003.
182. Garzón R, Calin GA, Croce CM. MicroRNAs in Cancer. *Annu Rev Med* 2009;**60**:167–179 DOI: 10.1146/annurev.med.59.053006.104707
183. Hanahan D, Weinberg RA. The hallmarks of cancer. *Cell* 2000;**100**:57–70.
184. Warburg, O. On the origin of cancer cells. *Science* 1956;**123**:309–314.
185. Jones RG, Thompson CB. *Genes Dev.* 2009;**23**:537–548. Web Jan. 11, 2013. http://genesdev.cshlp.org/content/23/5/537.full#sec-4

186. Croce CM. Oncogenes and cancer. *N Engl J Med* 2008;**358**:502–511.
187. Franovic A, Holterman CE, Payette J, et al. *Proc Natl Acad Sci USA* 2009;**106**:21306–21311. Web Jan 11, 2013. http://www.ncbi.nlm.nih.gov/pmc/articles/PMC2795516/#B1
188. O'Connor, C. Human chromosome translocations and cancer. *Nature Education* 2008;**1**:56.
189. NCG4.0: Network of Cancer Genes. Web 2 Jan. 2013. http://ncg.kcl.ac.uk/index.php
190. Chung CC, Magalhaes WCS, Gonzalez-Bosquet J, et al. Genome-wide association studies in cancer – current and future directions. *Carcinogenesis* 2010;**31**:111–120.
191. Croce CM. (2008) Op. cit.
192. Croce CM. (2008) Op. cit.
193. Croce CM. (2008) Op. cit.
194. Vogelstein B, Kinzler KW. Cancer genes and the pathways they control, *Nat Med* 2004;**10**:789–799.
195. Antoniou AC, Pharoah PDP, McMullan G, et al. A comprehensive model for familial breast cancer incorporating BRCA1, BRCA2 and other genes. *Br J Cancer* 2002;**86**:76–83. Web Jan 25, 2013. http://www.ncbi.nlm.nih.gov/pmc/articles/PMC2746531/
196. Lee RC, Feinbaum RL, Ambros V. The C. elegans heterochronic gene lin-4 encodes small RNAs with antisense complementarity to lin-14. *Cell* 1993;**75**:843–54.
197. Cheng CZ. MicroRNAs as Oncogenes and Tumor Suppressors *New Eng J Med* 2005;**353**:1768–1771. Web Jan 26, 2013. http://content.nejm.org/cgi/content/full/353/17/1768
198. Esquela-Kerscher A, Slack FJ. Oncomirs – microRNAs with a role in cancer. *Nat Rev Cancer* 2006;**6**:259–269.
199. Croce CM. Causes and consequences of microRNA dysregulation in cancer. *Nat Rev Genet* 2009;**10**:704–714. | doi:10.1038/nrg2634
200. Garzón R, Calin GA, and Croce CM. Op. cit.
201. Buermans HP, Ariyurek Y, van Ommen G, et al. New methods for next generation sequencing based microRNA expression profiling. *BMC Genomics* 2010;**11**:716.
202. Mraz M, Pospisilova S, Malinova K, et al. MicroRNAs in chronic lymphocytic leukemia pathogenesis and disease subtypes. *Leuk. Lymphoma* 2009;**50**:3:506–9.
203. Yan Li-X, Huang X-F, Shao Q, et al. MicroRNA miR-21 overexpression in human breast cancer is associated with advanced clinical stage, lymph node metastasis and patient poor prognosis. *RNA*. 2008;14:2348–2360. Web 12 Mar. 2013. http://rnajournal.cshlp.org/content/14/11/2348.full#sec-10
204. Jones PA, Baylin SB. The epigenomics of cancer. *Cell* 2007;**128**:683–692. http://dx.doi.org/10.1016/j.bbr.2011.03.031
205. Egger G, Liang G, Aparicio A, et al. Epigenetics in human disease and prospects for epigenetic therapy. *Nature* 2004;**429**;457–463. doi:10.1038/nature02625
206. Jones PA, Baylin SB. The fundamental role of epigenetic events in cancer. *Nat. Rev Genet* 2002;**3**: 415–428.
207. Ibidem.
208. Peedicayil J. Epigenetic therapy: A new development in pharmacology. *Indian J Med Res* 2006;**123**:17–24.
209. Sigalotti L, Fratta E, Coral S, et al. Epigenetic drugs as pleiotropic agents in cancer treatment: biomolecular aspects and clinical applications. *J Cell Physiol* 2007;**212**:330–44.
210. National Cancer Institute. FactSheet: Metastatic cancer. Web Feb. 4 2013. http://www.cancer.gov/cancertopics/factsheet/Sites-Types/metastatic
211. Cronin K, Feuer E, Wesley M, et al. Current estimates for 5 and 10 year relative survival. Statistical Research and Applications Branch, NCI, Technical Report #2003–04.
212. Ibidem.
213. Paget S. The distribution of secondary growths in cancer of the breast. *Lancet* 1889;**133**:571–3.
214. Hanahan D, Weinberg RA. Op. cit.
215. Horak CE, Lee JH, Marshall J-C, et al. The role of metastasis suppressor genes in metastatic dormancy. *APMIS* 2008;**116**:586–601. 10.1111/j.1600-0463.2008.01213.x

216. Fidler I, *Molecular biology of cancer: invasion and metastases*. In: V.T. DeVita, S. Hellman, S.A. Rosenberg (eds), Cancer principles and practice of oncology, Ed. 5, pp 135–152, New York: Lippincott-Raven, 1997.
217. Weigelt B, Glas AM, Wessels LF, et al. Gene expression profiles of primary breast tumors maintained in distant metastases. *Proc Natl Acad Sci USA* 2003;**100**:15901–5.
218. Kozlowski JM, Hart IR, Fidler IJ, Hanna N. A human melanoma line heterogeneous with respect to metastatic capacity in athymic nude mice. *J Natl Cancer Inst* 1984;**72**:913–7.
219. Ramis-Conde I, Drasdo D, Anderson ARA, et al. Modeling the Influence of the E-Cadherin-β-Catenin Pathway in Cancer Cell Invasion: A Multiscale Approach. *Biophys J* 2008;**95**:155–165. http://dx.doi.org/10.1529/biophysj.107.114678
220. Fidler I. Op. cit.
221. Wolf K, Friedl P. Mapping proteolytic cancer cell-extracellular matrix interfaces. *Clin Exp Metastasis* 2009;**26**:289–98. doi: 10.1007/s10585-008-9190-2
222. Bendas G, Borsig L. Cancer Cell Adhesion and Metastasis: Selectins, Integrins, and the Inhibitory Potential of Heparins. *Int J Cell Biol* 2012;**2012**: Article ID 676731. doi:10.1155/2012/676731
223. Desgrosellier JS and Cheresh DA. Integrins in cancer: biological implications and therapeutic opportunities. *Nat Rev Cancer* 2010;**10**:9–22.
224. Bendas G, Borsig L. Op. cit.
225. Brooks PC, Clark RAF, Cheresh DA, Requirement of vascular integrin α(v)β3 for angiogenesis, *Science* 1994;**264**:569–571.
226. Ley K, Laudanna C, Cybulsky CMI, et al. "Getting to the site of inflammation: the leukocyte adhesion cascade updated," *Nat Rev Immunol* 2007;**7**:678–689.
227. Guan-zhen Y, Ying C, Can-rong N, et al. Reduced protein expression of metastasis-related genes (nm23, KISS1, KAI1 and p53) in lymph node and liver metastases of gastric cancer. *Int J Exp Pathol* 2007;**88**:175–183. doi: 10.1111/j.1365-2613.2006.00510.x
228. Weinberg RA. Mechanisms of malignant progression. *Carcinogenesis* 2008;**29**:1092–1095.
229. Ibidem.
230. Li M, Teruya-Feldstein J, Weinberg RA. Tumour invasion and metastasis initiated by microRNA-10b in breast cancer. *Nature* 2006;**449**:682–688.
231. Zheng B, Liang L, Hyuang S, et al. MicroRNA-409 suppresses tumour cell invasion and metastasis by directly targeting radixin in gastric cancers. *Oncogene* 2012;**31**:4509–4516. doi:10.1038/onc.2011.581
232. Yoshida BA, Mitchell M, Sokoloff D, et al. Metastasis-suppressor genes: A review and perspective on an emerging field. *Oncol Spectrums* 2001;**2**:166–192.
233. Debies MT, Welch DR. Genetic basis of human breast cancer metastasis. *J Mammary Gland Biol Neoplasia* 2001;**6**:441–451.
234. Guan-zhen Y, Ying C, Can-rong N, et al. Op. cit.
235. Lee CS, Redshaw A, Boag G. nm23-H1 protein immunoreactivity in laryngeal carcinoma. *Cancer* 1996;**77**:2246–2250.
236. Liu H, Mao H, Fu X. Expression of Nm23 in breast cancer–correlation with distant metastasis and prognosis. *Zhonghua Zhong Liu Za Zhi* 2001;**23**:224–227.
237. Horak CE, Lee JH, Marshal J-C, et al. Op. cit.
238. Heimann R, Lan F, McBride R, et al. Separating favorable from unfavorable prognostic markers in breast cancer: the role of E-cadherin. *Nature* 1980;**283**:139–146.
239. Heimann R, Ferguson DJ, Hellman S. The relationship between nm23, angiogenesis, and the metastatic proclivity of node-negative breast cancer. *Cancer Res* 1998;**58**:2766–2771.
240. Horak CE, Lee JH, Marshal J-C, et al. Op. cit.
241. Heimann R, Lan F, McBride R, et al. Op. cit.
242. Guan-zhen Y, Ying C, Can-rong N, et al. Op. cit.
243. IARC monograph on the evaluation of carcinogenic risks to humans: Agents classified by the IARC Monographs, Volumes 1–106. Web Feb. 15, 2013. http://monographs.iarc.fr/ENG/Classification/index.php

244. Peto J, Cancer epidemiology. *Nature* 2001;**411**:390–395.
245. Trichopoulos D, Li LP, Hunter DJ. What causes cancer? *Sci Am* 1996;**275**:80–87.
246. Anand P, Kunnunmakara AB, Sundaram C, et al. Cancer is a preventable disease that requires major lifestyle changes. *Pharmaceutical Res* 2008;**25**:1–20. DOI: 10.1007/s1095-008-9661-9
247. Cancer Facts & Figures, 2012. The American Cancer Society. Atlanta, GA.
248. Cancer: Key Facts. Fact sheet N°297, Reviewed January 2013. WHO. Web 11 Mar. 2013. http://www.who.int/mediacentre/factsheets/fs297/en/
249. IARC Monographs Programme finds cancer hazards associated with shiftwork, painting and firefighting, Press release No 180, 5 December 2007. Web Feb 15, 2013. http://www.iarc.fr/en/media-centre/pr/2007/pr180.html
250. Hernandez LG, van Steeg H, Luijten M et al. Mechanisms of non-genotoxic carcinogens and importance of a weight of evidence approach. *Mutat Res* 2009;**682**:94–109. doi: 10.1016/j.mrrev.2009.07.002. Epub 2009 Jul 22.
251. Ibidem.
252. Fouad T. CDC: Obesity approaching tobacco as top preventable cause of death, 5 April 2004. Web. 12 Oct. 2010. http://www.doctorslounge.com/primary/articles/obesity_death/
253. Schmidt C. UV Radiation and Skin Cancer: The Science behind Age Restrictions for Tanning Beds. *Environ Health Perspect*. 2012;**120**:a308–a313.
254. Environmental and occupational cancers: Fact Sheet No 350, March 2011. World Health Organization. Web 22 Feb. 2013. http://www.who.int/mediacentre/factsheets/fs350/en/
255. Faguet GB. *The Affordable Care Act:* Op. cit.
256. Stewart SL, Cardinez CJ, Richardson LC, et al. Surveillance for Cancers Associated with Tobacco Use – United States, 1999–2004. MMWR: Surveillance Summaries. September 5, 2008:1–33. Web 17 Feb 2013. http://www.cdc.gov/mmwr/preview/mmwrhtml/ss5708a1.htm
257. International Agency for Research on Cancer. IARC monographs on the evaluation of carcinogenic risks to humans: tobacco smoke and involuntary smoking. Vol. 83. Lyon, France: *International Agency for Research on Cancer*, 2004.
258. Thun MJ, Carter BD, Feskanich D, et al. 50-Year Trends in Smoking-Related Mortality in the United States, *N Engl J Med* 2013;**368**:351–364 DOI: 10.1056/NEJMsa1211127
259. Cancer Facts & Figures, 2012. Op. cit.
260. U.S. Department of Health and Human Services. A Report of the Surgeon General: How tobacco smoke cause disease; What it means to you. Atlanta: U.S. Department of Health and Human Services, Centers for Disease Control and Prevention, National Center for Chronic Disease Prevention and Health Promotion, Office on Smoking and Health, 2010.
261. Smoking & Tobacco use. Centers for Disease Control and Prevention: Fast Facts. Web 17 Feb 2013. http://www.cdc.gov/tobacco/data_statistics/fact_sheets/fast_facts/index.htm
262. Faguet GB. *Pain Control and Drug Policy.* Op. cit.
263. A Report of the Surgeon General: How Tobacco Smoke Causes Disease – The Biology and Behavioral Basis for Smoking-Attributable Disease Fact Sheet. Web 20 Feb. 2013. http://www.surgeongeneral.gov/library/reports/tobaccosmoke/factsheet.html
264. DUUS Publication No 2010–1232, January 10, 2010. U.S. Department of Health and Human Services, Centers for Disease Control and Prevention, National Center fop Human Statistics, Web. 17 Oct. 2010. http://www.cdc.gov/nchs/data/hus/hus09.pdf#executivesummary
265. Clinical Guidelines on the Identification, Evaluation, and Treatment of Overweight and Obesity in Adults. NHLBI Obesity Education Initiative, NIH. Web. 3 Jun. 2010. http://www.nhlbi.nih.gov/guidelines/obesity/ob_gdlns.pdf
266. Finkelstein, EA, Trogdon, JG, Cohen, JW, and Dietz, W. Annual medical spending attributable to obesity: Payer- and service-specific estimates. *Health Aff* 2009;**28**:w822–w831.
267. Calle EE, Kaaks R. Overweight, obesity and cancer: epidemiological evidence and proposed mechanisms. *Nat Rev Cancer* 2004;**4**:579–591. Web Feb 23, 2013. http://www.sns.ias.edu/~vazquez/notes/papers/ref.metabolism.obesity.cancer.Calle_2004.pdf
268. Allison, D. B., Downey, M., Atkinson, R. L., et al., writing for TOS Obesity as a Disease Writing Group. Obesity as a Disease: A White Paper on Evidence and Arguments

Commissioned by the Council of The Obesity Society. *Obesity* 2008;**16**:1161–1177. doi: 10.1038/oby.2008.231
269. The Science of Drug Abuse and Addiction. The National Institute of Drug Abuse. Web 10 Feb 2009. http://archives.drugabuse.gov/about/welcome/aboutdrugabuse/chronicdisease/
270. Medical consequences of drug abuse. National Institute of Drug Abuse. Web Feb 23, 2013. http://www.drugabuse.gov/related-topics/medical-consequences-drug-abuse
271. Faguet GB. *Pain Control and Drug Policy.* Op. cit.
272. Schaler J. Addiction is a choice. Chicago: Open Court, 2000.
273. Faguet GB. *Pain Control and Drug Policy.* Op. cit.
274. Turnbaugh PJ, Hamady M, Yatsunenko T, et al. A core gut microbiome in obese and lean twins. *Nature* 2009;**457**:480–484.
275. Hildebrabdt MA, Hoffman C, Sherrill-Mix SA, et al. High-fat diet determines the composition of the murine gut microbiome independently of obesity. *Gastroenterology* 2009;**137**:1716–1724.
276. Faguet GB. *Pain Control and Drug Policy.* Op. cit.
277. American teens are less likely than European tees to use cigarettes and alcohol, but more likely to use illicit drugs. University of Michigan News Report, Jan 01, 2012. Web http://www.ns.umich.edu/new/releases/20420-american-teens-are-less-likely-than-european-teens-to-use-cigarettes-and-alcohol-but-more-likely-to-use-illicit-drugs
278. National Institute on Alcohol Abuse and Alcoholism. Overview on alcohol consumption: Moderate and binge drinking. Web Feb 24, 2013. http://www.niaaa.nih.gov/alcohol-health/overview-alcohol-consumption/moderate-binge-drinking
279. Substance Abuse and Mental Health Services Administration, Results from the 2010 National Survey on Drug Use and Health: Summary of National Findings, NSDUH Series H-41, HHS Publication No. (SMA) 11–4658. Rockville, MD: Substance Abuse and Mental Health Services Administration, 2011.
280. Boffetta P, Hashibe M. Alcohol and cancer. *Lancet Oncol* 2006;**7**:149–156.
281. Faguet GB. *Pain Control and Drug Policy.* Op. cit.
282. Reinarman C. Addiction as accomplishment: The discursive construction of disease *Informa Healthcare* 2005;**13**:307–320 doi:10.1080/16066350500077728
283. Faguet GB. *Pain Control and Drug Policy.* Op. cit.
284. Faguet GB. *The War on Cancer.* Op. cit.
285. Faguet GB. *Pain Control and Drug Policy.* Op. cit.
286. Cancer Facts & Figures, 2012. Op. cit.
287. Howlader N, Noone AM, Krapcho M, et al. (eds). SEER Cancer Statistics Review. 1975–2009. Bethesda (MD): National Cancer Institute, 2012.
288. Berenson A. A cancer drug's big price rise is cause for concern. *New York Times.* March 12, 2006:A1.
289. Cancer Facts & Figures, 2012. Op.cit.
290. Years of Life Lost in 2009 due to Major Causes of Death in U.S. Surveillance Epidemiology and End Results: Cancer statistics. Web Feb 25. 2013. http://seer.cancer.gov/csr/1975_2009_pops09/browse_csr.php?section=1&page=sect_01_zfig.20.html
291. Risk of developing/dying, both sexes: All cancer sites. Surveillance Epidemiology and End Results: Cancer statistics. Web Feb 25. 2013 http://seer.cancer.gov/csr/1975_2009_pops09/browse_csr.php?section=2&page=sect_02_table.12.html
292. Percy CL, Miller BA, Ries LAG. Effect of changes in cancer classification and the accuracy of death certificates on trends in cancer mortality. *Ann NY Acad Sci* 1990;**609**:87–97.
293. Wikipedia contributors, Cancer registry, *Wikipedia, The Free Encyclopedia.* Web Feb. 26, 2013. http://en.wikipedia.org/w/index.php?title=Cancer_registry&oldid=511975118
294. Cancer Facts & Figures – 2012, Op. cit.
295. SEER Cancer Statistics Review (CSR) 1975–2009. Overview. Table 1.11: Median Age of Cancer Patients at Diagnosis, 2005–2009 Web Feb 25. 2013. http://seer.cancer.gov/archive/csr/1975_2009_pops09/browse_csr.php?sectionSEL=1&pageSEL=sect_01_table.11.html
296. SEER Cancer Statistics Review (CSR) 1975–2009. Overview. Table 1.11. Op. cit.

297. Cancer Facts & Figures – 2013. Estimated number of new cancer cases and deaths by sex, US, 2013. The American Cancer Society. Atlanta, GA.
298. Landis SH, Murray T, Bolden S, et al. Cancer Statistics, 1999. *CA Cancer J Clin* 1999;**49**:8–31.
299. Lifetime Risk (Percent) of Being Diagnosed with Cancer by Site and Race/Ethnicity: Males, 18 SEER Areas, 2007–2009 (Table 1.15) and Females, 18 SEER Areas, 2007–2009 (Table 1.16). 2012. Web Mar. 5, 2013. http://seer.cancer.gov/csr/1975_2009_pops09/results_merged/topic_lifetime_risk_diagnosis.pdf
300. Siegel R, Naishadham D. Jemal A. Cancer statistics, 2013. *CA Cancer J Clin* 2013;**63**:11–30. doi: 10.3322/caac.21166
301. Cancer prevalence: How many people have cancer? American Cancer Society. Web Mar 7, 2013. http://www.cancer.org/cancer/cancerbasics/cancer-prevalence
302. SEER Stat Fact Sheets: Breast Cancer. Web Mar 8, 2013. http://seer.cancer.gov/statfacts/html/breast.html
303. SEER Stat Fact Sheets: Prostate Cancer. Web Mar 8, 2013. http://seer.cancer.gov/statfacts/html/prost.html
304. National Cancer Institute: PDQ® Genetics of Prostate Cancer. Bethesda, MD: National Cancer Institute. Date last revised: 2012-05-31. Web 8 Mar. 2013. http://cancer.gov/cancertopics/pdq/genetics/prostate/HealthProfessional
305. SEER Cancer statistics: Breast, Table 4:11 Annual incidence rates (In Situ cases). Web 11 Mar. 2013. http://seer.cancer.gov/csr/1975_2009_pops09/browse_csr.php?section=4&page=sect_04_table.11.html
306. Cancer Trends Progress Report – 2011/2012, Update. NCI, Web 15 Mar. 2013. http://progress-report.cancer.gov/doc_detail.asp?pid=1&did=2011&chid=106&coid=1029&mid=#trends
307. SEER Stat Fact Sheets. Cancer: (choose site). Web 18 Mar. 2013. http://seer.cancer.gov/statfacts/html/
308. American Cancer Society. Cancer Facts & Figures 2013. Atlanta: American Cancer Society; 2013. Web 15 Jan. 2013. http://www.scribd.com/doc/121800203/Cancer-Facts-and-Figures-2013
309. Ibidem.
310. SEER Fast Fact: Statistics stratified by cancer site. Web 19 Mar. 2013. http://seer.cancer.gov/faststats/selections.php?#Output
311. SEER 5-year relative survival (%). SEER Program, 2002–2008, both sexes by race and site. Web 21 Mar 2013. http://seer.cancer.gov/csr/1975_2009_pops09/browse_csr.php?section=1&page=sect_01_zfig.11.html
312. SEER Fast Stats. Statistics Stratified by Cancer Site. Op. cit.
313. Sexually-transmitted diseases: Human papillomavirus (HPV). CDC. Web 22 Mar. 2013. http://www.cdc.gov/std/HPV/pap/default.htm#sec3
314. Markowitz LE, Dunne EF, Saraiya M et al. Centers for Disease Control and Prevention (CDC); Advisory Committee on Immunization Practices (ACIP) (2007). Quadrivalent Human Papillomavirus Vaccine Recommendations of the Advisory Committee on Immunization Practices (ACIP). *MMWR. Recommendations and reports :* March 23, 2007 / 56(RR02); 1–24. Web 20 Mar. 2013. http://www.cdc.gov/mmwr/preview/mmwrhtml/rr5602a1.htm
315. Jones DS, Podolsky SH, and Greene JA. The Burden of Disease and the Changing Task of Medicine, *N Engl J Med* 2012;**366**:2333–2338
316. SEER Fast Stats. Statistics Stratified by Cancer Site. Op. cit.
317. OECD Indicators: Life expectancy at birth, 2009. Web 22 Mar. 2013. http://www.oecd-ilibrary.org/sites/health_glance-2011-en/01/01/g1-01-01.html?contentType=&itemId=/content/chapter/health_glance-2011-4-en&containerItemId=/content/serial/19991312&accessItemIds=/content/book/health_glance-2011-en&mimeType=text/html
318. Defining Cancer: National Cancer Institute. Web 23 Mar. 2013. http://www.cancer.gov/cancertopics/cancerlibrary/what-is-cancer
319. Arber E. Cell proliferation as a major risk for cancer: a concept of doubtful validity. *Cancer Res* 1995;**55**:3759–3762.

320. Rosenberg SA. Identification of cancer antigens: impact on development of cancer immunotherapies. *Cancer J Sci Am* 2000;6(Suppl 3):S200–207.
321. Reddy A, Kaelin G Jr. Using cancer genetics to guide the selection of anticancer drug targets. *Curr Opin Pharmacol* 2002;**2**:366–373.
322. DeVita VT, Moxley JH, Brace K, Frei E III. Intensive combination chemotherapy and X-irradiation in the treatment of Hodgkin's disease. *Proc Am Assoc Cancer Res* 1965;**6**:15.
323. Burnett FM. The concept of immunological surveillance, *Prog Exp Tumor Res* 1970;**13**:1–27.
324. Immune Surveillance. Eds RT Smith and M Landry. Academic Press, New York – London, 1970.
325. Nathanson L. Spontaneous regression of malignant melanoma: a review of the literature on incidence, clinical features, and possible mechanisms. *Natl Cancer Inst Monogr* 1976;**44**:67–76.
326. Mathé G, Amiel JL, Schwarzenberg L, et al. Active immunotherapy for acute lymphoblastic leukaemia. *Lancet* 1969;**1**:697–699.
327. Grasser I. Interferon and cancer: therapeutic prospects. *Rev Eur Etud Clin Biol* 1970;**15**:23–7.
328. Amery WK, Spreafico F, Rojas AF, et al. Adjuvant treatment with levamisole in cancer: a review of experimental and clinical data. *Cancer Treat Rev* 1977;**4**:167–94.
329. Rosenberg SA, Lotze MT, Muul LM, Et al. Observations on the systemic administration of autologous lymphokine-activated killer cells and recombinant interleukin-2 to patients with metastatic cancer. *N Engl J Med* 1985;**313**:1485–1492.
330. FactSheet: Biological therapies for cancer. National Cancer institute. Web 14 Apr 2013. http://www.cancer.gov/cancertopics/factsheet/Therapy/biological
331. Ibidem.
332. Ibidem.
333. Nagano Y, Kojima Y. Pouvoir immunisant du virus vaccinal inactivé par des rayons ultraviolets. *C. R. Seances Soc. Biol. Fil* (in French) 1954;**148**:1700–2.
334. Pieters T. Interferon and its first clinical trial: Looking behind the scenes. *Med Hist* 1993;**37**:270–295.
335. Cantell, K. *The Story of Interferon: The Ups and Downs in the Life of a Scientist*. River Edge, NJ. World scientific Publishing, 1998.
336. Nagata S, Taira H, Hall A, et al. Synthesis in E. coli of a polypeptide with human leukocyte interferon activity. *Nature* 1980;**284**:316–20.
337. Tan YH, Hong WJ. Gene expression in mammalian cells. US patent 6207146, 2001.
338. Nelkin, D. *Selling Science: How the press covers science and technology*, New York, W.H. Freeman & Company, 1995.
339. Rosenberg SA. Progress in human tumour immunology and immunotherapy. *Nature* 2001;**411**:380–384.
340. Dudley ME, Wunderlich JR, Robbins PF, et al. Cancer Regression and Autoimmunity in Patients After Clonal Repopulation with Antitumor Lymphocytes. *Science* 2002;**298**:850–854.
341. Schwartz RN, Stover L, Dutcher J. Managing toxicities of high-dose Interleukin-2. *Oncology* 2002;**16**:11–20.
342. Jager E, Knuth A. Clinical cancer vaccine trials. *Curr Opin Immunol* 2002;**14**:178–182.
343. Vaccines, Blood & Biologics: April 29, 2010 Approval Letter – Provenge. FDA. Web 14 Apr. 2013. http://www.fda.gov/BiologicsBloodVaccines/CellularGeneTherapyProducts/ApprovedProducts/ucm210215.htm
344. Kantoff PW, Higano CS, Shore ND, et al. Sipuleucel-T Immunotherapy for Castration-Resistant Prostate Cancer. *N Engl J Med* 2010;**363**:411–22.
345. Blattner W. Epidemiology of HTLV-1 and associated diseases. (Blattner W, ed.). In Human retrovirology: HTLV-1. New York: Raven Press, 1990, 251–265.
346. Gallo RC, Montagnier L. The chronology of AIDS research. *Nature*. 1987;**326**:435–6.
347. Crewdson J. In Gallo case, truth termed a casualty. *Chicago Tribune* 1 Jan. 1995. Web 17 Apr. 2013. http://www.virusmyth.com/aids/hiv/jcgallocase.htm

348. The Nobel Prize in Physiology or Medicine 2008: Harald zur Hausen, Françoise Barré-Sinoussi, Luc Montagnier, Web 10 Apr. 2103. http://www.nobelprize.org/nobel_prizes/medicine/laureates/2008/
349. Gallo RC, Montagnier L. The Discovery of HIV as the Cause of AIDS. *N Engl J Med* 2003; **349**:2283–2285.
350. Moore PS, Chang Y. Why do viruses cause cancer? Highlights of the first century of human tumour virology. *Nat Rev Cancer* 2010;**10**:878–889.
351. Epstein MA, Achong BG, Barr YM. Virus particles in cultured lymphoblasts from Burkitt's lymphoma. *Lancet* 1964;**15**:702–703.
352. Litter E, Baylis SA, Zeng Y, et al. Diagnosis of nasopharyngeal carcinoma by means of recombinant Epstein-Barr virus proteins. *Lancet* 1991;**337**:685–689.
353. Blumberg BS, London WT. Hepatitis B virus: Pathogenesis and prevention of primary cancer of the liver. *Cancer* 1982;**50**:2657–2665.
354. Miyoshi I, et al. Type C virus particles in a cord T-cell line derived by co-cultivating normal human cord leukocytes and human leukaemic T cells. *Nature* 1981;**294**, 770–771.
355. Durst M, Gissmann L, Ikenberg H. et al. A papillomavirus DNA from a cervical carcinoma and its prevalence in cancer biopsy samples from different geographic regions. *Proc Natl Acad Sci USA* 1983;**80**, 3812–3815.
356. Boshart M, Gismann L, Ikenberg H, et al. A new type of papillomavirus DNA, its presence in genital cancer biopsies and in cell lines derived from cervical cancer. *EMBO J* 1984;**3**:1151–1157.
357. Gallo RC, Montagnier L. Op. cit.
358. Choo QL, Kyo G, Weiner AJ, et al. Isolation of a cDNA clone derived from a blood-borne non-A, non-B viral hepatitis genome. *Science* 1989;**244**:359–362.
359. Chang, Y. et al. Identification of herpesvirus-like DNA sequences in AIDS-associated Kaposi's sarcoma. *Science* 1994;**265**:1865–1869.
360. Feng H, Shuda M, Chang Y, et al. Clonal integration of a polyomavirus in human Merkel cell carcinoma. *Science* 2008;**319**:1096–1100.
361. Dillman RO. Cancer immunotherapy. *Cancer Biother Radiopharma* 2011;**26**:1–64.
362. Kirkwood JM, Butterfield LH, Tarhini AA, et al. Immunotherapy of cancer in 2012. *CA Cancer J Clin* 2012;**62**:309–335. doi: 10.3322/caac.20132
363. *Hematologic Malignancies: Methods and techniques.* GB Faguet editor. Totowa NJ, The Humana Press, 2001.
364. Brisco MJ. *Quantifying residual leukemia by clone-specific polymerase chain reaction*, In: Hematologic Malignancies: Methods and techniques, GB Faguet editor, Totowa, NJ, The Humana Press, 2001.
365. Brisco MJ. Ibidem.
366. Outcomes Working Group, Health Services Research Committee, America Society of Clinical Oncology. Outcomes of cancer treatment for technology assessment and cancer treatment guidelines. *J Clin Oncol* 1996;**14**:671–679.
367. Guthrie F. XIII – On some derivatives from the olefines. *Q J Chem So* 1860;**12**:109–126. Web 25 Apr. 2013. http://pubs.rsc.org/en/Content/ArticleLanding/1860/QJ/qj8601200109
368. Encyclopedia of the First World War: Deaths from gas attacks, available online at http://www.spartacus.schoolnet.co.uk/FWWgasdeaths.htm
369. Krumbhaar EB. Role of the blood and the bone marrow in certain forms of gas poisoning. *JAMA* 1919;**72**:39–41.
370. Pappenheimer AM, Vance M. The effects of intravenous injections of Di-Chloroethylsulfide in rabbits, with special reference to its leukotoxic action. *J Exp Med* 1920;**31**:71–95.
371. Lynch VHW, SmithE K Marshall: On dichlorethylsulphide (mustard gas). I. The systemic effects and mechanism of action. *J. Pharmacol Exp Ther* 1919;**12**, 265.
372. Warthin AS, Weller CB. *The Medical Aspects of Mustard Gas Poisoning*. St. Louis, CV Mosby, 1919.
373. Flury F, Wieland H: Uber Kampfgasvergiftungen VII. Die pharmakologische Wirkung des Dichlorathylsulfids. Ztschr. f. d. ges *Exp Med* 1921;**13**:367.

References

374. Yoshida T. The Yoshida sarcoma, an ascites tumor. *Gann* 1949;**40**:1–20.
375. Shear MJ, Hartwell JL, Peters VB, et al. *Some aspects of a joint institutional research program on chemotherapy of cancer: current laboratory and clinical experiments with bacterial polysaccharide and with synthetic organic compounds.* In: Moulton FR, editor. Approaches to tumor chemotherapy. Washington, DC: AAAS; 1947. p. 236–84.
376. Berenblum I. Experimental inhibition of tumor induction by mustard gas and other compounds. *J Path Bact* 1935;**40**:549–558.
377. Einhorn J. Nitrogen mustard: The origin of chemotherapy for cancer. *Int J Radiat Oncol Biol Phys* 1985;**11**:1375–1378.
378. Christakis P. The Birth of Chemotherapy at Yale Bicentennial Lecture Series: Surgery Grand Round. *Yale J Biol Med* 2011;**84**:169–172.
379. Ibidem.
380. Ibidem.
381. Gillman A, Phillips F. The Biological Actions and Therapeutic Applications of the B-Chloroethyl Amines and Sulfides. *Science* 1946;**103**:409–436. Web 20 Apr. 2013. http://www.sciencemag.org/content/103/2675/409.full.pdf?ijkey=ef7e9bd9250d96143df96c63dcc498584aba87de&keytype2=tf_ipsecsha
382. Rhoads CP. The Edward Gamaliel Janeway Lecture: the sword and the ploughshare. J Mt Sinai Hosp. 1946;**13**:299–309.
383. Scislowski S. Not All of Us Were Brave, Toronto, CA, Dundurn Press, 1997
384. Hirsch J. An anniversary for cancer chemotherapy. *JAMA* 2006;**296**:1518–1520.
385. Pechura CM, Rall DP. Eds. *Veterans at Risk: The Health Effects of Mustard Gas and Lewisite.* Washington DC, National Academies Press, 1993.
386. Ibidem.
387. Southern G. Poisonous Inferno. Mustang, OK, Airlife Publishing, 2005.
388. Pechura CM, Rall DP. Op. cit.
389. Alexander SF. Medical report of the Bari Harbor Mustard casualties. *Mil Surgeon* 1947;**10**:2–17.
390. Berenblum I. Op. cit.
391. Goodman LS, Wintrobe MM, Dameshek W, et al. Nitrogen mustard therapy: use of methyl-bis (β-chloroethyl) amine hydrochloride and tris (β-chloroethyl)amine hydrochloride for Hodgkin's disease, lymphosarcoma, leukemia, and certain allied and miscellaneous disorders. *JAMA* 1946;**132**:126–32.
392. Jacobson LO, Spurr CL, Barron ES, et al. Studies of the effect of methyl methyl-*bis*-(β-chloroethyl) amine hydrochloride on neoplastic diseases and allied disorders of the hemopoietic system. *JAMA* 1946;**132**:263.
393. Karnofsky DA, Carver LF, Rhoads CF et al. *An evaluation of methyl-bis-(β-chloroethyl) amine hydrochloride (nitrogen mustards) in the treatment of lymphomas, leukemias, and allied diseases*, In: Moulton FR (ed): Approaches to cancer chemotherapy. Washington, DC, AAAS, 1947.
394. Rhoads CP. Report on a cooperative study of nitrogen mustard (HN_2) therapy of neoplastic disease. *Trans Assoc Am Physicians* 1947;**60**:110–117.
395. DeVita VT Jr, Serpick A. A combination chemotherapy in the treatment of Hodgkin's disease (HD). *Proc Am Assoc Cancer Res* 1967;**8**:13.
396. Shear MJ, Hartwell JL, Peters VB, et al. Op. cit.
397. Woods DD. The relation of p-aminobenzoic acid to the mechanism of action of sulphanilamide. *Br J Exp Pathol* 1940;**21**:74.
398. Fildes P. A rational approach to research in chemotherapy. *Lancet* 1940;**1**:995.
399. Seeger DR, Smith JM, Hultquist ME. Antagonist for pteroylglutamic acid. *J Am Chem Soc* 1947;**69**:2567.
400. Farber S, Diamond LK, Mercer RD et al. Temporary remissions in acute leukemia in children produced by the folic acid antagonist, 4-aminopteroylglutamic acid (Aminopterin). *N Engl J Med* 1948;**238**:787.

401. Hertz R, Lewis J, Lipsett M. Five years' experience with chemotherapy of metastatic choriocarcinoma and related trophoblastic tumors in women. *Am J Obstet Gynecol* 1961;**82**:631–640.
402. Seeger DR, Cosulich DB, Smith JM Jr, et al. Analogs of pteroylglutamic acid III. 4-amino derivatives. *J Am Chem Soc* 1949;**71**:1753–1758.
403. Burchenal JH, Murphy ML, Ellison RR, et al. Clinical evaluation of a new antimetabolite, 6-mercaptopurine, in the treatment of leukemia and allied diseases. *Blood* 1953;**8**:965.
404. Murphy ML, Tan TC, Ellison RR, et al. Clinical evaluation of chloroquine and thioguanine. *Proc Am Assoc Cancer Res* 1955;**2**:36.
405. Morton M. *Serendipity in Modern Medical Breakthroughs*. New York, NY Arcade Publishing, March 2007.
406. Rettig R. *Cancer Crusade*. Op. cit.
407. Boyd, MR. *The NCI In Vitro Anticancer Drug Discovery Screen; Concept, Implementation and Operation 1985–1995*. In: Teicher BA (Ed.): Cancer Drug Discovery and Development, Vol. 2; Drug Development; Preclinical Screening, Clinical Trial and Approval, Totowa NJ, The Humana Press, 1997, pp. 23–43.
408. Introduction, DTP, NCI. Web 3 May 2013. http://dctd.cancer.gov/ProgramPages/dtp/default.htm
409. Ibidem.
410. Bainbridge WS. *The cancer problem*. New York, MacMillan, 1914.
411. Sikora K, Advani S, Koroltchouk V, et al. Essential drugs for cancer therapy: A World Health Organization Consultation. *Ann Oncol* 1999;**10**:385–390.
412. Ibidem.
413. WHO Model List of Essential Medicines – 17th List (March 2011): Antineoplastic, Immunosuppressives, and Medicines used in Palliative Care. Web 6 May 2013. http://whqlibdoc.who.int/hq/2011/a95053_eng.pdf
414. Woglom WH. *General review of cancer therapy*, In: Moulton FR (ed): Approaches to tumor chemotherapy. Washington, DC AAAS, 1947, p. 1–10.
415. Hitchings GH, Elion GB. The chemistry and biochemistry of purine analogs. *Ann NY Acad Sci* 1954;**60**:195–9.
416. Heidelberger C, Chaudhuari NK, Danenberg P, et al. Fluorinated pyrimidines. A new class of tumor inhibitory compounds. *Nature* 1957;**179**:663–6.
417. Hertz R, Lewis J, Lipsett M. Op. cit.
418. Woglom, WH Op. cit.
419. Tannock I. Cell kinetics and chemotherapy: a critical review. Cancer Treat Rep 62:1117–1133, 1978.
420. Ibidem.
421. Skipper HE. Historic milestones in cancer biology: A few that are important to cancer treatment (revisited). *Semin Oncol* 1979;**6**:506–514.
422. Ibidem.
423. Mendelsohn ML. The growth fraction: a new concept applied to tumors. *Science* 1960;**132**:1496.
424. Goldie JH, Coldman AJ. A mathematical model for relating the drug sensitivity of tumors to their spontaneous mutations rate. *Cancer Treat Rep* 1979;**63**:1727–1733.
425. Laird AK. Dynamics of growth in tumors and normal organisms, *Natl Cancer Inst Monogr* 1969;**30**:15–28.
426. Bonadonna G, Rossi A, Valagussa BS. Adjuvant CMF in operable breast cancer: Ten years later. *World J Surg* 1985;**5**:95–115.
427. Chute JP, Chen T, Feigal E, et al: Twenty years of phase III trials for patients with extensive-stage small-cell lung cancer: Perceptible progress. *J Clin Oncol* 1999;**17**:1794–1801.
428. Breathnach OS, Freidlin B, Concley B, et al. Twenty-Two Years of Phase III Trials for Patients With Advanced Non–Small-Cell Lung Cancer: Sobering Results. *JCO* 2001:**19**:1734–1742.

429. Karnofsky DA, Abelmann WH, Craver LF, et al. The use of nitrogen mustards in the palliative treatment of carcinoma. *Cancer* 1948;**1**:634–656.
430. Kennedy BJ. The snail's pace of lung carcinoma chemotherapy. *Cancer* 1998;**82**:801–803.
431. Schiller J, Harrington D, Belani CP, et al. Comparison of four chemotherapy regimens for advanced non-small-cell lung cancer. *N Engl J Med* 2002;**346**:92–8.
432. Soon YY, Stokler MR, Askie LA, et al. Duration of Chemotherapy for Advanced Non–Small-Cell Lung Cancer: A Systematic Review and Meta-Analysis of Randomized Trials. *JCO* 2009;**27**:3277–3283.
433. Da Silvera Lima JP, Viera dos Santos L, Chen Sasse E, et al. Optimal duration of first-line chemotherapy for advanced non-small cell lung cancer: A systematic review with meta-analysis. *Eur J Cancer* 2009;**45**:601–607.
434. SEER. Cancer Statistics: Lung & Bronchus; 5-year relative and period survival (SCC/NSCC). Web 25 Mar. 2013. http://seer.cancer.gov/csr/1975_2009_pops09/browse_csr.php?section=15&page=sect_15_table.13.html
435. Dranitsaris G, Cottrell W, Evans WK. The cost and cost-effectiveness of treating non-small cell lung cancer. *Curr Opin Oncol* 2002;**14**:375–83.
436. Martin DS, Gelhorn A. Combinations of chemical compounds in experimental cancer chemotherapy. *Cancer Res* 1951;**11**:35.
437. Skipper HE. *Nucleotide metabolism and cancer chemotherapy*, In: Rebuck JW, Bethell FH, Monto RW, Eds: The Leukemias: Etiology, Pathophysiology, and Treatment. New York, Academic Press, 1957, p 541.
438. Freireich EJ, Karon M, Frei E III. Quadruple combination therapy (VAMP) for acute lymphoblastic leukemia of childhood. *Proc Am Assoc Cancer Res* 5:**20**, 1964.
439. Holland JF. Hopes for tomorrow versus realities of today: therapy and prognosis in acute lymphocytic leukemia of childhood. *Pediatrics* 1970;**45**:191–3.
440. DeVita VT, Serpick A. Combination chemotherapy in the treatment of advanced Hodgkin's disease. *Proc Am Assoc Cancer Res* 1967;**8**:13.
441. Devita VT Jr, Simon RM, Hubbard SM et al. Curability of advanced Hodgkin's disease with chemotherapy: Long-term follow-up of MOPP-treated patients at the National Cancer Institute (NCI). *Ann Intern Med* 1980;**92**:586–595.
442. Donohue JP, Einhorn LH, Perez JM. Improved management of non-seminomatous testis tumors. *Cancer* 1978;**42**:2903–8.
443. Surbone A and DeVita VT Jr. Dose intensity. The neglected variable in clinical trials. *Ann NY Acad Sci* 1993;**698**:279–288.
444. Hryaiuk WA, Figueredo A, Goodyear M. Application of dose intensity to problems in chemotherapy of breast and colon cancer. *Semin Oncol* 1987;**14**:3–11.
445. Waxman S, Anderson KC. History of the development of arsenic derivatives in cancer therapy. *Oncologist* 2001;**6**:3–10.
446. Aublanc JB. Dissertation sur le cancer présentée et soutenue à l'Ecole de médecine de Paris, le 16 pluviôse an XI, par JB Aublanc. PhD diss., imp. Farge, 1803, pg 40.
447. Overview of HSCT in Europe: 2010. European Group for Blood and Marrow Transplantation. Web 14 May 2013. http://www.ebmt.org/Contents/Research/TransplantActivitySurvey/Results/Pages/Results.aspx
448. Ibidem.
449. Stephenson J. Bone marrow/Stem cells: No edge in breast cancer. *JAMA* 1999;**281**:1641–1642.
450. Stadtmauer EA et al. Conventional-dose chemotherapy compared with high-dose chemotherapy plus autologous hematopoietic stem-cell transplantation for metastatic breast cancer. Philadelphia Bone Marrow Transplant Group. *N Engl J Med* 2000;**342**:1069–1076.
451. Editorial. Retraction for Baxwoda et al 13 (10):2483. *J Clin Oncol* 2001;**19**:2973.
452. Farquhar C, Basser R, Marjoribanks J, et al. High dose chemotherapy and autologous bone marrow or stem cell transplantation versus conventional chemotherapy for women with early

poor prognosis breast cancer (Cochrane Review). In: *The Cochrane Library*, Issue e, 2004. Chichester, UK: John Wiley & Sons, ltd.
453. Overview of HSCT in Europe: 2010. Op.cit.
454. Center for International Blood and Marrow Transplant, a contractor for the C.W. Bill Young Cell Transplantation Program operated through the U. S. Department of Health and Human Services, Health Resources and Services Administration, Healthcare Systems Bureau. U.S. Transplant Data by Center Report, Breast cancer, Number of Transplants Reported for Breast cancer From 2008 – 2011. Web 15 May 2013. http://bloodcell.transplant.hrsa.gov/research/transplant_data/us_tx_data/data_by_disease/national.aspx
455. Ibidem.
456. Bhatnagar B, Badros AZ. Controversies in Autologous Stem Cell Transplantation for the Treatment of Multiple Myeloma. http://dx.doi.org/10.5772/54115
457. Kolb HJ, Socie G, Duell T, et al. Malignant neoplasms in long-term survivors of bone marrow transplantation. Late Effects Working Party of the European Cooperative Group for Blood and Marrow Transplantation and the European Late Effect Project Group. Ann Intern Med 1999;**131**:738–744.
458. Wingard JR, Majhail NS, Brazauskas R, et al. Long-Term Survival and Late Deaths After Allogeneic Hematopoietic Cell Transplantation. *J Clin Oncol* 2011;**29**:2230–2239.
459. Ibidem.
460. Ibidem.
461. Döhner H, Estey EH, Amadori S, et al. Diagnosis and management of acute myeloid leukemia in adults: recommendations from an international expert panel, on behalf of the European LeukemiaNet *Blood* 2010;**115**:453–474.
462. Pui C-H, Evans WE. Acute lymphoblastic leukemia. *N Engl J Med* 1998;**339**:605–615.
463. Villela L, Bolaños-Meade J. Acute Myeloid Leukaemia: Optimal Management and Recent Developments. *Drugs* 2011;**71**:1537–1550.
464. Ortiz-Tudela E, Mteyrek A, Ballesta A, et al. *Handb Exp Pharmacol.* 2013;**217**:261–288. doi: 10.1007/978-3-642-25950-0_11
465. Hrushesky, WJM. The Rationale for Non-Zero-Order Drug Delivery Using Automatic, Computer-Based Drug Delivery Systems (Chronotherapy). *J Biol Resp Modifiers* 1987;**6**:587–598.
466. Perry MC (Ed). *The chemotherapy source book*. Baltimore, MD, Williams and Wilkins; 1st edition, 1992.
467. Eriguchi M, Levi F, Yanagie HT, et al. Chronotherapy for cancer. Biomed Phamacother. 2003;**57**(Suppl 1):92s–95s.
468. Kagan EM. Cancer and the clock: chronotherapy's struggle for legitimacy. DSpace@MIT Web 18 May 2013. http://dspace.mit.edu/handle/1721.1/39436
469. Cancer Treatment Centers of America: Chronotherapy. Web 19 May 2013. http://www.cancercenter.com/conventional-cancer-treatment/chemotherapy/chronotherapy.cfm
470. Druker BJ, Talpaz M, Resta DJ, et al, Efficacy and safety of a specific inhibitor of the BCR-ABL tyrosine kinase in chronic myeloid leukemia. *N Engl J Med* 2001;**344**:1031–1037.
471. Target cancer therapies. NCI: Fact sheet. Web 24 May 2013. http://www.cancer.gov/cancertopics/factsheet/Therapy/targeted
472. Chen MH, Kerkel R, Force T. Mechanisms of cardiomyopathy associated with tyrosine kinase inhibitor cancer therapeutics. *Circulation* 2008;**118**:84–95.
473. Gorre, M. E. et al. Clinical resistance to STI-571 cancer therapy caused by BCR-ABL gene mutation or amplification. *Science* 2001;**293**:876–880.
474. Target cancer therapies. NCI: Fact sheet. Op. cit.
475. Sawyers C. Targeted cancer therapy. *Nature* 2004;**432**:294–297.
476. Smith SL. Ten years of Orthoclone OKT3 (muromonab-CD3): a review. *Journal of transplant coordination : official publication of the North American Transplant Coordinators Organization (NATCO)* 1996 (3):109–119.
477. Faguet GB, Agee JF. Monoclonal antibodies against the Chronic Lymphocytic Antigen cCLLa: Characterization and sensitivity. *Blood* 1987;**70**:437–443.

478. Silverman GJ. Anti-CD20 therapy and autoimmune disease: therapeutic opportunities and evolving insights. *Front Biosci* 2007;**12**:2194–2206.
479. Slamon DJ, Clark GM, Wong SG, et al. Human breast cancer: correlation of relapse and survival with amplification of the *HER-2/neu* oncogene. *Science* 1987;**235**:177–182.
480. Adams GP, Weiner LM. Monoclonal antibody therapy of cancer. *Nat Biotechnol* 2005;**23**:1147–1157.
481. Kreitman RJ. Immunotoxins for Targeted Cancer Therapy. *AAPSJ* 2006;**8**:E532–E551.
482. Faguet GB, Agee JF: Four Ricin chain A-based immunotoxins directed against the common chronic lymphocytic leukemia antigen (cCLLa): In vitro characterization. *Blood* 1993;**82**:536–543.
483. A-dmDT390-bisFv (UCHT1) Immunotoxin Therapy for Patients With T-cell Diseases, Clinical Trials.gov. Web 10 Jun 2013. http://clinicaltrials.gov/show/NCT00611208
484. Bird BR, Swain SM. Review Cardiac toxicity in breast cancer survivors: review of potential cardiac problems. *Clin Cancer Res* 2008;**14**:14–24.
485. Richardson PG, Mitsiades C, Hideshima T, Anderson KC. Bortezomib: proteasome inhibition as an effective anticancer therapy. *Annu Rev Med* 2006;**57**:33–47.
486. Holden SN, Eckhardt SG, Basser R, et al. Clinical evaluation of ZD6474, an orally active inhibitor of VEGF and EGF receptor signaling, in patients with solid, malignant tumors. *Ann Oncol* 2005;**16**:1391–7.
487. Campiglio M, Normanno N, Ménard S. Re: Effect of epidermal growth factor receptor inhibitor on development of estrogen receptor-negative mammary tumors. *J Natl Cancer Inst* 2004;**96**:715.
488. Weinstein IB. Cancer. Addiction to oncogenes – the Achilles heal of cancer. *Science* 2002;**297**:63–64.
489. Flores J. Específico nuevamente descubierto en el reyno de Goatemala para la curacion the horrible mal de cancro y otros mas frecuentes, Cadiz, 1783.
490. Achim M. Lagartijas Medicinales: Remedios Americanos y debates científicos en la ilustración. Web 8 Dec 2012. http://www.cneq.unam.mx/cursos_diplomados/diplomados/anteriores/medio_superior/diplo_oaxcts/12_matl_dida/mod8/Lagartijas%20medicinales,%20Miruna%20Achim.pdf
491. Ibidem.
492. Maunoir CT. *Nouvelle méthode pour traiter le sarcocele sans extirper le testicule.* Genève, 1820.
493. Boehm-Viswanathan T. Is angiogenesis inhibition the Holy Grail of cancer therapy? *Curr Opin Oncol* 2000;**12**:89–94.
494. Bennett JH. On cancerous and cancroid growths, Edinburgh, Sutherland & Knox, 1849, p 237.
495. Arnot J. Practical illustrations of the remedial efficacy of a very low anesthetic temperature. I. in cancer, *Lancet* 1850;**56**:257–259.
496. Zaffaroni N, Fiorentini G, De Giorgi U. Hyperthermia and hypoxia: New developments in anticancer chemotherapy. *Eur J Surg Oncol* 2001;**27**:340–342.
497. Greve JW. Alternative techniques for the treatment of colon carcinoma metastases in the liver: current status in The Netherlands. *Scand J Gastroenterol* 2001;**234**:77–81.
498. Mala T, Edwin B, Gladhaug I, et al. Magnetic-resonance-guided percutaneous cryoablation of hepatic tumors. *Eur J Surg* 2001;**167**:610–617.
499. Ecclesiastes 1:9. (1611 King James Version).
500. Faguet GB. *The War on Cancer.* Op. cit.
501. Helke F. Book Review. The War on Cancer: An anatomy of failure. Medical Veritas: *The journal of Medical Truth*, 2007;**4**:1540–1541. Web 23 Apr. 2013. http://www.medicalveritas.com/images/vol4issue2Book3.pdf
502. Gerson C. Gerson Institute. Web 20 Apr. 2013. http://gerson.org/gerpress/about-us/
503. Gerson Institute. Web 20 Apr. 2013. http://gerson.org/gerpress/the-gerson-therapy/
504. Complementary and Alternative Medicine, Annual report 2011. National Cancer Institute. Web 21 May 2103. http://cam.cancer.gov/cam_annual_report_fy11.pdf

505. Sporn MB. The war on cancer. *Lancet* 1996;**347**:1377–1381.
506. DeVita VT. The War on cancer has a birthday, and a present. *J Clin Oncol* 1997;**15**:867–869.
507. Sporn MB. Op. cit.
508. Jemal A, Ward E, Thun M. Declining Death Rates Reflect Progress against Cancer. *PLoS ONE* March 09, 2010. doi:10.1371/journal.pone.0009584
509. Kantarjian H. The Price of Drugs for Chronic Myeloid Leukemia (CML); A Reflection of the Unsustainable Prices of Cancer Drugs: From the Perspective of a Large Group of CML Experts. *Blood* 2013;**121**:4439–4442.
510. Bach PB. Limits on Medicare's Ability to Control Rising Spending on Cancer Drugs. *N Engl J Med* 2009;**360**:626–633.
511. Kantarjian H. Op. cit.
512. Bailar JC, Gornik HL. Cancer undefeated. *N Engl J Med* 1997;**336**:1569–1574.
513. Faguet GB. *The War on Cancer*. Op. cit.
514. World Oncology Forum: Are we winning the war on cancer? Web 1 June 2013. http://www.eso.net/varie/wof.html
515. Cavalli F. An appeal to world leaders. *Lancet* 2013;**381**:425–426.
516. STOP CANCER NOW! On this World Cancer Day 2013, participants of the World Oncology Forum raise the alarm about the increasing devastation caused by cancer across the world. Web 1 Jun 2013. www.eso.net/images/Allegati/statementenglish.pdf
517. *Sustaining progress against cancer in an era of cost containment: Discussion Paper*. Kean M, Lessor T. (Eds). Cambridge, MA: Feinstein Kean Healthcare; June 2012. Web 16 Jul. 2013. http://turningthetideagainstcancer.org/sustaining-progress-discussion-paper.pdf
518. SEER Cancer statistics: Breast, Table 4:11 Op. cit.
519. Special Report: Measurement of Progress Against Cancer. Extramural Committee to Assess Measures of Progress Against Cancer. *J Natl Cancer Inst* 1990;**82**:825–835.
520. Wu J, Josepj SO, Muggia FM. Targeted Therapy: Its Status and Promise in Selected Solid Tumors, Part I. *Oncology* 2012;**26**:1–12.
521. Cancer Statistics 2013: A presentation from the American Cancer Society. Web 3 Sept. 2013. http://www.cancer.org/research/cancerfactsstatistics/cancerfactsfigures2013/cancer-statistics-2013-slide-presentation.pdf
522. Cancer Facts & Figures: American Cancer Society. Web 20 Jan. 2013. http://www.cancer.org/acs/groups/content/@nho/documents/document/2008cafffinalsecuredpdf.pdf
523. Cancer Trends, Progress Report: 2011/2012. Web 20 Jan. 2013. http://progressreport.cancer.gov/highlights.asp
524. Andersen LD, Remington P, Trentham-Dietz A, et al. Assessing a decade of progress in cancer control. *The Oncologist* 2002;**7**:200–204.
525. Kuenstner S, Langelotz C, Budach V, et al. The comparability of quality of life scores. a multitrait multimethod analysis of the EORTC QLQ-C30, SF-36 and FLIC questionnaires. *Eur J Cancer* 2002;**38**:339–48.
526. Slevin ML, Stubbs L, Plant HJ, et al. Attitudes to chemotherapy: comparing views of patients with cancer with those of doctors, nurses, and general public. *BMJ* 1990;**300**:1458–1460.
527. Kiebert G, Wait S, Beernhard J, et al. Practice and Policy of measuring quality of life and health economics in cancer trials: A survey among co-operative trial groups. *Qual Life Res* 2000;**9**:1073–1080.
528. Bailar JC 3rd, Smith EM. Progress against cancer? *N Engl J Med* 1986;**314**:1226–1232.
529. Bailar JC, Gornik HL. Op. cit.
530. Sporn MB. Op. cit.
531. Epstein SS. *The Politics of Cancer Revisited*. Hankins, NY, East Ridge Press, 1998.
532. NCI Mission Statement. Web 3 Jan. 2013. http://www.cancer.gov/aboutnci/overview/mission
533. NCI's Divisions and Centers. Web 3 Jan. 2013. http://www.cancer.gov/aboutnci/organization#NCI+Divisions+and+Centers

534. National Cancer Institute: 2011 Fact Book. Web 26 Jun. 2013. Web http://obf.cancer.gov/financial/attachments/11Factbk.pdf
535. Ibidem.
536. CTEP. Op. cit.
537. CTEP. Major Ongoing Initiatives: Clinical Trials Cooperative Group Program; Clinical Trials Cooperative Groups. Web 28 Jun. 2013. http://dctd.cancer.gov/ProgramPages/ctep/major_ctcgp.htm
538. Community Clinical Oncology Program Network: History and Vision. Web 29 Jun. 2013. http://ccop.cancer.gov/about/history-vision
539. Louis PCA. *Essays in Clinical Instruction*. London, UK: P. Martin; 1834.
540. Louis PCA. Research into the effects of blood-letting in some inflammatory diseases and on the influence of tartarized antimony and vessication in pneumonitis. *Am J Med Sci* 1836;**18**:102–111.
541. Bollet AJ. Pierre Louis: the numerical method and the foundation of quantitative medicine. *Am J Med Sci* 1973;**266**:92–101.
542. Warner JH. *Attitudes to Foreign Knowledge*. In: The Therapeutic Perspective: Medical practice, Knowledge, and Identity in America 1820–1835. Cambridge MA, Harvard University Press 1986.
543. Rangachari PK. Evidence-based medicine: A French wine with a Canadian label?. *J R Soc Med* 1997;**90**:280–284.
544. Hill AB. The clinical trial. *N Engl J Med* 1952; **247**:113–119.
545. NIH. CLinicalTriald.gov. Web 30 Jun. 2013. http://clinicaltrials.gov
546. Zelen M. *Theory and practice of clinical trials*. In: Holland-Frei Cancer Medicine. 5th edition. Bast RC Jr, Kufe DW, Pollock RE, et al., Ed., Hamilton, ON, BC Decker; 2000.
547. FDA's Drug Review Drug Review Steps Simplified. Web 30 Jun. 2013. http://www.fda.gov/Drugs/ResourcesForYou/Consumers/ucm289601.htm
548. Jüni P, Altman DG, Egger M. Assessing the quality of controlled clinical trials. *BMJ*, 2001;**323**:42–48.
549. Altman DG, Bland JM. Treatment allocation in controlled trials: why randomize? *BMJ* 1999;**318**:1209.
550. SEER, 5-year survival distant stage, both sexes. Web 1 Jul. 2013. http://seer.cancer.gov/csr/1975_2009_pops09/browse_csr.php?section=9&page=sect_09_table.08.html
551. Zelen M. Op. cit.
552. Faguet GB, Davies HC. Survival in Hodgkin's disease: The role of immunocompetence and other major risk factors. *Blood* 1982;**59**:938–945.
553. Ibidem.
554. Zelen M. Op. cit.
555. Breathnach O, Freidlin B, Conley B, et al. Twenty-two years of phase III trials for patients with advanced non-small-cell lung cancer: sobering results. *J Clin Oncol* 2000;**19**:1734–1742.
556. EORTC Clinical Trials: Target accrual. Web 2 Jul. 2013. http://www.eortc.org/clinical-trials
557. Fisher B, Costantino JP, Wickerham DL, et al. Tamoxifen for prevention of breast cancer: Report of the National Surgical Adjuvant Breast and Bowel Project P-1 Study. *J Natl Cancer Inst* 1998;**90**:1371–1388.
558. Levine M, Moutquin JM, Walton R, et al; Canadian Task Force on Preventive Health Care and the Canadian Breast Cancer Initiative's Steering Committee on Clinical Practice Guidelines for the Care and Treatment of Breast Cancer Chemoprevention of breast cancer. A joint guideline from the Canadian Task Force on Preventive Health Care and the Canadian Breast Cancer Initiative's Steering Committee on Clinical Practice Guidelines for the Care and Treatment of Breast Cancer. *Can Med Assoc J* 2001;**164**:1681–1690.
559. Breast cancer risk assessment tool. Web 2 Jul. 2013. http://www.cancer.gov/bcrisktool/
560. Powles T, Eeles R, Ashley S, et al. Interim analysis of the incidence of breast cancer in the Royal Marsden Hospital tamoxifen randomized chemoprevention trial. *Lancet* 1998;**352**:98–101.
561. Veronesi U, Maisonneuve P, Sacchini V, et al. Tamoxifen for breast cancer among hysterectomised women. *Lancet* 2002;**359**:1122–1124.

562. Cuzick J, Forbes J, Edwards R, et al.: First results from the International Breast Cancer Intervention Study (IBIS-I): A randomized prevention trial. *Lancet* 2002;**360**:817–24.
563. Vogel VG, Costantino JP, Wickerham DL, et al. Update of the National Surgical Adjuvant Breast and Bowel Project Study of Tamoxifen and Raloxifene (STAR) P-2 Trial: Preventing Breast Cancer. *Cancer Prev Res* (Phila) 2010;**3**:696–706.
564. How much did the STAR study cost? Star trial FAQ. The Fox Chase Cancer Center. Web Jul. 2013. http://www.fccc.edu/prevention/studies/chemo/starTrial/faq.html#12
565. Cuzick J. Future possibilities in the prevention of breast cancer: Breast cancer prevention trials. *Breast Cancer Res* 2000;**2**:258–263.
566. Jaffe ER, Kaushansky K. The American Society of Hematology: a success at age 50. *Blood* 2008;**111**:11–15.
567. About Board-Certified Doctors, ABMS-MOC. Web 5 Jul 2013. http://www.certificationmatters.org/about-board-certified-doctors/about-board-certification.aspx
568. American Board of Internal Medicine: Policies and Procedures for Certification. Web 5 Jul. 2013. http://www.abim.org/pdf/publications/Policies-and-Procedures-Certification-July-2013.pdf
569. DeVita VT, Lawrence TS, Rosenberg SA. *Cancer: Principles & Practice of Oncology.* Philadelphia PA, Lippincott Williams & Wilkins, 2011.
570. ASCO: 2012 Annual Meeting Attendee Demographics. Web 5 Jul. 2013. http://chicago2013.asco.org/2012-annual-meeting-attendee-demographics
571. ASCO: Abstract submission statistics. Web 5 Jul. 2013. http://chicago2013.asco.org/abstract-submission-statistics
572. Chastek B, Harley C, Kallich J, et al. Health Care Costs for Patients With Cancer at the End of Life. J Oncol Pract, November 2012;**8**:75s–80s. Web 7 Jul. 2013. http://jop.ascopubs.org/content/8/6S/75s.full
573. Pasternak S. End-of-Life Care Constitutes Third Rail of U.S. Health Care Policy Debate. The Medicare News Group, June 03, 2013. Web 7 Jul. 2013. http://www.medicarenewsgroup.com/context/understanding-medicare-blog/understanding-medicare-blog/2013/06/03/end-of-life-care-constitutes-third-rail-of-u.s.-health-care-policy-debate
574. Riley GF, Lubitz JD. Long term trends in Medicare payments in the last year of life. *Health Serv Res* 2010;**45**:565–576.
575. Johnson DH. Evolution of cisplatin-based chemotherapy in non-small cell lung cancer: a historical perspective and the eastern cooperative oncology group experience. *Chest* 2000;**117**:133S–137S.
576. Faguet GB, Davis HC: Regression analysis in medical research. *Sout Med J* 1984;**77**:722–725.
577. Coiffier B, Lepage E, Brière J, et al. CHOP chemotherapy plus rituximab compared with CHOP alone in elderly patients with diffuse large- B-cell lymphoma. *N Engl J Med* 2002;**346**:235–242.
578. Cheson BD. CHOP plus Rituximab – Balancing Facts and Opinion. *N Engl J Med* 2002;**346**:280–282.
579. Emanuel EJ, Dubler NN. Preserving the physician-patient relationship in the era of managed care. *JAMA* 1995;**273**:323–329.
580. Council of Ethical and Judicial Affairs, American Medical Association: Ethical issues in managed care. *JAMA* 1995;**273**:330–335.
581. Gray BH. *The profit motive and patient care: The changing accountability of doctors and hospitals.* Cambridge, MA Harvard University, 1991.
582. Baker LC. Acquisition Of MRI Equipment By Doctors Drives Up Imaging Use And Spending. *Health Aff* 2010;**29**:2252–2259.
583. Babiarz LS, Yousem DM, Parker L, et al. Utilization Rates of Neuroradiology across Neuroscience Specialties in the Private Office Setting: Who Owns or Leases the Scanners on Which Studies Are Performed. *Am Neuroradiol.* 2012;**33**:143–48.

584. Gazelle SG, Halpern EF, RyAn HS, et al. Utilization of Diagnostic Medical Imaging: Comparison of Radiologist Referral versus Same-Specialty Referral. *Radiology* 2007;**245**:517–522.
585. Barr TR, Towle EL. National Oncology Practice Benchmark, 2011 Report on 2010 Data. *J Oncol Practice* 2011;**7**:67s–82s. doi: 10.1200/JOP.2011.000402
586. Kurowski B. Six key challenges in oncology disease management. *Dis Manag* 1998;**1**:99.
587. Smyth A. Reimbursement issues for the oncologist. *Oncol Reimburs* 1993;**1**:1–4.
588. Kane L. Medscape Oncologist Compensation Report: 2012 results. Web 12 Jul. 2013. http://www.medscape.com/features/slideshow/compensation/2012/oncology
589. Barr TR, Towle EL. Op. cit.
590. Ibidem.
591. Kane L. Op. cit.
592. Smith TJ, Girtman J, Riggins J. Why Academic Divisions of Hematology/Oncology Are in Trouble and Some Suggestions for Resolution. *J Clin Oncol* 2001;**19**:260–264.
593. Holcombe RF. Mission-Focused, Productivity-Based Model for Sustainable Support of Academic Hematology/Oncology Faculty and Divisions. *J Oncol Practice* 2010:**6**:74–79.
594. Crawford J, Caserta C, Roila F. Hematopoietic growth factors: ESMO Clinical Practice Guidelines for the applications. *Ann Oncol* 2010;**21**(Suppl 5):v248–v251.
595. Stadtmauer EA, O'Neill A, Goldstein LJ, et al. Conventional-dose chemotherapy compared with high-dose chemotherapy plus autologous hematopoietic stem-cell transplantation for metastatic breast cancer. Philadelphia Bone Marrow Transplant Group. *N Engl J Med* 2000;**342**:1069–1076.
596. Brody H. Medicine's Ethical Responsibility for Health Care Reform – The Top Five List. *N Engl J Med*, 2010;**362**:283–285.
597. Faguet, GB. *The Affordable Care Act*. Op. cit.
598. Brody H. Op. cit.
599. Jena AB, Seabury S, Lakdawalla K, et al. Malpractice Risk According to Physician Specialty. *N Engl J Med*, 2011;**365**:629–636.
600. Studdert DM, Mello MM, Sage WM, et al. Defensive medicine among high-risk specialist physicians in a volatile malpractice environment. *JAMA*, 2005;**293**:2609–2617. Web. 23 Oct. 2010. http://www.rmi.gsu.edu/rmi/faculty/klein/RMI_3500/Readings/Other/MM_DefensiveMedicine.pdf
601. Grillo-Lopez, AJ. USA's healthcare reform: Why it will not work. *Expert Rev Anticancer Ther* 2010;**10**(2):121–122. doi: 10.1586/era.09.180
602. Faguet G. *Pain Control and Drug Policy*. Op. cit.
603. DeFrances CJ, Smith SK, Langan PA, et al., Civil Jury Cases and Verdicts in Large Counties. U.S. Department of Justice: Office of Justice Programs, July 1995. Web. 27 Aug. 2011. http://bjs.ojp.usdoj.gov/content/pub/pdf/cjcavilc.pdf
604. McQuillan LJ, Abramyan H, Archie AP, et al. *Jackpot Justice: The True Cost of America's Tort System*. San Francisco, CA. *Pacific Research Institute*, 2007.
605. Merenstein D. Winners and Losers. *JAMA* 2004;**291**:1696–1697.
606. The Litigation Industry, Manhattan Institute for Policy Research. Web. 13 Jul. 2013. http://www.manhattan-institute.org/html/clp.htm
607. Editorials. Peer review: reform or revolution. *BMJ* 1997;**315**:759–760.
608. Editorials. Measuring the social impact of research. *BMJ* 2001;**323**:528.
609. Kabat GC, Anderson ML, Heo M, et al. Adult Stature and Risk of Cancer at Different Anatomic Sites in a Cohort of Postmenopausal Women. Cancer *Epidemiol Biomarkers Prev.* 2013;**22**:1353–1363.
610. Ibidem.
611. Meyers M. *Prize Fight: The Race and the Rivalry to be the First in Science*. New York, NY Palgrave Macmillan, June, 2012.
612. Eisenhofer G. Scientific productivity: Waning importance for career development of today's scientists? Web 10 Jul 2004. http://his.com/~graeme/pandp.html

613. National Surgical Adjuvant Breast and Bowel Project. Web 15 Jul. 2013. http://www.nsabp.pitt.edu
614. SWOG. Leading Cancer Research: About us. Web 15 Jul. 2013. http://www.swog.org/Visitors/AboutUs.asp
615. Austin D, Baker C. Pharmaceutical R&D and the evolving market for prescription drugs. http://www.cbo.gov/sites/default/files/cbofiles/ftpdocs/106xx/doc10681/10-26-drugr&d.pdf
616. The Pharmaceutical industry helps strengthened the U.S. economy. Web 16 Jul. 2013. http://www.phrma.org/economic-impact
617. PhRMA. Nearly 1,000 medicines in development to help patients in their fight against cancer. Web16Jul.2013.http://www.phrma.org/media/releases/nearly-1000-medicines-development-help-patients-their-fight-against-cancer
618. The Pharmaceutical industry helps strengthened the U.S. economy. Op. cit.
619. Grabowski H, Vernon J. Returns to R&D on new drug introductions in the 1980s. *J Health Econom* 1994;**13**:383–406.
620. Harris G, Carey B. Researchers fail to reveal full drug pay, *New York Times*, June 8, 2008.
621. Nguyen D, Ornstein C, Weber T. Dollars for docs: What drug companies are paying your doctor, Nov 17, 2010. Web. 23 Nov. 2010. http://projects.propublica.org/docdollars/
622. Campbell EG, Pham-Kanter G, PhD; Vogeli C, et al. Physician Acquiescence to Patient Demands for Brand-Name Drugs: Results of a National Survey of Physicians. *JAMA Intern Med.* 2013;173:237–9 doi:10.1001/jamainternmed.2013.1539
623. Faguet, GB. *The Affordable Care Act*. Op. cit.
624. Goozner M. Rise of the Machines, The Fiscal Times February 11, 2010. Available at: http://www.thefiscaltimes.com/Articles/2010/02/11/Rise-Of-The-Machines.aspx?p=1. Accessed March 20, 2011.
625. Kantarjian H. Op. cit.
626. Faguet, GB. *The Affordable Care Act*. Op. cit.
627. Pharmaceutical research and manufacturers of America, available online at http://www.phrma.org/
628. Djulbegovic B, Lacevic M, Cantor A, et al. The uncertainty principle and industry-sponsored research. *Lancet* 2000;**356**:635–638.
629. Blumenthal D, Campbell EG, Anderson MS, et al. Withholding research results in academic life science: Evidence from a national survey of faculty *JAMA* 1997;**277**:1224–1228.
630. Schulman KA, Seils DM, Timbie JW, et al. A national survey of provisions in clinical-trial agreements between medical schools and industry sponsors. *N Engl J Med* 2002;**347**:1335–1341.
631. MacDonald MM, Hoffman-Goetz L. A retrospective study of the accuracy of cancer information in Ontario daily newspapers. *Can J Public Health* 2002;**93**:142–145.
632. National Institute of Health. Medicine in the Media: The Challenge of Reporting on Medical Research Symposium. Rockville, MD, June 23–25, 2002.
633. Saporito B. The Conspiracy To End Cancer: A team-based, cross-disciplinary approach to cancer research is upending tradition and delivering results faster. *Time Magazine*, April 01, 2013.
634. Editorial. Have we lost are way? *Lancet* 1993;**341**:343–344.
635. Kübler-Ross E. *On death and dying: What the dying have to teach doctors, nurses, clergy, and their own families*. New York, NY, Touchstone, 1997.
636. Loge JH, Kaasa S, Hytten K. Disclosing the cancer diagnosis: the patients' experiences. *Eur J Cancer* 1997;**33**:878–882.
637. Jenkins V, Fallowfield L, Saul J. Information needs of patients with cancer: results from a large study in UK cancer centers. *Br J Cancer* 2001;**84**:48–51.
638. Parker PA, Baile WF, de Moor C, et al. Breaking bad news about cancer patients' preferences for communications. *J Clin Oncol* 2001;**19**:2049–2056.
639. Schwartz K. A patient's story. The Boston Globe, July 16, 1995. Web 23 Jul. 2013. http://www.theschwartzcenter.org/docs/patient_story.pdf

640. Bruera E, Neumann CM, Mazzocato C, et al. Attitudes and beliefs of palliative care physicians regarding communication s with terminally ill cancer patients. *Palliat Med* 2000;**14**:287–298.
641. Grassi L, Giraldi T, Messina EG, et al. Physicians attitudes to and problems with truth-telling to cancer patients. *Support Care Cancer* 2000;**8**:40–50.
642. Fallowfield LJ, Jenkins VA, Beveridge HA. Truth may hurt but deceit hurts more: communication in palliative care. *Palliat Med* 2002;**16**:297–302.
643. Kaplowitz SA, Campo S, Chiu WT. Cancer patients' desires for communication of prognosis information. *Health Commun* 2002;**14**:221–41.
644. Faguet GB. *The War on Cancer*. Op. cit.
645. Slevin ML, Stubbs L, Plant HJ, et al. Attitudes to chemotherapy: comparing views of patients with cancer with those of doctors, nurses, and general public. *BMJ* 1990;**300**:1458–1460.
646. Carlsson M. Cancer patients seeking information from sources outside the health care system. *Support Care Cancer* 2000;**8**:453–457.
647. Cassileth BR, Zupkis RV, Sutton-Smith K, et al. Information and participation preferences among cancer patients. *Ann Intern Med* 1980;**92**:832–836.
648. Gattellari M, Butow PN, Tattersall MH. Informed consent: what did the doctor say? *Lancet* 1999;**353**:1713.
649. Kübler-Ross E. Op. cit.
650. Coulter A. Partnerships with patients: the pros and cons of shared clinical decision making. *J Health Service Res Policy* 1997;**2**:112–121.
651. Charles C, Whelam T, Gafni A. What do we mean by partnership in making decisions about treatment? *BMJ* 1999;**319**:780–782.
652. Degner LF, Krsitjanson LJ, Bowman D, et al. Information needs and decisional preferences in women with breast cancer. *JAMA* 1997;**277**:1485–1492.
653. Institute of Medicine. *Crossing the quality chasm: a new health system for the 21st century*. Washington, DC: National Academies Press; 2001.
654. Hewitt M, Simone JV (Ed) *Ensuring quality cancer care. National Cancer Policy Board*. Institute of Medicine and Commission On Life Sciences. National Research Council:. Washington, DC, National Academy Press, 1999.
655. Schnider EC, Epstein AM. Developing a System to Assess the Quality of Cancer Care: ASCO's National Initiative on Cancer Care Quality (table 2). *JCO* 2004;**22**:2985–2991.
656. Quality Oncology Practice Initiative: Summary of measures Spring 2013. Web 28 Jul. 2013. http://qopi.asco.org/Documents/QOPISpring13MeasuresSummary_001.pdf
657. NCCN Clinical Practice Guidelines in Oncology. Web 17 Aug. 2013. http://www.nccn.org/professionals/physician_gls/f_guidelines.asp
658. Faguet GB. *Pain Control and Drug Policy*.
659. NCI's simplified informed consent: Recommendations. Web 29 Jul. 2013. http://www.cancer.gov/clinicaltrials/conducting/simplification-of-informed-consent-docs/page2
660. World Medical Association declaration of Helsinki. Web 28 Jul. 2013. http://history.nih.gov/research/downloads/helsinki.pdf
661. National Commission for the Protection of Human Subjects of Biomedical and Behavioral Research. The Belmont Report. Washington, DC: DHEW Publication No. 0578–0012, 1978. Web 2 Aug. 2013. http://www.hhs.gov/ohrp/humansubjects/guidance/belmont.html
662. Permissible Medical Experiments. *Trials of War Criminals before the Nuremberg Military Tribunals under Control Council Law No. 10: Nuremberg October 1946–April 1949*. Washington DC, U.S. Government Printing Office (n.d.), vol. 2, pp. 181–182.
663. Owen E. *Time Daily* Center for Disease Control and Prevention. U.S. Pubic Health Service Syphilis Study at Tuskegee: Presidential Apology, May 16, 1997. Web 2 Aug. 2013. http://www.cdc.gov/tuskegee/clintonp.htm
664. DOE Openness: Human Radiation Experiments: ACHRE Report. Chapter 5: The Manhattan district Experiments; the first injection. Washington, D.C., Superintendent of Documents

U.S. Government Printing Office, June 1998. Web 2 Aug. 2013. http://www.hss.energy.gov/healthsafety/ohre/roadmap/achre/chap5_2.html
665. Eyal, Nir, Informed Consent, *The Stanford Encyclopedia of Philosophy* (Fall 2012 Edition), Edward N. Zalta (ed.). Web 3 Aug. 2013. http://plato.stanford.edu/entries/informed-consent/
666. National Commission for the Protection of Human Subjects of Biomedical and Behavioral Research. Op. cit.
667. Hewlett S. Consent to clinical trials: preliminary study of the views of prospective participants. *J Med Ethics* 1996;**22**:232–7.
668. Bok S. Shading the truth and seeking informed consent for research purposes. *Kennedy Inst Ethics J* 1995;**5**:1–17.
669. Evans M. Justified deception? The single blind placebo in drug research. *J Med Ethics* 2000;**26**:188–93.
670. Leighl N, Gattleari M, Butow P, et al. Discussing adjuvant cancer therapy. *J Clin Oncol* 2001;**19**:1768–1778.
671. Yardley SJ, Davis CL, Sheldon F. Receiving a diagnosis of lung cancer: patients' interpretations, perceptions and perspectives. *Palliat Med* 2001, **15**:379–86.
672. Wolf SM, Paradise J, Caga-Anan C. The Law of Incidental Findings in Human Subjects Research: Establishing Researchers' Duties. *J Law Med Ethics* 2008;**36**:361–383.
673. Gottlieb S. FDA censures NEJM editor. *BMJ* 2000;**320**:1562.
674. Crewdson J. Op. cit.
675. Cook-Deegan RM. Do research moratoria work? National Bioethic Advisory Commission. Cloning human beings. Vol II, Commissioned Papers. Rockville, MD. 1997.
676. Editorial. Retraction. *J Clin Oncol* 2001. Op. cit.
677. Habeck M. Clinical research comes under scrutiny. *Lancer Oncol* 2001 Oct 2 (10):588.
678. SSKRP attorneys in the news. Class action suit against Fred Hutchinson Cancer Center sends shock waves through clinical trials community. Web 3 Aug. 2013. http://www.sskrplaw.com/lawyer-attorney-1478109.html
679. Faguet GB. *The War on Cancer*. Op. cit.
680. Zier LS, Burack JH, Mico G, et al. Surrogate Decision Makers' Responses to Physicians' Predictions of Medical Futility. *Chest* 2009;**136**:110–117.
681. Gabbay E, Calvo-Broce J, Meyer KB, et al. The Empirical Basis for Determinations of Medical Futility. *J Gen Intern Med* 2010;**25**:1083–1089.
682. Chastek B, Harley C, Kallich J, et al. Health Care Costs for Patients With Cancer at the End of Life. *JOP* 2012;**8**:75s–80s.
683. Morden NE, Chang CH, Jacobson JO, et al. End-Of-Life care for Medicare Beneficiaries with cancer is highly intensive overall and varies widely. *Health Aff* 2012;**31**:786–796.
684. Blackhall LJ. Must we always use CPR? *N Engl J Med* 1987;**317**:1281–1285.
685. Paris JJ, Crone RK, Reardon F. Physicians' refusal of requested treatment. *N Engl J Med* 1990;**322**:1012–1015.
686. Goldberg GR, Meier DE. A Swinging Pendulum: Comment on "On Patient Autonomy and Physician Responsibility in End-of-Life Care" *Arch Intern Med* 2011;**171**:854. doi:10.1001/archinternmed.2011.173
687. Leadbetter R. Danaus. Encyclopedia Mythica. Web 8 Aug. 2013. http://www.pantheon.org/articles/d/danaus.html
688. AMA Code of Medical Ethics: Opinion 2.037 – Medical Futility in End-of-Life Care. Web 8 Aug. 2013. http://www.ama-assn.org/ama/pub/physician-resources/medical-ethics/code-medical-ethics/opinion2037.page
689. Caplan AL. Odds and ends: trust and the debate over medical futility. *Ann Intern Med* 1996;**125**:688–689.
690. Scneiderman LJ, Jecker NS, Jonsen AR. Medical futility: its meaning and ethical implications. *Ann Intern Med* 1990;**112**:949–954.
691. Caplan AL. Op. cit.
692. Schneiderman LJ, Jecker NS, Jonsen AR. Medical futility: Response to critics. *Ann Inter Med* 1996;**125**:669–674.

693. Berry DA, Broadwater G, Klein JP, et al. High-dose versus standard chemotherapy in metastatic breast cancer: comparison of Cancer and Leukemia Group B trials with data from the Autologous Blood and Marrow Transplant Registry. *J Clin Oncol* 2002;**20**:743–750.
694. Transplant Data by Center Report, Breast cancer, Number of Transplants Reported for Breast cancer From 2008 – 2011. Web 15 May 2013. http://bloodcell.transplant.hrsa.gov/research/transplant_data/us_tx_data/data_by_disease/national.aspx
695. Powles TJ, Coombes RC, Smith IE, et al. Failure of chemotherapy to prolong survival in a group of patients with metastatic breast cancer. *Lancet* 1980;**1**:580–582.
696. Breathnach O, Freidlin B, Conley B, et al. Twenty-two years of phase III trials for patients with advanced non-small-cell lung cancer: sobering results. *J Clin Oncol* 2000;**19**:1734–1742.
697. Berry DA, Broadwater G, Klein JP, et al. Op. cit.
698. Mettu NB, Hurwitz H, Hsu DS. Use of Molecular Biomarkers to Inform Adjuvant Therapy for Colon Cancer. *Oncology* 2013;**27**:746–54. Web 20 Sept. 2013. http://www.cancernetwork.com/colorectal-cancer/content/article/10165/2152538?cid=intraarticle
699. Van Loon K, Venook AP. Biomarkers in Colon Cancer: The Chasm Between Expectations and Reality. Oncology 2013 Vol 27 No. 8. Web 20 Sept. 2013. http://www.cancernetwork.com/colorectal-cancer/content/article/10165/2152548
700. Califano, JA Jr., Physician-Assisted Living, *America,* November 14, 1998, pp. 10–12.
701. UNESCO: The Routes of Santiago de Compostela in France, available online at http://whc.unesco.org/sites/868-loc.htm
702. Saunders C. The evolution of hospices. Free inquiry. Winter 1991/92:19–23.
703. A controlled trial to improve care for seriously ill hospitalized patients. The Study to Understand Prognoses and Preferences for Outcomes and Risks of Treatments (SUPPORT). The SUPPORT Principal Investigators. *JAMA* 1995;**274**:1591–1598.
704. Califano, JA Jr. Op. cit.
705. World Health Organization. Cancer pain relief and palliative care. Geneva, Switzerland: World Health Organization; 1990:11–12.
706. Clinical Practice Guidelines: Statement on Clinical Practice Guidelines for Quality Palliative Care. American Academy of Hospice and Palliative Medicine June 2006. Web 11 Sept. 2013. http://www.aahpm.org/Practice/default/quality.html
707. United States Senate Special Committee on Aging: Death with Dignity: A inquiry into related public issues, Part 1. Web 11 Sept. 2013. http://www.aging.senate.gov/publications/871972.pdf
708. Ibidem.
709. Saunders CM. *The Management of Terminal Illness*. London: Hospital Medicine Publications; 1967.
710. Faguet GB. *The War on Cancer*. Op. cit.
711. Jemal A, Ward E, Thun M (2010). Op. cit.
712. Simard EP, MPH, Ward EM, Siegel R. Cancers with increasing incidence trends in the United States: 1999 through 2008. *CA Cancer J Clin* 2012;**62**:118–128.
713. NCI: Cancer. Changing the Conversation: An annual plan and budget proposal for fiscal year 2012. Web 17 Sept. 2013. http://www.cancer.gov/PublishedContent/Files/aboutnci/budget_planning_leg/plan-archives/nci_plan.pdf#page=12
714. Wolin KY, Carson K, Colditz GA. Obesity and Cancer. *The Oncologist* 2010;**15**:556–565.
715. Cancer Facts & Figures, 2012. The American Cancer Society. Atlanta, GA.
716. CDC: Smoking and tobacco-related mortality. Web 17 Sep. 2013. http://www.cdc.gov/tobacco/data_statistics/fact_sheets/health_effects/tobacco_related_mortality/index.htm
717. Tobacco and related Health-R&D approach. Report to R&D Committee of the Philip Morris Inc, by Dr. H. Wakeman. New York Office, November 15, 1961.
718. Wingo PA, Lynn AG, Ries MS, et al: Annual report to the nation on the status of cancer, 1973–1996, with a special section on lung cancer and tobacco smoking. *J Natl Cancer Inst* 1999;**91**:675–690.
719. Greelee RT, Hill-Harmon MB, Murray T, et al. Cancer statistics, 2001 *CA Cancer J Clin* 2001;**51**:15–27.

720. Klein EA, Thompson IM Jr, Tangen CM, et al. Vitamin E and the risk of prostate cancer: the Selenium and Vitamin E Cancer Prevention Trial (SELECT). *JAMA* 2011;**306**:1549–1956.
721. Markowitz LE, Dunne EF, Saraiya M et al. Centers for Disease Control and Prevention (CDC); Advisory Committee on Immunization Practices (ACIP) (2007). "Quadrivalent Human Papillomavirus Vaccine: Recommendations of the Advisory Committee on Immunization Practices (ACIP)". *MMWR. Recommendations and reports : Morbidity and mortality weekly report. Recommendations and reports / Centers for Disease Control* **56** (RR-2):1–24.
722. Fisher B, Costantino JP, Wickerham DL, et al. Op. cit.
723. Loeb S, Carter HB, Berndt S, et al. Is Repeat Prostate Biopsy Associated with a Greater Risk of Hospitalization? *J Urol* 2012;**187**:e831–e832.
724. Ibidem.
725. Chodak GW, Thisted RA, Gerber GS, et al. Results of conservative management of clinically localized prostate cancer. *N Engl J Med* 1994;**330**: 242–248.
726. U.S. Preventive Services Task Force Screening for Prostate Cancer: Current Recommendation. Web 22 Sept. 2013. http://www.uspreventiveservicestaskforce.org/prostatecancerscreening.htm
727. Nelson HD, Tyne K, Naik A, et al.: Screening for breast cancer: an update for the U.S. Preventive Services Task Force. *Ann Intern Med* 2009;**151**:727–737.
728. Elmore JG, Barton MB, Moceri VM, et al.: Ten-year risk of false positive screening mammograms and clinical breast examinations. *N Engl J Med* 1998;**338**:1089–1096.
729. Hubbard RA, Kerlikowske K, Flowers CI, et al.: Cumulative probability of false-positive recall or biopsy recommendation after 10 years of screening mammography: a cohort study. *Ann Intern Med* 2012;**155**:481–492.
730. Rosenberg RD, Hunt WC, Williamson MR, et al.: Effects of age, breast density, ethnicity, and estrogen replacement therapy on screening mammographic sensitivity and cancer stage at diagnosis: review of 183,134 screening mammograms in Albuquerque, New Mexico. *Radiology* 1998;**209**:511–518.
731. NCI. Cancer Prevention Overview. Web 17 Sept 2013. http://www.cancer.gov/cancertopics/pdq/prevention/overview/HealthProfessional
732. NCI. Cancer Screening Overview. Web 17 Sept 2013. http://www.cancer.gov/cancertopics/pdq/screening/overview/patient
733. Curry J, Byers T, Hewitt M, editors. Fulfilling the potential of cancer prevention and early detection. Washington, DC, The National Academies Press 2003.
734. Cancer Prevention & Early detection: Facts & figures – 2012. American Cancer Society Inc. Atlanta, GA. Web 17 Sept 2013. http://www.cancer.org/acs/groups/content/@epidemiology-surveilance/documents/document/acspc-033423.pdf
735. Faguet, GB. *The Affordable Care Act*. Op. cit.
736. Environmental Working Group. EWG Farm subsidies: Tobacco subsidies. Web 19 Sept 2013. http://farm.ewg.org/progdetail.php?fips=00000&progcode=tobacco
737. Twombly R. Tobacco Settlement Seen as Opportunity Lost To Curb Cigarette Use. *J Natl Cancer Inst* 2004;**96**: 730–732.
738. WHO: Cancer prevention. Web 19 Sept 2013. http://www.who.int/cancer/prevention/en/
739. WHO: Early detection of cancer. Web 19 Sept. 2013. http://www.who.int/cancer/detection/en/
740. WHO Framework Convention on Tobacco Control. Web 17 Sept. 2013. http://www.who.int/cancer/prevention/tobacco_implementation/fctc/en/index.html
741. Faguet GB. *The War on Cancer*. Op. cit.
742. Beauchamp TL, Childress JF. *Principles of biomedical ethics. 3rd ed.* New York, Oxford University Press, 1989.
743. Gillion R. Medical ethics: Four principles plus attention to scope. *Br J Med* 1994;**309**:184–187.
744. Faguet GB. *The War on Cancer*. Op. cit.
745. Van Loon K, Venook AP. Op.cit.
746. Faguet GB. *The Affordable Care Act*. Op. cit.

747. United States. Congress. Senate. Committee on Labor and Public Welfare. Subcommittee on Health., (1971). Op cit.
748. Faguet GB, Agee JF. Monoclonal antibodies against the chronic lymphocytic leukemia antigen cCLLa: Characterization and Reactivity. *Blood* 1987;70:437–443.
749. Faguet GB, Satya-Prakash KL, Agee JF. Cytochemical, cytogenetic, immunophenotypic and tumorigenic characterization of two hairy cell lines. *Blood* 1988;71:422–429.
750. Faguet GB, Agee JF. Transplantation of human hairy cell leukemia in radiation preconditioned nude mice: Characterization of the model by histologic, histochemical, phenotypic and tumor kinetic studies. *Blood* 1988;71:1517–1517.
751. Faguet GB, Agee JF. Four Ricin chain A-based immunotoxins directed against the common chronic lymphocytic leukemia antigen (cCLLa): In vitro characterization. *Blood* 1993;82:536–543.
752. Faguet GB, Agee JF. The chronic lymphocytic leukemia antigen (cCLLa) as immunotherapy target: Pharmacokinetics and biodistribution of two divalent, ricin-based immunotoxins in xenografted athymic mice. *Leuk Lymphoma* 1997.**25**:509–520.
753. Wilt TJ, Brawer MK, Jones KM, et al. Radical Prostatectomy versus Observation for Localized Prostate Cancer. *N Engl J Med 2012*;**367**:203–213.
754. Jenq G, Tinetti ME. Changes in End-of-Life care during the last decade: More not better. *JAMA* 2013;**309**:470–7.
755. Ibidem.

Index

A
Abbasid Caliphate, 21
ACS. *See* American Cancer Society (ACS)
Aëtius of Amidenus, 19, 20
Ægineta, P., 19, 20
Alternate methods, 131, 132
American Board of Internal Medicine
 (ABIM), 155, 156
American Board of Medical Specialties
 (ABMS), 155, 156
American Cancer Society (ACS), 4–6,
 85–88, 91, 92, 103, 135,
 197, 201
American College of Surgeons (ACoS), 84
American Society for the Control of Cancer, 4
American Society of Hematology (ASH), 155,
 157, 178
Ancient Egypt, 13–19
 Sakkara pyramid, 13
Apollo program, 201
Archigenes of Apamea, 17
Aselli, G., 24
ASH. *See* American Society
 of Hematology (ASH)
Astruc, J., 24
Avenzoar, 21
Avicenna, 21

B
Baby boomers, 95
Bacteria-cancer link hypothesis
 colon cancer, 30
 MALT, 30
Bard, L., 28
Bateson, W., 43

Bayle, G.L., 26
Becquerel, H., 31
Bennett, J.H., 130
BMSC transplantation
 allogeneic & autologous, 119
 GVHD, 119
Boveri, T., 28
Broca, P.P., 26
Byzantium, 23

C
Califano, J., 187
Cancer
 adrenal, 59, 63
 bladder, 50, 58, 67, 91, 178,
  194, 207
 breast
  BRCA1, 56, 59, 60
  BRCA2, 59, 60
  BRCA3, 60
  Erb-B2, 55, 57
 cervical, 25, 55, 58, 93,
  105, 195
 colorectal, 55, 60, 61, 71, 91, 125, 128,
  140, 207
 embryonal, 59
 endocrine and thyroid, 55
  RET, 55
 endometrial, 59, 74, 75, 153
 esophageal, 21, 61, 67, 75, 77
 gastric, 30, 58, 59, 61, 67, 75
 glioblastoma, 58, 61, 125
 glioma, 59
 hamartoma, 59
 head & neck, 61

Cancer (*cont.*)
  Hodgkin, 86, 207
  invasion-metastasis cascade
      (*see* Invasion-metastasis cascade)
  invasive, 87, 88, 90, 114, 135, 138
  leiomyomas
      BCL, 51, 52
      CTCL, 126
      mycosis fungoides, 126–127
      Sézari syndrome, 126
  leukemias
      acute lymphoid, 120
      acute myeloid, 86, 121
      chronic lymphocytic, 35, 61, 86
      chronic myeloid (*see* Chronic myeloid)
      hairy cell leukemia, 104
  liver, 58, 61, 140, 192
  local, 25, 27, 64, 93
  lung cancer
      NSCLC, 116–118, 160
      SCLC, 118
  lymphoma, 30, 35, 45, 54, 55, 57, 58, 61,
      86, 88, 106, 120, 121, 125, 126,
      128, 131, 160, 161, 168, 178
      immunoglobulin heavy chain locus,
          55, 57
  medulloblastoma, 58, 59
  meningioma, 59
  metastatic, 13, 65, 107, 135, 138, 181,
      186, 200
  neuroblastoma, 53, 57, 58, 120
  osteosarcoma, 59
  ovarian, 40, 58–61
  pancreas, 25, 57–59, 61, 72, 93, 140, 178,
      192, 194
  paragangliomas, 59
  parathyroid, 59
  pituitary, 59
  prostate, 35, 58, 61, 65, 85–89, 93, 104,
      106, 111, 112, 127, 136, 137, 178,
      182, 194, 196, 203, 208
  renal, 59, 72
      Wilms', 59
  retinoblastomas, 36, 54, 56, 59, 60, 85
  sarcoma, 27, 33, 50, 58, 59
  skin
      basal cell, 59, 86, 88
      dermatofibrosarcoma protuberans, 57, 125
      melanoma, 58, 59, 61, 66, 71, 86, 88,
          92, 104, 112, 131, 140, 178, 192
      squamous cell carcinomas, 32, 57
  stomach, 21, 58, 59, 72, 86, 90, 91
Cancer cell lines, 112
  NCI-60, 112

Cancerous dinosaurs
  desmoplastic fibromas, 13
  hemangiomas, 13
  osteoblastomas, 13
Cancer prevention trials
  BCPT, 153
  IBIS-I, 153
  MORE, 153
  SELECT, 194
  STAR, 153, 154
Cancer-promoting, 24, 60, 67,
      101, 194
Cancer treatment
  alternate methods
      current, 131
      historical, 129
      OCCAM list, 133
  Biological Response Modifiers, 103
  chemotherapy (cell-kill)
      (*see* Chemotherapy (cell-kill))
  chemotherapy drugs (current), 51,
      123, 125, 162
  chemotherapy intensification
      BMSC transpplantation (*see* BMSC
          transplantation)
      dose intensity, 118–119
      PBSC transpplantation (*see* PBSC
          transplantation)
  chemotherapy modalities
      first line, 185, 187,
          203, 205
      salvage, 164, 200
      second line, 164, 185, 205
  chemotherapy regimens
      CHOP, 160, 161
      COMLA, 160
      ESAP, 160
      MACOP-B, 160
      m-BACOP, 160
      MOPP, 118
      PVB, 118
      VAMP, 118
  chronotherapy, 122, 123
  clinical trials
      Phase I, 126, 149, 150
      Phase II, 126, 150
      Phase III, 116, 117, 150–153,
          159, 160
      deaths, 70, 78, 83, 86, 87, 90, 91,
          95, 116, 135, 136, 139,
          178, 192–194, 196, 198,
          200, 207, 209
  early detection
      CT-scan, 196

molecular methods (*see* Molecular detection)
MRI, 196, 197
facts & figures, 86–88, 92
human cancer viruses (*see* Human cancer viruses)
incidence, 84–86, 89–91, 140, 153, 191, 195, 207
National Program of Cancer Registries (NPCR), 84
North American Association of Central Cancer Registries (NAACCR), 84, 86
outcomes
  cost, 106, 107, 136, 191
  cure, 181
  DFS, 177
  Overall, 135, 136
  QOL, 106, 138, 141, 177, 181
  remission, 106, 107
  5-year survival, 107, 117, 139, 140, 177, 181
  YPLL, 72, 78
prevalence
  APC, 95
  Connecticut Registry, 88
probability of
  developing, 87–88, 95
  dying, 87–88
radiation, 33, 54, 63
surgery, 203
Surveillance, Epidemiology and End Results (SEER), 84, 118
targeted therapeutics
  MoAbs (*see* MoAbs)
  other types, 125
trends in cancer incidence and mortality, 89–91
Carcinogens
  genotoxic, 69, 71
  Group 1 (*see* Group 1 Carcinogens)
  Group 2A, 69
  Group 2B, 69
  non-genotoxic, 69, 71
Cell lines
  NCI-60, 112
Celsus, A.C., 17
Center for Disease Control & Prevention, 71
Chemotherapy (cell-kill)
  cell cycle dependent, 102
  cell cycle independent
    Busulfan, 102
    Chlorambucil, 102
    Melphalan, 102
  G1-and G2-phase dependent
    Asparaginase/Bleomycin, 102
    Corticosteroids, 102
    Topotecan, 102
  M-phase dependent
    Podophyllotoxins, 102
    Taxanes, 102
    Vinca alkaloids, 102
  S-specific
    antimetabolites, 102
    anti-purines, 102
Chevalier, C., 27
Chronic myeloid, 86
  bcr/abl, 54, 55
Circulating tumor cells (CTC), 54
Clinical researchers and publications, 166–167
Community Clinical Oncology Program (CCOP), 8, 147, 148
Copernicus, N., 23
Correns, C., 43
Cruveilhier, J., 26
CTCGP (Clinical Trials Cooperative Group Program)
  ACOSOG, 147
  CALGB, 147
  COG, 147
  ECOG, 147
  EORTC, 147, 153
  GOG, 147
  NCCTG, 147
  NCIC CTG, 147
  NSABP, 147, 153, 167
  RTOG, 147
  SWOG, 147, 167
Cura famis, 130
Cure rates, 30, 65, 118, 122, 131, 138, 175, 200, 207

D

Darwin, C., 42
Death rates, 33, 91, 95, 104, 120, 135, 136, 138, 140, 193, 194, 207
Delpech, J., 26
Developmental Therapeutics Program (DTP), 112, 113
De Vries, H., 43
Dickens, C., 135
Differentiation markers
  CD3, 126
  CD20, 126

Differentiation markers (*cont.*)
    CD-25, 126
    CD33, 126
    CD52, 126
Donné, A., 130

E
Early Medical centers
    Bologna, 21, 22
    Montpellier, 21, 22
    Paris, 22
    Studium of Salerno, 22
    Viaticum, 22
Early-stage diagnosis, 17, 89, 91, 136, 138, 191, 207
Eastern Roman (Byzantine) Empire, 19, 20
Ehrlich, P., 112, 126, 202
Emirate of Granada, 21
Endocrine-modifiers, 71
Epigenetics, 38, 62, 106
Ethical medical care, 185

F
Fallopius, G., 23
Ferdinand II of Aragón, 22
Fibiger, J.A.G., 29
Food & Drug Administratio (FDA), 30, 104, 105, 107, 113, 115, 123–126, 128, 136, 148, 149, 165, 168, 170, 180, 181, 197, 201, 208

G
Galen of Pergamum
    De tumoribus praeter naturam
        Karkinomas, 19
        Karkinos, 19
    De tumoribus secondum naturam, 19
    De tumoribus supra naturam, 20
General Parran, T.J. Jr., 4
Genes
    Abbot Napp, F.C., 41
    activation of genes
        CIP1/p21, 50
        WAF1, 50
    allosomes, 44, 45
        hemophilia A, 45
    apoptosis
        Apo2L/DR4, 51
        Apo2L/DR5, 51
        Apo3L/DR3, 51
        Bad, 51

BAG, 51
Bak, 51
Bax, 51
Bax/Bax, 51
Bax/Bcl-2, 51
Bcl-2, 51
Bcl-10, 51
Bcl-2/Bad, 51
Bcl-2/Bcl-2, 51
Bcl-w, 51
Bcl-x, 51
Bcl-XL, 51
Bcl-XS, 51
Bid, 51
Bik, 51
Bim, 51
Blk, 51
extrinsic, 51, 52
FasL/FasR L, 51
granzyme pathways, 51, 52
intrinsic, 51, 52
Perforin, 51, 52
TNF, 51
TNF-α/TNFR1, 51
autosomes, 44, 45
    sickle cell anemia, 45
codons, 44
    AUG, 44
cystic fibrosis gene, 37
    Tsui, L.-C., 37
deletions, 45, 55, 59, 61
    DiGeorge syndrome, 45
DNA methylation, 62
DNA repair genes, 36, 55, 60, 101, 208
    GADD45, 50
DNA viruses, 55
the double Helix
    Crick, F.A., 38, 39
    Franklin, R., 38, 39
    Pauling, L., 38
    Watson, J.D., 38, 39
    Wilkins, M.H., 38, 39
E2F1, 49
EGF, 48, 57
exons, 43, 44
FGF, 48, 57
Franz, F., 42
Gatekeepers
    mutated *Rb1*, 50
    RB1, 49, 54–56, 59, 60
    TP53, 49, 50, 59, 60
histone modifications, 62
IGF, 48

introns, 43, 44
Mendel, Johann
    cross-pollination, 42, 43
    dominant elements, 42, 43
    recessive elements, 43
MicroRNA genes, 61
multiple copies
    Down syndrome, 45
    trisomy 12, 45
Nestler, K., 42
nucleotide bases, 36, 37
oncogenes, 58
Parkinson's disease gene, 37
    Nussbaum, R., 37
PDGF, 48
Phase progression genes, 50
    14-3-σ, 50
phases (G_0, G_1, S, and G_2), 48
polymorphism, 36
pRB, 49, 50
    RNA-associated, 62
    telomeres, 50, 52, 53
        TTAGGG & AATCCC, 52
    transcription, 43, 44, 49, 57,
        62, 115
translocations
    Burkitt's lymphoma, 45, 57
    del(16)(q22), 45
    t(8;14), 45
    t(9;22), 45
    t(14;18), 45, 52
    t(15;17), 45
tumor suppressor genes, 59
Genetics, 9, 29, 38, 42, 43, 61, 62, 64, 65, 83,
    106, 135, 146, 156, 191
Gerson diet, 129, 131, 132
Gilman, A., 108
Godinot, J., 25
    first cancer hospital, 25
Goldie-Coldman, 116
Gompertzian growth pattern, 116
Goodman, L., 108
Greece & Rome, 14–19
Group 1 Carcinogens
    infectious agents
        HBV, 70, 105, 194, 209
        HPV-16, 25, 93, 105
        HPV-18, 93, 105, 195
    lifestyle factors
        alcoholism, 76–79, 194, 195, 209
        obesity, 70
        physical inactivity, 70
        poor nutrition, 70
        tobacco smoking, 70
    medical treatment
        chemotherapy, 33, 69
        X-rays, 33, 69, 111
    non-infectious agents
        air pollution (diesel exhaust), 69
        asbestos and formaldehyde, 69
        natural elements (UV light, radon gas),
            69
Growth factors
    HRAS, 58
    KRAS, 58
    NRAS, 58
Guthrie, F., 107

H
Halsted, W.S., 24
Hannover, A., 27
Harvard University, 5
Harvey, W., 24, 130
Health system
    Affordable Care Act, xv
    Medicaid, 170, 176
    Medicare, 136, 163, 169, 170, 176
Hill, J., 25, 32
Hippocrates of Kos
    Aphorisms, 15
    Asclepius, 15
    Hygieia, 15
    karkinomas, 17, 19
    Panacea, 15
Holmes, O.W., 28
Hospice vs acute care
    Aikenhead, M., 188
    Daughters of Charity, 188
    Garnier, J., 188
    Kubler-Ross, E., 188, 190
    Saunders, D.C.M., 188
Human cancer viruses
    List, 105
    vaccines
        Cervarix®, 93, 105
        Gardasil®, 93, 105
        HBV, 194
        HCV, 194
Human Genome Project
    Collins, F., 37
    Venter, J.C., 37
    whole-genome shotgun, 37

I
Ibn Al-Nafis, 21
Ichikawa, K., 32

Immune suppressors, 71
Incidence, 25, 26, 71, 84–87, 89–92, 117, 121, 136–138, 140, 151, 153, 191–195, 197, 207, 209
IND, 149
Informed consent, 150, 177, 180, 181
Institutional review board (IRB), 149, 180
Invasion-metastasis cascade
    β-catenins, 65
    E-cadherins, 65–67
    integrins
        α5β1, 66
        α6β4, 66
        αvβ3, 66
        αvβ5, 66
    metastasis-promoting genes
        ERBB2, 67
        MMP11, 67
        MTA1, 67
        WDNM-1, 67
        WDNM-2, 67
    metastasis-suppressor genes
        BRMS1, 67
        CTGF, 67
        KAI1, 67
        KiSS1, 67
        MKK4, 67
        MKK7, 67
        MSGs KISS1, 67
        nm23, 67
        RhoGDI2, 67
        SMAD7, 67
        SSeCKS, 67
    selectins
        E-selectins, 66
        L-selectins, 66
        P-selectins, 66
Isabel the catholic, 22

J
Jackson, D. Sr., 4
Jansen, Z., 27

K
Knockout mice, 53
Knudson, A., 108
Köhler, G., 126
Kojima, 103
König, F., 27

L
Lagartija cures, 130
Lawmakers, 3
Le Dran, H.F., 24
Leonides of Alexandria, 20
Lifestyles, 53, 69–71, 74, 76, 78, 86, 140, 193
Lindskog, G., 108
Lister, J., 30
Long, C.W., 30
Louis, P.C.A., 148
Lymphocytes
    T-lymphocytes, 48, 104, 119, 126
        cytotoxic, 51

M
Macrophages, 51, 103
Manhattan project, 201
Master Settlement Agreement (MSA), 198
McCoy, G.W., 4
Medical futility
    ends
        physiological, 185
        psychological, 185
    odds, 184
Medicine-as-a-business
    the chemotherapy concession, 161–164
        lifestyle-factors, 53, 69, 76
    overutilization of services, 161–164
Mendelsohn's growth fraction, 116
Milstein, C., 126
MoAbs
    Campath®, 126, 136
    cCLLa, 204
    Herceptin®, 126, 127
    Myelotarg®, 126
    OKT3®, 126
    Rituxan®, 126, 127
Molecular biology, 9, 28, 130, 135, 146
Molecular detection
    cytogenetics, 106
    flow cytometry, 106, 196
    fluorescence in-situ hybridization, 106
    microarrays, 106
    PCR, 106, 125
    spectral karyotype, 106
Morgagni, G.B., 25
Müller, J., 27
Mummies, 14
    Ptolemaic, 14

Mustard gas
  JD, 108
  nitrogen mustard, 83, 102, 107–111, 114, 117, 118

N
Nagano, 103
National Cancer Act (1937), 5, 33
National Cancer Act (1971)
  Farber, S., 6, 7, 112
  Kennedy, E., 8
  Landers, A., 7
  Lasker, M.W., 5, 7, 201
  President Nixon, 8, 141, 192, 207
NationaL Cancer Institute (NCI)
  Detrick, F., 8
  Extramural Research Program
    DCB, 145
    DCCPS, 145
    DCP, 145
    DCTD, 145, 147
    DEA, 146
  hollow-fibers, 112
  Intramural Research Program
    CCR, 146, 147
    DCEG, 146
  mission statement, 9
National Institute of Drug Addiction (NIDA), 75
National Institutes of Health
  Cancer Centers Program Network, 146–147
  CCRCG, 146
  CRFG, 146
  PPG, 146
Nestorius, 21

O
Oribasius of Pergamum, 19, 20
Osler, W., 149, 164
Outcome benchmarks, 138, 177

P
Paget, J., 27, 64, 65
Paradigm shift in cancer management
  early detection, 191–198
    developing better cancer screening tests, 196, 197
  Holistic management of advanced cancer
    a Manhattan-like search for new cancer agents, 201
    restructuring the treatment of advanced-stage cancer, 202–205
    reviving the art of End of Life care, 205–206
  prevention
    alcoholism, 193–195
    carcinogenic viruses, 193–195
    obesity, 193–195
    targeting smoking, 194
    ultraviolet light, 194
Paré, A., 22
Pasteur, L., 130
Pauling, L., 32, 38
PBSC transplantation
  autologous & allogeneic, 119
  GVHD, 119, 121
Peller, S., 29
P450 enzymes, 71
Percivall Pott, 25, 32
Peter Bent Brigham Hospital, 7
Petit, J.-L., 24
Peyrilhe, B., 24
Pharmaceutical companies (PhRMA)
  blockbuster drugs, 136, 168, 195, 209
  direct-to-consumer TV advertising, 169
  drug marketing to doctors, 168
Physician-patient interaction
  disclosure
    the belmont report, 179, 180
    in clinical trials, 178–181
    in the community setting, 174–178
  end of life care, 188, 189
    hospice vs acute care (*see* Hospice vs acute care)
  ethical medical care
    autonomy and justice, 199, 209
    beneficence, 199, 201, 206, 209, 210
    non-maleficence, 185, 199, 201, 209
  informed & shared model, 175
  medical futility (*see* Medical futility)
  paternalistic, 175, 178
Pierre & Marie Curie, 31
  polonium, 31, 32
  radium, 31, 32
Prevention, 30, 70, 71, 75, 78, 83, 84, 90, 93, 105, 135–138, 141, 146, 149, 153, 176, 193–198, 209
Providers, 71, 123, 129, 157, 161, 168, 176

Public health service, 4, 84, 148, 149
   office of cancer investigations, 111
   U.S. Department of Health and Human Services
      centers for disease control and prevention, 71, 86
      report of the surgeon general, 5

R
Ramazzini, B., 25
Raspail, F.V., 28
RB1 (mutated)
   bladder cancer, 50
   childhood retinoblastoma, 50
   osteogenic sarcoma, 50
Recamier, J., 25
Remak, R., 27
René Descartes, 23
   cogito ergo sum, 24
Rhazes, 21
Röentgen, W.C., 31
Rous, P., 32
   rous sarcoma virus, 33, 55, 57
Russian Federation, 96

S
SEER. *See* Surveillance Epidemiology and End Results (SEER)
Side effects, 114, 118, 120, 122, 127, 150, 151, 159, 164, 175, 180, 195
Skipper, H.E., 115, 116
Standard of care
   medical malpractice, 164–166
      deep-pocket defendants, 165
      oncologist compensation, 162
      trial lawyers, 165, 166
      litigation industry, 166
Storck, 130
Sub-Saharan Africa, 95
Surveillance Epidemiology and End Results (SEER), 84, 93, 117, 118

T
Targeted therapeutics, 107, 123–128, 136, 138, 141, 151, 168
Time Magazine, 103, 171
Treatment by cold, 130
Tumor antigens, 195
   CEA, 195
   HER-2, 195
   MAGE, 195
   MART, 195
   MUC-1, 195
   PSA, 195–197, 203
Tumor promoters, 71
Tumor-specific immunity, 102
Tuskegee, 179

U
US Bureau of the Census, 95
U.S. Congress, 6, 33
   House Health Subcommittee, 112
U.S. National Library of Medicine, 40
US Presidents
   Johnson, Lyndon, 6
   Nixon, Richard, 6, 8, 141, 192, 207

V
van Helmont, J.B., 23
Velpeau, A.A.L.M., 27
Vesalius, A., 18
Vincent, C., 27
Virchow, R., 27
von Hohenheim, W.B., 24
von Rokitansky, C., 27
von Tschermak, E., 43
von Waldeyer-Hartz, H., 27

W
War(s)
   Civil war, 83
   Korean, 83
   Vietnam, 83
   WWI, 32, 33, 83, 107, 110
      Mustard gas, 33, 107, 110
   WWII (*See* World War II (WWII))
The War on Cancer, 9, 96, 97, 105, 113, 131, 135, 137, 138, 141, 146, 149, 158, 172, 202, 207, 208
Western Europe, 22, 23, 96, 188
WHO. *See* World Health Organization (WHO)
Winternitz, M., 108
WOF. *See* World Oncology Forum (WOF)
World Health Organization (WHO), 35, 70, 84, 113, 114, 141, 189, 198
   essential & non essential drugs, 113, 114
World Oncology Forum (WOF), 136, 137

World War II (WWII)
  Bari
    Alexander, Stewart Francis (Lt. Col.), 110
    Basilica di San Nicola, 109
    Churchill, Winston S., 110
    Coningham, Sir Arthur (Vice-Marshal), 109
    General Eisenhower, Dwight D., 110
    Kesselring, Albert, 109
    Luftwaffe, 109
    M47A1 mustard gas bombs, 110
    Teuber, Lieutenant Gustav, 109
    U.S.S. John Harvey, 110
    von Richthofen, Wolfram, 109

Y

Yamagiwa, K., 32
5-Year survival, 89, 90, 92, 93, 107, 117, 121, 132, 138–140, 177, 181, 186, 192, 195, 200, 207